Handbook of Antimicrobial Therapy

Selected Articles from *Treatment Guidelines*
with updates from *The Medical Letter*®

Published by

The Medical Letter, Inc.
1000 Main Street
New Rochelle, New York 10801-7537

800-211-2769
914-235-0500
Fax 914-632-1733
www.medicalletter.org

18th Edition

Contents

Introduction

The Medical Letter, Inc. is a nonprofit company founded in 1958 by Arthur Kallet, the co-founder of Consumers Union, and Dr. Harold Aaron, with the goal of providing healthcare professionals with objective, independent analyses of both prescription and over-the-counter drugs. In addition to its newsletters, *The Medical Letter on Drugs and Therapeutics* and *Treatment Guidelines from The Medical Letter*, the company also publishes handbooks and software on topics such as adverse drug interactions and antimicrobial therapy. It is supported solely by subscription fees and accepts no advertising, grants or donations.

The Medical Letter on Drugs and Therapeutics offers comprehensive drug evaluations of virtually all new drugs and reviews of older drugs when important new information becomes available on their usefulness or adverse effects. Occasionally, *The Medical Letter* publishes an article on a new non-drug treatment or a diagnostic aid. *Treatment Guidelines from The Medical Letter* consists of review articles of drug classes for treatment of major indications. A typical issue contains recommendations for first choice and alternative drugs with assessments of the drugs' effectiveness, safety and cost. *The Medical Letter* is published every other week and *Treatment Guidelines* is published once a month. Both are intended to meet the needs of the busy healthcare professional who wants unbiased, reliable and timely information on new drugs and comprehensive reviews of treatments of choice for major indications. Both publications help healthcare professionals make decisions based on the best interests of their patients, rather than the commercial interests of the pharmaceutical industry.

The editorial process used for Medical Letter publications relies on a consensus of experts to develop prescribing recommendations. An expert consultant or one of our editors prepares the preliminary report on a drug (for *The Medical Letter*) or drugs for particular indications (for *Treatment Guidelines*) in terms of their effectiveness, adverse effects and possible alternatives. Both published and available unpublished studies are carefully examined, paying special attention to the results of controlled clinical trials. The preliminary draft is sent to members of the Advisory Board of The Medical Letter, consultants who have clinical and experimental experience with the drug or type of drug or disease under review, the FDA and sometimes the CDC. The article is edited in-house by our editorial staff and the final publication is considered a crucial resource for members of the healthcare community to consult when they are overwhelmed by advertisements and personal visits from sales representatives of the pharmaceutical industry.

The Medical Letter, Inc., is based in New Rochelle, NY. For more information call (800) 211-2769 or go to www.medicalletter.org.

ANTIBACTERIAL DRUGS:
A BRIEF SUMMARY FOR QUICK REFERENCE

AMINOGLYCOSIDES — Aminoglycosides are effective against many gram-negative bacteria, but not gram-positives or anaerobes. They are often used together with a ß-lactam antibiotic such as ampicillin, ticarcillin, piperacillin, a cephalosporin, imipenem or aztreonam. They may be ototoxic and nephrotoxic, especially in patients with diminished renal function.

Amikacin *(Amikin)* — Amikacin is often effective for treatment of infections caused by gram-negative strains resistant to gentamicin and tobramycin, including some strains of *Pseudomonas aeruginosa* and *Acinetobacter*. It is generally reserved for treatment of serious infections caused by amikacin-susceptible gram-negative bacteria known or suspected to be resistant to the other aminoglycosides. Like other aminoglycosides, its distribution to the lungs is limited and when used to treat gram-negative bacilli that cause pneumonia it should be combined with another agent to which the organism is susceptible, such as a ß-lactam. It has also been used concurrently with other drugs for treatment of some mycobacterial infections.

Gentamicin (*Garamycin*, and others) — Useful for treatment of many hospital-acquired infections caused by gram-negative bacteria. Strains of gram-negative bacilli resistant to gentamicin are often susceptible to amikacin or to one of the third-generation cephalosporins, cefepime, or imipenem or meropenem. Gentamicin is also used with penicillin G, ampicillin or vancomycin for treatment of endocarditis caused by susceptible enterococci.

Kanamycin (*Kantrex*, and others) — Active against some gram-negative bacilli (except *Pseudomonas* or anaerobes), but most centers now use gentamicin, tobramycin or amikacin instead. Kanamycin can be useful concurrently with other drugs for treatment of tuberculosis.

Antibacterial Drugs: A Brief Summary for Quick Reference

Neomycin — A drug that can cause severe damage to hearing and renal function and has the same antibacterial spectrum as kanamycin. Parenteral formulations have no rational use because of their toxicity. Deafness has also followed topical use over large areas of skin, injection into cavities such as joints, and oral administration, especially in patients with renal insufficiency.

Streptomycin — Streptomycin has been displaced by gentamicin for treatment of gram-negative infections, but it is still sometimes used concurrently with other drugs for treatment of tuberculosis and is occasionally used with penicillin, ampicillin or vancomycin to treat enterococcal endocarditis.

Tobramycin (*Nebcin*, and others) — Similar to gentamicin but with greater activity *in vitro* against *Pseudomonas aeruginosa* and less activity against *Serratia*. In clinical use, it is not certain that it is significantly less nephrotoxic than gentamicin.

AMINOSALICYLIC ACID (PAS) — Used in antituberculosis regimens for many years, its distressing gastrointestinal effects caused many patients to stop taking it prematurely. An enteric-coated oral formulation *(Paser)* is more tolerable, and is used occasionally in combination with other drugs in treating tuberculosis due to organisms resistant to first-line drugs.

AMOXICILLIN (*Amoxil*, and others) — See Penicillins

AMOXICILLIN/CLAVULANIC ACID (*Augmentin*, and others) — See Penicillins

AMPICILLIN (*Principen*, and others) — See Penicillins

AMPICILLIN /SULBACTAM (*Unasyn*) — See Penicillins

AZITHROMYCIN (*Zithromax*, and others) — See Macrolides

AZTREONAM *(Azactam)* — A parenteral monobactam (ß-lactam) antibiotic active against most aerobic gram-negative bacilli, including *Pseudomonas aeruginosa*, but not against gram-positive organisms or anaerobes. Aztreonam has little cross-allergenicity with penicillins and cephalosporins.

BACITRACIN — A nephrotoxic drug used in the past to treat severe systemic infections caused by staphylococci resistant to penicillin G. Its use is now restricted mainly to topical application.

CAPREOMYCIN *(Capastat)* — A second-line antituberculosis drug.

CARBAPENEMS
Imipenem/Cilastatin *(Primaxin)* — The first carbapenem, imipenem, has an especially broad antibacterial spectrum. Cilastatin sodium inhibits renal tubular metabolism of imipenem. This combination may be especially useful for treatment of serious infections in which aerobic gram-negative bacilli, anaerobes, and *Staphylococcus aureus* (but not oxacillin-resistant strains) might all be involved. It is active against many gram-negative bacilli that are resistant to third- and fourth-generation cephalosporins, aztreonam and aminoglycosides. Resistance to imipenem in *Pseudomonas aeruginosa* occasionally develops during therapy. It has been rarely associated with seizures particularly with high doses in elderly patients.

Meropenem *(Merrem)* — A carbapenem for parenteral use similar to imipenem/cilastatin. It may have less potential than imipenem for causing seizures.

Doripenem *(Doribax)* — Doripenem has a spectrum of activity similar to imipenem/cilastatin. *In vitro*, it is more active than imipenem and meropenem against *P. aeruginosa* and is active against some pseudomonal isolates resistant to the other carbapenems; the clinical significance of this *in vitro* activity is unknown. It may have less potential than imipenem for causing seizures.

Ertapenem (*Invanz*) — Ertapenem has a longer half-life but narrower antibacterial spectrum than imipenem, meropenem and doripenem. It is more active against some extended-spectrum ß-lactamase-producing gram-negative bacilli, but less active against gram-positive cocci, *Pseudomonas aeruginosa* and *Acinetobacter* spp. For empiric treatment of intra-abdominal, pelvic and urinary tract infections and community-acquired pneumonia, it offers no advantage over older drugs other than once-daily dosing.

CARBENICILLIN — See Penicillins

CEPHALOSPORINS — All cephalosporins except ceftazidime have good activity against most gram-positive cocci, and all cephalosporins are active against many strains of gram-negative bacilli. All cephalosporins are inactive against enterococci and oxacillin-resistant staphylococci. These drugs are often prescribed for patients allergic to penicillin, but such patients may also have allergic reactions to cephalosporins. Rare, potentially fatal immune-mediated hemolysis has been reported, particularly with ceftriaxone and cefotetan.

The cephalosporins can be classified into four "generations" based on their activity against gram-negative organisms. All first-generation drugs have a similar spectrum, including many gram-positive cocci (but not enterococci or oxacillin-resistant *Staphylococcus aureus*), *Escherichia coli*, *Klebsiella pneumoniae*, and *Proteus mirabilis*. Among the first-generation parenteral cephalosporins, **cefazolin** (*Ancef*, and others) is less painful on intramuscular injection than **cephapirin** (*Cefadyl*, and others). The first-generation parenteral cephalosporins are usually given intravenously, and cefazolin is most frequently used because of its longer half-life.

The second-generation cephalosporins have broader *in vitro* activity against gram-negative bacteria. **Cefamandole** *(Mandol)* has increased activity against *Haemophilus influenzae* and some gram-negative bacilli, but is occasionally associated with prothrombin deficiency and bleeding. **Cefoxitin** *(Mefoxin)* has improved activity against *Bacteroides fragilis*, *Neisseria gonorrhoeae* and some aerobic gram-negative bacilli. **Cefotetan** *(Cefotan)* has a spectrum of activity similar to that of cefoxitin; it has a side chain that has rarely been associated with prothrombin deficiency and bleeding. **Cefuroxime** *(Zinacef, Kefurox)*, another second-generation cephalosporin, has a spectrum of activity similar to cefamandole. Cefuroxime and cefamandole are less active than third-generation cephalosporins against penicillin-resistant strains of *Streptococcus pneumoniae*. **Cefonicid** *(Monocid)* has a longer half-life than the other second-generation cephalosporins, but is less active against gram-positive organisms and less active than cefoxitin against anaerobes.

The third-generation cephalosporins, **cefotaxime** *(Claforan)*, **cefoperazone** *(Cefobid)*, **ceftizoxime** *(Cefizox)*, **ceftriaxone** *(Rocephin)* and **ceftazidime** *(Fortaz, and others)*, and the fourth-generation cephalosporin, **cefepime** *(Maxipime)*, are more active than the second-generation cephalosporins against enteric gram-negative bacilli, including nosocomially acquired strains resistant to multiple antibiotics. These agents are highly active against *Haemophilus influenzae* and *Neisseria gonorrhoeae*, including penicillinase-producing strains. Except for ceftazidime, they are moderately active against anaerobes, but often less so than metronidazole, chloramphenicol, clindamycin, cefoxitin, cefotetan, ampicillin/sulbactram, piperacillin/tazobactam, ticarcillin/clavulanic acid, or carbapenems. Ceftazidime has poor activity against gram-positive organisms and anaerobes. Cefotaxime, ceftizoxime, ceftriaxone and cefepime are the most active *in vitro* against gram-positive organisms, but ceftizoxime has poor activity against *Streptococcus pneumoniae* that are intermediate or highly resistant to penicillin. Cefoperazone, which can cause bleeding, is less active than other third-generation cephalosporins against many gram-negative bacilli, but more active than cefotaxime, ceftizoxime or ceftriaxone against *Pseudomonas aeruginosa*. Ceftazidime and cefepime have the greatest activity among the cephalosporins against *Pseudomonas aeruginosa*. Cefepime has somewhat greater activity against enteric gram-negative bacilli than the third-generation cephalosporins. The third-generation cephalosporins and cefepime are expensive, but are useful for treatment of serious hospital-associated gram-negative infections when used alone or in combination with aminoglycosides such as gentamicin, tobramycin or amikacin. Gram-negative bacteria that produce "broad spectrum" ß-lactamases are resistant to first-generation cephalosporins, but are usually sensitive to second and third generation cephalosporins. However, gram-negative bacilli that produce "extended spectrum ß-lactamases", particularly some *Klebsiella* strains and those that produce chromosomally-encoded ß-lactamases, are usually resistant to first, second and third-generation cephalosporins. These organisms are often hospital-associated. Cefipime may be more active than the third-generation cephalosporin against these strains, but imipenem and meropenem are most consistently active against them. Cefotaxime and ceftriaxone are often used for treatment of meningitis. Ceftriaxone has been widely used for single-dose treatment of gonorrhea.

Cephalexin (*Keflex*, and others), **cephradine** (*Velosef*, and others), and **cefadroxil** (*Duricef*, and others) are well-absorbed oral cephalosporins with first-generation antimicrobial activity; cephradine is also available for parenteral use. **Cefaclor** (*Ceclor*, and others), **cefuroxime axetil** (*Ceftin*), **cefprozil** (*Cefzil*) and **loracarbef** (*Lorabid*) are oral second-generation agents with increased activity against *Haemophilus influenzae* and *Moraxella catarrhalis*. **Cefixime** (*Suprax*), an oral cephalosporin with activity against gram-positive organisms similar to that of first-generation cephalosporins except for its poor activity against staphylococci; against gram-negative bacteria, it has greater activity than second-generation cephalosporins. It is useful for single-dose oral treatment of gonorrhea. **Cefpodoxime proxetil** (*Vantin*), **cefdinir** (*Omnicef*) and **cefditoren pivoxil** (*Spectracef*) are oral cephalosporins similar to cefixime, but with greater activity against methicillin-susceptible staphylococci. **Ceftibuten** *(Cedax)* is an oral cephalosporin similar to cefixime in its gram-negative activity and poor activity against staphylococci, but it has only inconsistent activity against *Streptococcus pneumoniae.*

Ceftobiprole is an investigational broad-spectrum cephalosporin with activity against MRSA. It may soon be available.

CHLORAMPHENICOL (*Chloromycetin*, and others) — An effective drug for treatment of meningitis, epiglottitis, or other serious infections caused by *Haemophilus influenzae*, severe infections with *Salmonella typhi*, for some severe infections caused by *Bacteroides* (especially those in the central nervous system), and for treatment of vancomycin-resistant *Enterococcus*. Chloramphenicol is often an effective alternative for treatment of pneumococcal or meningococcal meningitis in patients allergic to penicillin, but some strains of *Streptococcus pneumoniae* are resistant to it. Because it can cause fatal blood dyscrasias, chloramphenicol should be used only for serious infections caused by susceptible bacteria that cannot be treated effectively with less toxic agents.

CINOXACIN (*Cinobac***, and others) — See Quinolones**

CIPROFLOXACIN (*Cipro***, and others) — See Fluoroquinolones**

CLARITHROMYCIN (*Biaxin,*** and others) — See Macrolides**

CLINDAMYCIN (*Cleocin*, and others) — A derivative of lincomycin with a similar antibacterial spectrum, clindamycin can cause severe diarrhea and pseudomembranous colitis. It is one of the alternative drugs for anaerobic infections outside the central nervous system, and can also be used as an alternative for treatment of some staphylococcal infections in patients allergic to penicillins. Strains of *S. aureus* that are sensitive to clindamycin, but resistant to erythromycin become rapidly resistant to clindamycin when it is used. Clindamycin is also used concurrently with other drugs to treat *Pneumocystis carinii* pneumonia and toxoplasmosis.

Clindamycin may be beneficial in treatment of necrotizing fasciitis due to Group A streptococcus but, because of the possibility of resistance to clindamycin, it should be used in combination with penicillin G.

CLOFAZIMINE *(Lamprene)* — An oral agent used with other drugs for treatment of leprosy.

CLOXACILLIN — See Penicillinase-resistant Penicillins

COLISTIMETHATE *(Coly-Mycin)* — See Polymyxins

CYCLOSERINE *(Seromycin*, and others) — A second-line antituberculosis drug.

DAPTOMYCIN *(Cubicin)* — A cyclic lipopeptide antibiotic that is effective for treating complicated skin and soft tissue infections and methicillin-sensitive and methicillin-resistant *S. aureus* bacteremia, including right-sided endocarditis. It is rapidly bactericidal against gram-positive bacteria by causing membrane depolarization. Its anti-bacterial activity includes oxacillin-sensitive and resistant, and vancomycin-sensitive and resistant *S. aureus* and coagulase-negative staphylococci, streptococci and vancomycin-sensitive and resistant enterococci. Rarely, *S. aureus* strains with decreased susceptibility to daptomycin have emerged during treatment of *S. aureus* endocarditis with daptomycin. Some strains of *S. aureus* that have emerged with reduced susceptibility to vancomycin during treament with vancomycin, have shown reduced susceptibility to daptomycin. It is administered intravenously once daily and is excreted unchanged in urine; dose adjustments are required when given to individuals with severe renal insufficiency. Adverse effects include the potential for skeletal muscle damage, with rare reversible CPK elevations. More severe muscle effects, which were seen in preclinical studies, do not seem to occur at the currently approved doses; higher doses may increase the potential for rhabdomyolysis. Daptomycin should not be used to treat pneumonia because it is inactivated by surfactant.

DEMECLOCYCLINE *(Declomycin)* — See Tetracyclines

DICLOXACILLIN *(Dycill*, and others) — See Penicillinase-resistant Penicillins

DIRITHROMYCIN *(Dynabac)* — See Macrolides

DORIPENEM *(Doribax)* — See Carbapenems

DOXYCYCLINE *(Vibramycin*, and others) — See Tetracyclines

ERTAPENEM *(Invanz)* — See Carbapenems

ERYTHROMYCIN *(Erythrocin*, and others) — See Macrolides

ERYTHROMYCIN-SULFISOXAZOLE *(Pediazole*, and others) — See Macrolides

ETHIONAMIDE *(Trecator-SC)* — A second-line antituberculosis drug.

ETHAMBUTOL *(Myambutol)* — Often used in antituberculosis regimens, it can cause optic neuritis.

FLUOROQUINOLONES — Fluoroquinolones are synthetic anti-bacterial agents with activity against gram-positive and gram-negative organisms. With the increased use of fluoroquinolones, resistant organisms have become more frequent, especially among strains of *Staphylococcus aureus* and *Pseudomonas aeruginosa*. Resistance among *Streptococcus pneumoniae* strains has begun to emerge but is still rare, especially in the US. None of these agents is recommended for use in children or pregnant women. All can cause gastrointestinal disturbances and, less commonly central nervous system toxicity. Tendon effects and hypersensitivity reactions, including vasculitis, serum sickness-like reactions and anaphylaxis, occur rarely. Hypo- and hyper-glycemia can also occur rarely.

Ciprofloxacin (*Cipro*, and others) — Used for oral or intravenous treatment of a wide variety of gram-positive and gram-negative bacterial infections in adults, including those due to oxacillin-susceptible and resistant staphylococci, *Haemophilus influenzae*, *Neisseria*, enteric pathogens and other aerobic gram-negative bacilli, and *Pseudomonas aeruginosa*, but not anaerobes. Newer fluoroquinolones such as levofloxacin, gatifloxacin, gemifloxacin and moxifloxacin are preferred for treatment of gram-positive coccal infections such as those caused by *S. pneumoniae* and *S. aureus*. Ciprofloxacin is useful for treatment of urinary tract infections caused by enteric gram-negative bacilli or *Pseudomonas aeruginosa*. Oral ciprofloxacin has been effective in treating patients with neutropenia and fever who are at low risk for mortality. Ciprofloxacin is now one of the preferred prophylactic agents for contacts of patients with meningococcal disease. It is also used for prophylaxis after *Bacillus anthracis* (Anthrax) exposure. Emergence of resistance in staphylococcal and *Pseudomonas* strains and other gram-negative organisms is increasingly encountered.

Levofloxacin *(Levaquin)*, **moxifloxacin** *(Avelox)* and **gemifloxacin** *(Factive)* — More active than ciprofloxacin or ofloxacin against gram-positive organisms, such as *Streptococcus pneumoniae*, including strains highly resistant to penicillin, and *Staphylococcus aureus*. Like other fluoroquinolones, they are active against *Legionella pneumophila*, *Chlamydia spp.*, *Mycoplasma pneumoniae*, *Haemophilus influenzae* and *Moraxella catarrhalis*. All are effective for many community-acquired respiratory infections. Levofloxacin and moxifloxacin are less active than ciprofloxacin *in vitro* against enteric gram-negative bacilli and *Pseudomonas aeruginosa*, but have been effective in treating urinary tract infections and other systemic infections caused by these organisms. Levofloxacin and moxifloxacin have been used to treat some oxacillin-sensitive and oxacillin-resistant *S. aureus* infections, although resistance is increasing. Levofloxacin, moxifloxacin, ofloxacin or ciprofloxacin are sometimes used as second-line anti-tuberculous drugs in combination with other agents. Moxifloxacin has been used more frequently for treatment of tuberculosis than the other fluoroquinolones. Levofloxacin is more effective for treatment of *Legionella pneumophila* than azithromycin. The use of fluoroquinolones has been associated with the recent increase in severe cases of *C. difficile* colitis. Levofloxacin and moxifloxacin are available for both oral and parenteral use. Gemifloxacin is only available for oral use. Levofloxacin and moxifloxacin have rarely been associated with torsades de pointes arrhythmia. Gemifloxacin has produced more rashes than other fluoroquinolones.

Gatifloxacin — Gatifloxacin has been associated with hypergylcemia and hypoglycemia more often than the other fluoroquinolones and it is no longer available.

Lomefloxacin *(Maxaquin)* — An oral once-a-day fluoroquinolone promoted for treatment of urinary tract infections and bronchitis, but pneumococci and other streptococci are resistant to the drug.

Norfloxacin *(Noroxin)* — An oral fluoroquinolone for treatment of urinary tract infections due to Enterobacteriaceae, *Enterococcus* or *Pseudomonas aeruginosa*.

Ofloxacin *(Floxin,* and others) — An oral and intravenous fluoroquinolone similar to ciprofloxacin but less active against *Pseudomonas*. Ofloxacin can be used for single-dose treatment of gonorrhea and for seven-day treatment of chlamydial infections. It is sometimes used as a second-line anti-tuberculous drug in combination with other agents.

FOSFOMYCIN *(Monurol)* — Can be used as a single-dose oral agent with moderate effectiveness for treatment of uncomplicated urinary tract infections caused by many strains of enteric gram-negative bacilli, enterococci and some strains of *Staphylococcus saphrophyticus*, but generally not *Pseudomonas*. It is much more expensive than trimethoprim/sulfamethoxazole.

FURAZOLIDONE *(Furoxone)* — An oral nonabsorbable antimicrobial agent of the nitrofuran group that inhibits monoamine oxidase (MAO). The manufacturer recommends it for treatment of bacterial diarrhea. Its safety has been questioned (oral administration induces mammary tumors in rats) and other more effective drugs are available.

GATIFLOXACIN *(Tequin)* — See Fluoroquinolones (has been withdrawn)

GEMIFLOXACIN *(Factive)* — See Fluoroquinolones

GENTAMICIN *(Garamycin*, and others) — See Aminoglycosides

IMIPENEM/CILASTATIN *(Primaxin)* — See Carbapenems

ISONIAZID *(Nydrazid*, and others) — A major antituberculosis drug that can cause fatal hepatitis. **Rifampin-isoniazid-pyrazinamide** *(Rifater)* and **rifampin-isoniazid** *(Rifamate)* are fixed-dose combinations for treatment of tuberculosis.

KANAMYCIN (*Kantrex*, and others) — See Aminoglycosides

LEVOFLOXACIN *(Levaquin)* — See Fluoroquinolones

LINCOMYCIN *(Lincocin)* — Similar to clindamycin in antibacterial activity and adverse effects. Rarely indicated for treatment of any infection because it is less active than clindamycin.

LINEZOLID *(Zyvox)* — An oxazolidinone bacteristatic antibiotic available in both an oral and intravenous formulation. It is active against *Enterococcus faecium* and *E. faecalis* including vancomycin-resistant enterococcal infections. Linezolid is also active against oxacillin-resistant *Staphylococcus aureus*, *S. epidermidis* and penicillin-resistant *Streptococcus pneumoniae*. Reversible thrombocytopenia has occurred, especially with therapy for more than 2 weeks. A serotonin syndrome has been observed in patients taking linezolid together with a selective serotonin receptor inhibitor. Emergence of resistance has been observed with enterococcal and *S. aureus* strains.

LOMEFLOXACIN *(Maxaquin)* — See Fluoroquinolones

MACROLIDES

Azithromycin *(Zithromax)* — A macrolide antibiotic that has much less gastrointestinal toxicity than erythromycin and is not associated with drug interactions with the CYP3A cytochrome P-450 enzyme systems. A single dose has been effective for treatment of urethritis and cervicitis caused by *Chlamydia* and for treatment of trachoma. Azithromycin is useful in treating *Mycoplasma pneumoniae, Chlamydia pneumoniae* and *Legionella pneumophila* pneumonias, as well as some respiratory infections due to *Streptococcus pneumoniae, Haemophilus influenzae* or *Moraxella catarrhalis*. However, an increasing number of *S. pneumoniae* strains have become resistant to the macrolides and azithromycin should not be used alone to treat pneumococcal pneumonia unless the causative strain is known to be sensitive to the macrolides. Azithromycin alone is effective for prevention of *Mycobacterium avium* infections, and combined with other drugs, such as ethambutol, rifabutin or ciprofloxacin, it is effective for treatment.

Clarithromycin *(Biaxin)* — A macrolide antibiotic similar to azithromycin, but with a shorter half-life. It is somewhat more active than azithromycin against gram-positive organisms and less active against gram-negative organisms. Clarithromycin is effective for prevention of *Mycobacterium avium* infections and, combined with other drugs, for treatment of both *M. avium* and *Helicobacter pylori*. It has more adverse drug interactions than azithromycin. Clarithromycin is a strong inhibitor of CYP3A4 and can increase the serum concentrations of many drugs. It prolongs the QT interval and may rarely be associated with torsades de pointes, a potentially fatal arrhythmia. The risk is increased with concurrent use of other drugs that prolong the QT interval.

Dirithromycin *(Dynabac)* — Similar to erythromycin; it can be given once a day.

Erythromycin (*Erythrocin*, and others) — Used especially for respiratory tract infections due to pneumococci or Group A streptococci in patients allergic to penicillin, for pneumonia due to *Mycoplasma pneumoniae* or *Chlamydia spp.*, and for treatment of infection caused by *Legionella pneumophila*, erythromycin has few adverse effects except for frequent gastrointestinal disturbances but many drug interactions involving the CYP3A cytochrome P-450 system. Erythromycin given orally or intravenously may rarely be associated with torsades de pointes, a potentially fatal arrhythmia; risk of torsades is increased by concurrent use of CYP3A inhibitors and other drugs that prolong the QT inverval. Use in young infants has rarely been associated with hypertrophic pyloric stenosis. The estolate formulation *(Ilosone)* can cause cholestatic jaundice. Erythromycin is not recommended for treatment of serious staphylococcal infections, even when the organisms are susceptible to the drug *in vitro*, because of potential for rapid development of resistance. Strains of *Streptococcus pneumoniae* and Group A streptococci resistant to erythromycin have become more frequent and the drug should not be used alone to treat community-acquired pneumonia when pneumococcus is likely, unless susceptibility of the organism has been established.

Erythromycin/Sulfisoxazole (*Pediazole*, and others) — A combination of 100 mg of erythromycin ethylsuccinate and 300 mg sulfisoxazole acetyl per half-teaspoon for oral treatment of acute otitis media.

MEROPENEM *(Merrem)* — See Carbapenems

METHENAMINES (*Mandelamine*, and others) — Oral drugs that can sterilize an acid urine. They are used for prophylaxis of chronic or recurrent urinary tract infections, but trimethoprim/sulfamethoxazole is more effective.

METHICILLIN — See Penicillinase-resistant Penicillins

METRONIDAZOLE (*Flagyl*, and others) — Available in oral form for treatment of trichomoniasis, amebiasis, giardiasis and *Gardnerella vaginalis* vaginitis, metronidazole is also available for intravenous treatment of anaerobic bacterial infections. Good penetration of the blood-brain barrier may be an advantage in treating central-nervous-system infections due to *Bacteroides fragilis*. Metronidazole is frequently used for treatment of pseudomembranous enterocolitis due to *Clostridium difficile*. However, vancomycin given orally is more effective in serious cases. It is sometimes used in combination with other drugs to treat *H. pylori* infection.

MINOCYCLINE (*Minocin*, and others) — See Tetracyclines

MOXIFLOXACIN (*Avelox*) — See Fluoroquinolones

NAFCILLIN (*Nafcil*, and others) — See Penicillinase-resistant Penicillins

NALIDIXIC ACID (*NegGram*, and others) — See Quinolones

NEOMYCIN — See Aminoglycosides

NITROFURANTOIN (*Macrodantin*, and others) — This oral agent is used for prophylaxis or treatment of urinary tract infections, especially those resistant to other agents. Because of its potential toxicity, nitrofurantoin should not be used when renal function is markedly diminished. Nausea and vomiting are often troublesome, and peripheral neuropathy, pulmonary reactions and severe hepatotoxicity may occur.

NORFLOXACIN *(Noroxin)* — See Fluoroquinolones

OFLOXACIN *(Floxin)* — See Fluoroquinolones

OXACILLIN — See Penicillinase-resistant Penicillins

PENICILLINS

Natural Penicillins — Penicillin remains the drug of choice for Group A streptococcal infections and for treatment of syphilis and some other infections. Clindamycin may be beneficial for treatment of Group A streptococcal necrotizing fasciitis, but it should be combined with penicillin G because of increasing resistance to clindamycin in Group A streptococcus. *Streptococcus pneumoniae* strains frequently show intermediate or high-level resistance to penicillin. Penicillin is effective for fully sensitive strains, and high doses of penicillin, cefotaxime or ceftriaxone are effective for pneumonia due to strains with intermediate sensitivity; vancomycin is added for highly resistant strains, especially for meningitis.

Aminopenicillins:

Amoxicillin *(Amoxil, and others)* — An oral semisynthetic penicillin similar to ampicillin, it is better absorbed and may cause less diarrhea. Amoxicillin is at least as effective as oral ampicillin for the treatment of most infections, with the exception of shigellosis. High doses (at least 3000 mg/day) have been successful in treating pneumococcal respiratory infections caused by strains with reduced susceptibility to penicillin.

Amoxicillin/Clavulanic Acid *(Augmentin, and others)* — The ß-lactamase inhibitor, potassium clavulanate, extends amoxicillin's spectrum of activity to include ß-lactamase-producing strains of *Staphylococcus aureus*, *Haemophilus influenzae*, *Moraxella catarrhalis* and many strains of enteric gram-negative bacilli, including anaerobes such as *Bacteroides* spp. This combination may be useful for oral treatment of bite wounds, otitis media, sinusitis and some lower respiratory tract and urinary tract infections, but it can cause a higher incidence of diarrhea and other gastrointestinal symptoms than amoxicillin alone, and less costly alternatives are available. An oral extended-release form of *Augmentin (Augmentin XR)* containing a higher content of amoxicillin in each tablet (1000 mg) has been successful in treating acute bacterial sinusitis and community-acquired pneumonia caused by strains of pneumococci with reduced susceptibility to penicillin, but high dose amoxicillin which costs much less can also be used.

Ampicillin (*Principen*, and others) — This semisynthetic penicillin is as effective as penicillin G in pneumococcal, streptococcal and meningococcal infections, and is also active against some strains of *Salmonella*, *Shigella*, *Escherichia coli* and *Haemophilus influenzae* and many strains of *Proteus mirabilis*. The drug is not effective against penicillinase-producing staphylococci or ß-lactamase-producing gram-negative bacteria. Rashes are more frequent with ampicillin than with other penicillins. Taken orally, ampicillin is less well absorbed than amoxicillin.

Ampicillin/Sulbactam *(Unasyn)* — A parenteral combination of ampicillin with the ß-lactamase inhibitor sulbactam, which extends the antibacterial spectrum of ampicillin to include ß-lactamase-producing strains of *Staphylococcus aureus* (but not those resistant to oxacillin), *Haemophilus influenzae, Moraxella catarrhalis, Neisseria* and many gram-negative bacilli, including *Bacteroides fragilis*, but not *Pseudomonas aeruginosa, Enterobacter* or *Serratia*. It may be useful for treatment of gynecological and intra-abdominal infections. Some strains of *Acinetobacter* resistant to all other antibiotics may respond to high doses of ampicillin/sulbactam in combination with polymyxins.

Penicillinase-Resistant Penicillins: The drugs of choice for treatment of infections caused by penicillinase-producing staphylococci that are methicillin-sensitive, they are also effective against penicillin-sensitive pneumococci and Group A streptococci. For oral use for methicillin-sensitive *S. aureus* infections, **dicloxacillin** is preferred; for severe infections, a parenteral formulation of **nafcillin** or **oxacillin** should be used. **Methicillin** is no longer marketed in the US. Strains of *Staphylococcus aureus* or *epidermidis* that are resistant to these penicillins ("oxacillin-resistant") are also resistant to cephalosporins, and carbapenems. Infections caused by these strains should be treated with vancomycin, with or without rifampin and/or gentamicin, or with linezolid or daptomycin. Neither ampicillin, amoxicillin, carbenicillin, piperacillin nor ticarcillin is effective against penicillinase-producing staphylococci.

Extended-Spectrum Penicillins:

Carbenicillin *(Geocillin)* — The oral indanyl ester of carbenicillin; it does not produce therapeutic blood levels, but can be used for treatment of urinary tract infections, including those due to susceptible gram-negative bacilli such as *Pseudomonas aeruginosa* that may be resistant to other drugs.

Piperacillin *(Pipracil)* — A penicillin for parenteral treatment of gram-negative bacillary infections. It is similar to ticarcillin in antibacterial activity, but covers a wider spectrum, particularly against *Klebsiella pneumoniae* and *Bacteroides fragilis*. Its *in vitro* activity against *Pseudomonas* is greater than that of ticarcillin, but increased clinical effectiveness in *Pseudomonas* infections has not been demonstrated. Piperacillin is also active against some gram-positive cocci, including streptococci and some strains of *Enterococcus*. For treatment of serious gram-negative infections, it should generally be used in combination with an aminoglycoside such as gentamicin, tobramycin or amikacin.

Piperacillin/Tazobactam *(Zosyn)* — A parenteral formulation combining piperacillin with tazobactam, a ß-lactamase-inhibitor. The addition of the ß-lactamase inhibitor extends the spectrum of piperacillin to include ß-lactamase producing strains of staphylococci and some gram-negative bacilli, including *Bacteroides fragilis*. Infections caused by gram-negative bacilli that produce "extended spectrum" ß-lactamase are often resistant to piperacillin/tazobactam, those that produce chromosomal ß-lactamase are always resistant. The combination of the two drugs is usually no more active against *Pseudomonas aeruginosa* than piperacillin alone.

Ticarcillin *(Ticar)* — A penicillin similar to carbenicillin. Large parenteral doses of this semisynthetic penicillin can cure serious infections caused by susceptible strains of *Pseudomonas*, *Proteus* and some other gram-negative organisms. *Klebsiella* are generally resistant. Ticarcillin is also active against some gram-positive cocci, including streptococci and some strains of *Enterococcus*. It is often given together with another drug such as gentamicin, tobramycin or amikacin for treatment of serious systemic infections. It is less active than ampicillin, amoxicillin or piperacillin against strains of *Streptococcus pneumoniae* with reduced susceptibility to penicillin and against enterococci.

Ticarcillin/Clavulanic Acid *(Timentin)* — A parenteral preparation combining ticarcillin with potassium clavulanate, a ß-lactamase inhibitor. The addition of the ß-lactamase inhibitor extends the antibacterial spectrum of ticarcillin to include ß-lactamase producing strains of *Staphylococcus aureus*, *Haemophilus influenzae*, and some enteric gram-negative bacilli, including *Bacteroides fragilis*. The combination is usually no more active against *Pseudomonas aeruginosa* than ticarcillin alone.

POLYMYXINS B AND E (polymyxin B – various generics; polymyxin E – *Coly-Mycin*; colistimethate; colistin sulfate) — The polymyxins are used topically in combination with other antibiotics for treatment of infected wounds and otitis externa. They should generally not be used parenterally because safer and more effective alternatives are available. However, some strains of gram-negative bacilli (particularly *Klebsiella*, *Pseudumonas aeruginosa* and *Acinetobacter)* resistant to all other available antibiotics have been treated with one of the polymyxins; for infections caused by *Acinetobacter,* sulbactam (in the form of ampicillin/ sulbactam) is often added.

PYRAZINAMIDE — An antituberculosis drug now often used in the initial treatment regimen. Rifampin-isoniazid-pyrazinamide *(Rifater)* is a fixed-dose combination for treatment of tuberculosis.

QUINOLONES

Nalidixic Acid *(NegGram,* and others) — An oral drug active *in vitro* against many gram-negative organisms that commonly cause urinary tract infections. Development of resistance by initially susceptible strains is rapid, however, and clinical results are much less favorable than would be expected from sensitivity testing alone. Nalidixic acid can cause severe adverse effects, including visual disturbances, intracranial hypertension, and convulsions. Other drugs are generally preferred for treatment of urinary tract infections.

Cinoxacin *(Cinobac,* and others) — An oral drug similar to nalidixic acid for treatment of urinary tract infections.

QUINUPRISTIN/DALFOPRISTIN *(Synercid)* — Two streptogramin antibacterials marketed in a fixed-dose combination for parenteral use. The combination is active against vancomycin-resistant *Enterococcus faecium* (but not *E. faecalis*) as well as *Staphylococcus aureus*, *Streptococcus pneumoniae* and *S. pyogenes*. Adverse effects include frequent thrombophlebitis at the infusion site (it is best given through a central venous catheter) and arthralgias and myalgias. It has a number of drug interactions. The availability of linezolid and daptomycin as alternates have lead to infrequent use of quinupristin/dalfopristin.

RETAPAMULIN *(Altabax)* — A topical pleuromutilin antibiotic approved for treatment of impetigo caused by methicillin-susceptible *S. aureus* and Group A streptococci *(S. pyogenes)*.

RIFABUTIN *(Mycobutin)* — Similar to rifampin, rifabutin is used to prevent and treat tuberculosis and disseminated *Mycobacterium avium* infections in patients with AIDS. It has fewer drug interactions than rifampin.

RIFAMPIN *(Rifadin, Rimactane)* — A major drug for treatment of tuberculosis. To prevent emergence of resistant organisms, it should be used together with other antituberculosis drugs. It is sometimes used concurrently with other drugs for treatment of *Mycobacterium avium* infections in AIDS patients. Rifampin is also useful for prophylaxis in close contacts of patients with sulfonamide-resistant meningococcal disease and for prophylaxis in children who are close contacts of patients with *Haemophilus influenzae* meningitis. Rifampin is a potent inducer of CYP3A enzymes and may increase the metabolism of the many drugs, particularly some protease inhibitors. **Rifampin-isoniazid-pyrazinamide** *(Rifater)* and **rifampin-isoniazid** *(Rifamate)* are fixed-dose combinations for treatment of tuberculosis.

RIFAPENTINE *(Priftin)* — A long-acting analog of rifampin used in the treatment of tuberculosis. Studies of its effectiveness are limited. Until more data become available, rifampin is preferred.

RIFAXIMIN *(Xifaxan)* — A non-absorbed oral antibiotic derived from rifampin, it is about as effective as ciprofloxacin for treatment of traveler's diarrhea, which is mostly caused by *E. coli*. It is not effective against gastrointestinal infections associated with fever or blood in the stool or those caused by *Campylobacter jejuni*. It has fewer adverse effects and drug interactions than systemic antibiotics, but should not be taken during pregnancy. Hypersensitivity reactions have been reported.

SPECTINOMYCIN *(Trobicin)* — A single-dose alternative for treatment of urogenital or anal gonorrhea. It is effective for penicillin-resistant infections and for patients who are allergic to penicillin. Spectinomycin is not effective against syphilis.

STREPTOMYCIN — See Aminoglycosides

SULFONAMIDES — Previously used for acute, uncomplicated urinary tract infections sulfonamides are now rarely used because of the increasing frequency of sulfonamide-resistance among gram-negative bacilli and the availability of fluoroquinolone and trimethoprim/sulfamethoxazole. When used, a soluble oral sulfonamide such as sulfisoxazole (*Gantrisin*, and others) is preferred.

TELITHROMYCIN *(Ketek)* — A ketolide antibiotic, derived from erythromycin, it is only approved for oral treatment of mild to moderate community-acquired pneumonia in adults. Telithromycin is often active against most strains of *S. pneumoniae* that are resistant to penicillin and macrolides (erythromycin, clarithromycin and azithromycin). It can cause serious, even fatal, hepatotoxicity, exacerbation of myasthenia gravis, visual disturbances, and it is expensive. It is a strong inhibitor of CYP3A enzymes and can cause potentially dangerous increases in serum concentrations of substrates, including simvastatin (*Zocor*, and others), lovastatin (*Mevacor*, and others), atorvastatin *(Lipitor)* and midazolam (*Versed*, and others). Like clarithromycin and erythromycin it may prolong the QT inverval and should not be taken concurrently with other drugs that prolong the QT interval. Medical Letter consultants advise against its use.

TETRACYCLINES — **Doxycycline** (*Vibramycin*, and others), **oxytetracycline** *(Terramycin)*, and **minocycline** (*Minocin*, and others) are available in both oral and parenteral formulations; **tetracycline** and **demeclocycline** *(Declomycin)* are available only for oral use. Parenteral tetracyclines can cause severe liver damage, especially when given to patients with diminished renal function or in pregnancy. **Doxycycline** requires fewer doses and causes less gastrointestinal disturbance than other tetracyclines. It can be used for prophylaxis after *Bacillus anthracis* (anthrax) exposure. Doxycycline and other tetracyclines are effective in treating pneumonia caused by *Mycoplasma pneumoniae*, *Chlamydia pneumoniae* and *Legionella* species and are commonly used to treat Lyme disease in adults and urethritis, cervicitis, proctitis or pelvic inflammatory disease when caused by *Chlamydial* species. **Minocycline** may be useful for prophylactic treatment of close contacts of patients with meningococcal infection, but it frequently causes vomiting and vertigo.

TIGECYCLINE (*Tygacil*) — The first glycylcycline, tigecycline is FDA-approved for parenteral treatment of complicated intra-abdominal infections and complicated skin and skin structure infections in adults. It has a broad spectrum of antimicrobial activity, including activity against methicillin-resistant *S. aureus* (MRSA) and some multiply resistant gram-negative bacilli.

TOBRAMYCIN (*Nebcin*, and others) — See Aminoglycosides

TRIMETHOPRIM (*Proloprim*, and others) — An agent marketed only for oral treatment of uncomplicated urinary tract infections caused by gram-negative bacilli. Frequent use has the potential for producing organisms resistant not only to this drug but also to trimethoprim/sulfamethoxazole.

TRIMETHOPRIM/SULFAMETHOXAZOLE (*Bactrim, Septra*, and others) — A combination of a folic acid antagonist and a sulfonamide, useful especially for oral treatment of urinary tract infections, shigellosis, otitis media, traveler's diarrhea, bronchitis, *Pneumocystis carinii* pneumonia and methicillin-resistant *S. aureus* (MRSA) infections. An intravenous preparation is available for treatment of serious infections. Allergic reactions are common, especially in HIV-infected patients. It may occasionally produce elevation of serum creatinine, hyperkalemia and renal insufficiency.

VANCOMYCIN (*Vancocin*, and others) — An effective alternative to the penicillins for endocarditis caused by *Streptococcus viridans* or *Enterococcus*, for severe staphylococcal infections, and for penicillin-resistant *S. pneumoniae* infections. An increasing number of strains of enterococci (especially *E. faecium*), however, are resistant to vancomycin. Some strains of *S. aureus* have reduced susceptibility to vancomycin or are highly resistant. Linezolid or daptomycin may be used to treat infections caused by these strains of enterococci or *S. aureus*. Vancomycin is the most frequently used for treatment of infections caused by oxacillin-resistant *Staphylococcus aureus* and *epidermidis*, but for strains that are oxacillin-sensitive, nafcillin or oxacillin are more effective. For serious infections caused by *S. aureus* or enterococci higher than the traditional doses of 15 mg/kg every 12 hours IV for adults with normal renal function are being advocated by some consultants, but improved efficacy of such regimens has not yet been demonstrated and such higher dose regimens increase the incidence of nephrotoxicity, especially when combined with the use of aminoglycosides.

Oral treatment with vancomycin is more effective in treating severe antibiotic-associated colitis due to *Clostridium difficile*, compared to metronidazole.

PATHOGENS MOST LIKELY TO CAUSE INFECTIONS IN SPECIFIC ORGANS AND TISSUES

In many acute and most chronic infections, the choice of antimicrobial therapy can await the results of appropriate cultures and antimicrobial susceptibility tests. In acute life-threatening infections such as meningitis, pneumonia or bacteremia, however, and in other infections that have reached a serious stage, waiting 24 to 48 hours can be dangerous, and the choice of an antimicrobial agent for initial use must be based on tentative identification of the pathogen. Knowing the organisms most likely to cause infection in specific tissues, together with evaluation of gram-stained smears and familiarity with the antimicrobial susceptibility patterns of organisms prevalent in the hospital or community, permits a rational choice of initial treatment.

In the table below, bacteria, fungi, viruses and other pathogens are listed in estimated order of the frequency with which they cause acute infection, but these frequencies are subject to annual, seasonal and geographical variation. The order of pathogens may also vary depending on whether the infections are community or hospital-acquired, and whether or not the patient is immunosuppressed. This listing is based both on published reports and on the experience of Medical Letter consultants. Organisms not listed here may also be important causes of infection.

TABLE OF BACTERIA, FUNGI, AND SOME VIRUSES MOST LIKELY TO CAUSE ACUTE INFECTIONS

BLOOD (SEPTICEMIA)
Newborn Infants
1. *Streptococcus* Group B
2. *Escherichia coli* (or other gram-negative bacilli)
3. *Listeria monocytogenes*
4. *Staphylococcus aureus*
5. *Streptococcus pyogenes* (Group A)

6. Enterococcal spp.
7. *Streptococcus pneumoniae*

Children
1. *Streptococcus pneumoniae*
2. *Neisseria meningitidis*
3. *Staphylococcus aureus*
4. *Streptococcus pyogenes* (Group A)
5. *Haemophilus influenzae*
6. *Escherichia coli* (or other gram-negative bacilli)

Adults
1. *Staphylococcus aureus*
2. *Escherichia coli* (or other enteric gram-negative bacilli)
3. *Streptococcus pneumoniae*
4. Enterococcal spp.
5. Non-enteric gram-negative bacilli
    (*Pseudomonas, Acinetobacter, Aeromonas*)
6. *Candida* spp. and other fungi
7. *Staphylococcus epidermidis*
8. *Streptococcus pyogenes* (Group A)
9. Other streptococci (non-Group A and not Lancefield-groupable)
10. *Bacteroides* spp.
11. *Neisseria meningitidis*
12. *Neisseria gonorrhoeae*
13. *Fusobacterium* spp.
14. Mycobacteria
15. *Rickettsia* spp.
16. *Ehrlichia* spp.
17. *Brucella* spp.
18. *Leptospira* spp.

MENINGES
1. Viruses (enterovirus, herpes simplex, HIV, arbovirus, lymphocytic choriomeningitis [LCM] virus, mumps and others)

2. *Neisseria meningitidis*
3. *Streptococcus pneumoniae*
4. *Streptococcus* Group B (infants less than two months old)
5. *Escherichia coli* (or other gram-negative bacilli)
6. *Haemophilus influenzae* (in children)
7. *Streptococcus pyogenes* (Group A)
8. *Staphylococcus aureus* (with endocarditis or after neurosurgery, brain abscess)
9. *Mycobacterium tuberculosis*
10. *Cryptococcus neoformans* and other fungi
11. *Listeria monocytogenes*
12. Enterococcal spp. (neonatal period)
13. *Treponema pallidum*
14. *Leptospira* spp.
15. *Borrelia burgdorferi*
16. *Toxoplasma gondii*

BRAIN AND PARAMENINGEAL SPACES
1. Herpes simplex (encephalitis)
2. Anaerobic streptococci and/or *Bacteroides* spp. (cerebritis, brain abscess, and subdural empyema)
3. *Staphylococcus aureus* (cerebritis, brain abscess, epidural abscess)
4. *Haemophilus influenzae* (subdural empyema)
5. Arbovirus (encephalitis)
6. Mumps (encephalitis)
7. *Toxoplasma gondii* (encephalitis)
8. Human immunodeficiency virus (HIV)
9. *Mycobacterium tuberculosis*
10. *Nocardia* (brain abscess)
11. *Listeria monocytogenes* (encephalitis)
12. *Treponema pallidum*
13. *Cryptococcus neoformans* and other fungi
14. *Borrelia burgdorferi*
15. Other viruses (varicella-zoster [VZV], cytomegalovirus [CMV], Ebstein-Barr [EBV] and rabies)

16. *Mycoplasma pneumoniae*
17. *Taenia solium* (neurocysticercosis)
18. *Echinococcus* spp. (echinococcosis)
19. *Strongyloides stercoralis* hyperinfection
20. *Angiostrongylus cantonensis*
21. Free-living amoeba (*Naegleria*, *Acanthameoba* and *Balamuthia* spp.)

ENDOCARDIUM

1. *Staphylococcus aureus*
2. Viridans group of *Streptococcus*
3. Enterococcal spp.
4. *Streptococcus bovis*
5. *Staphylococcus epidermidis*
6. *Candida albicans* and other fungi
7. Gram-negative bacilli
8. *Streptococcus pneumoniae*
9. *Streptococcus pyogenes* (Group A)
10. *Corynebacterium* spp. (especially with prosthetic valves)
11. *Haemophilus*, *Actinobacillus*, *Cardiobacterium hominis* or *Eikenella* spp.

BONES (OSTEOMYELITIS)

1. *Staphylococcus aureus*
2. *Salmonella* spp. (or other gram-negative bacilli)
3. *Streptococcus pyogenes* (Group A)
4. *Mycobacterium tuberculosis*
5. Anaerobic streptococci (chronic)
6. *Bacteroides* spp. (chronic)

JOINTS

1. *Staphylococcus aureus*
2. *Streptococcus pyogenes* (Group A)
3. *Neisseria gonorrhoeae*
4. Gram-negative bacilli
5. *Streptococcus pneumoniae*

6. *Neisseria meningitidis*
7. *Haemophilus influenzae* (in children)
8. *Mycobacterium tuberculosis* and other *Mycobacteria*
9. Fungi
10. *Borrelia burgdorferi*

SKIN AND SUBCUTANEOUS TISSUES
Burns
1. *Staphylococcus aureus*
2. *Streptococcus pyogenes* (Group A)
3. *Pseudomonas aeruginosa* (or other gram-negative bacilli)

Skin infections
1. *Staphylococcus aureus*
2. *Streptococcus pyogenes* (Group A)
3. Dermatophytes
4. *Candida* spp. and other fungi
5. Herpes simplex or zoster
6. Gram-negative bacilli
7. *Treponema pallidum*
8. *Borrelia burgdorferi*
9. *Bartonella henselae* or *quintana*
10. *Bacillus anthracis*

Decubitus Wound infections
1. *Staphylococcus aureus*
2. *Escherichia coli* (or other gram-negative bacilli)
3. *Streptococcus pyogenes* (Group A)
4. Anaerobic streptococci
5. *Clostridia* spp.
6. Enterococcal spp.
7. *Bacteroides* spp.

Traumatic and Surgical Wounds
1. *Staphylococcus aureus*

2. Anaerobic streptococci
3. Gram-negative bacilli
4. *Clostridia* spp.
5. *Streptococcus pyogenes* (Group A)
6. Enterococcal spp.

EYES (Cornea and Conjunctiva)
1. Herpes and other viruses
2. *Neisseria gonorrhoeae* (in newborn)
3. *Staphylococcus aureus*
4. *Streptococcus pneumoniae*
5. *Haemophilus influenzae* (in children), including biotype *aegyptius* (Koch-Weeks bacillus)
6. *Moraxella lacunata*
7. *Pseudomonas aeruginosa*
8. Other gram-negative bacilli
9. *Chlamydia trachomatis* (trachoma and inclusion conjunctivitis)
10. Fungi

EARS
Auditory Canal
1. *Pseudomonas aeruginosa* (or other gram-negative bacilli)
2. *Staphylococcus aureus*
3. *Streptococcus pyogenes* (Group A)
4. *Streptococcus pneumoniae*
5. *Haemophilus influenzae* (in children)
6. Fungi

Middle Ear
1. *Streptococcus pneumoniae*
2. *Haemophilus influenzae* (in children)
3. *Moraxella catarrhalis*
4. *Streptococcus pyogenes* (Group A)
5. *Staphylococcus aureus*
6. Anaerobic streptococci (chronic)

7. *Bacteroides* spp. (chronic)
8. Other gram-negative bacilli (chronic)
9. *Mycobacterium tuberculosis*

PARANASAL SINUSES
1. *Streptococcus pneumoniae*
2. *Haemophilus influenzae*
3. *Moraxella catarrhalis*
4. *Streptococcus pyogenes* (Group A)
5. Anaerobic streptococci (chronic sinusitis)
6. *Staphylococcus aureus* (chronic sinusitis)
7. *Klebsiella* spp. (or other gram-negative bacilli)
8. *Mucor* spp., *Aspergillus* spp. (especially in diabetics and immunosuppressed patients)

MOUTH
1. Herpes viruses
2. *Candida* spp.
3. *Leptotrichia buccalis* (Vincent's infection)
4. *Bacteroides* spp.
5. Mixed anaerobes
6. *Treponema pallidum*
7. *Actinomyces*

THROAT
1. Respiratory viruses
2. *Streptococcus pyogenes* (Group A)
3. *Neisseria meningitidis* or *gonorrhoeae*
4. *Leptotrichia buccalis*
5. *Candida* spp.
6. *Corynebacterium diphtheriae*
7. *Bordetella pertussis*
8. *Haemophilus influenzae*
9. *Fusobacterium necrophorum*

LARYNX, TRACHEA, AND BRONCHI

1. Respiratory viruses
2. *Streptococcus pneumoniae*
3. *Haemophilus influenzae*
4. *Streptococcus pyogenes* (Group A)
5. *Corynebacterium diphtheriae*
6. *Staphylococcus aureus*
7. Gram-negative bacilli
8. *Fusobacterium necrophorum*

PLEURA

1. *Streptococcus pneumoniae*
2. *Staphylococcus aureus*
3. *Haemophilus influenzae*
4. Gram-negative bacilli
5. Anaerobic streptococci
6. *Bacteroides* spp.
7. *Streptococcus pyogenes* (Group A)
8. *Mycobacterium tuberculosis*
9. *Actinomyces, Nocardia* spp.
10. Fungi
11. *Fusobacterium necrophorum*

LUNGS
Pneumonia

1. Respiratory viruses (influenza virus A and B, adenovirus, respiratory syncytial virus, parainfluenza virus, rhinovirus, enteroviruses, cytomegalovirus, Epstein-Barr virus, varicella-zoster virus, measles virus, herpes simplex virus, hantavirus and coronavirus [SARS])
2. *Mycoplasma pneumoniae*
3. *Streptococcus pneumoniae*
4. *Haemophilus influenzae*
5. Anaerobic streptococci, fusospirochetes
6. *Bacteroides* spp.

7. *Staphylococcus aureus*
8. *Klebsiella* spp. (or other gram-negative bacilli)
9. *Legionella pneumophila*
10. *Chlamydia pneumoniae* (TWAR strain)
11. *Streptococcus pyogenes* (Group A)
12. *Rickettsia* spp.
13. *Mycobacterium tuberculosis*
14. *Pneumocystis carinii*
15. Fungi (especially *Aspergillus* species in immunosuppressed patients)
16. *Moraxella catarrhalis*
17. *Legionella micdadei (L. pittsburgensis)*
18. *Chlamydia psittaci*
19. *Fusobacterium necrophorum*
20. *Actinomyces* spp.
21. *Nocardia* spp.
22. *Rhodococcus equi*
23. *Bacillus anthracis* (mediastinitis)
24. *Yersinia pestis*

Abscess
1. Anaerobic streptococci
2. *Bacteroides* spp.
3. *Staphylococcus aureus*
4. *Klebsiella* spp. (or other gram-negative bacilli)
5. *Streptococcus pneumoniae*
6. Fungi
7. *Actinomyces, Nocardia* spp.

GASTROINTESTINAL TRACT
1. Gastrointestinal viruses
2. *Campylobacter jejuni*
3. *Salmonella* spp.
4. *Escherichia coli*
5. *Shigella* spp.

Pathogens

6. *Yersinia enterocolitica*
7. *Entamoeba histolytica*
8. *Giardia lamblia*
9. *Staphylococcus aureus*
10. *Vibrio cholerae*
11. *Vibrio parahaemolyticus*
12. Herpes simplex (anus)
13. *Treponema pallidum* (rectum)
14. *Neisseria gonorrhoeae* (rectum)
15. *Candida* spp.
16. *Clostridium difficile*
17. *Cryptosporidium parvum*
18. Cytomegalovirus (CMV)
19. Human immunodeficiency virus (HIV)
20. *Mycobacterium avium* complex
21. *Helicobacter pylori*
22. *Tropheryma whippelii*

URINARY TRACT
1. *Escherichia coli* (or other gram-negative bacilli)
2. *Staphylococcus aureus* and *epidermidis*
3. *Neisseria gonorrhoeae* (urethra)
4. Enterococcal spp.
5. *Candida* spp.
6. *Chlamydia* spp. (urethra)
7. *Treponema pallidum* (urethra)
8. *Trichomonas vaginalis* (urethra)
9. *Ureaplasma urealyticum*

FEMALE GENITAL TRACT
Vagina
1. *Trichomonas vaginalis*
2. *Candida* spp.
3. *Neisseria gonorrhoeae*
4. *Streptococcus pyogenes* (Group A)

5. *Gardnerella vaginalis* and associated anaerobes
6. *Treponema pallidum*

Uterus
1. Anaerobic streptococci
2. *Bacteroides* spp.
3. *Neisseria gonorrhoeae* (cervix)
4. *Clostridia* spp.
5. *Escherichia coli* (or other gram-negative bacilli)
6. Herpes simplex virus, type II (cervix)
7. *Streptococcus pyogenes* (Group A)
8. *Streptococcus,* Groups B and C
9. *Treponema pallidum*
10. *Actinomyces* spp. (most common infection of intrauterine devices)
11. *Staphylococcus aureus*
12. Enterococcal spp.
13. *Chlamydia trachomatis*
14. *Mycoplasma hominis*

Fallopian Tubes
1. *Neisseria gonorrhoeae*
2. *Escherichia coli* (or other gram-negative bacilli)
3. Anaerobic streptococci
4. *Bacteroides* spp.
5. *Chlamydia trachomatis*

MALE GENITAL TRACT
Seminal Vesicles
1. Gram-negative bacilli
2. *Neisseria gonorrhoeae*

Epididymis
1. *Chlamydia*
2. Gram-negative bacilli

3. *Neisseria gonorrhoeae*
4. *Mycobacterium tuberculosis*

Prostate Gland
1. Gram-negative bacilli
2. *Neisseria gonorrhoeae*

PERITONEUM
1. Gram-negative bacilli
2. Enterococcal spp.
3. *Bacteroides* spp.
4. Anaerobic streptococci
5. *Clostridia* spp.
6. *Streptococcus pneumoniae*
7. *Streptococcus* Group

CHOICE OF
Antibacterial Drugs

Original publication date – May 2007
Since the original publication of this article footnote #17 has been changed to reflect new information.

Information about empirical treatment of bacterial infections, emerging trends in antimicrobial resistance, new drugs and new data about older drugs continue to become available. Usual pathogens and empiric treatment for some common types of infections are summarized in the text and a table listing the drugs of choice and alternatives for each pathogen begins on page 56. The recommendations made here are based on the results of susceptibility studies, clinical trials and the opinions of Medical Letter consultants.

INFECTIONS OF SKIN, SOFT TISSUE AND BONE

SKIN AND SOFT TISSUE — Uncomplicated skin and skin structure infections in immunocompetent patients are most commonly due to *Staphylococcus aureus, Streptococcus pyogenes* (group A) or *Streptococcus agalactiae* (group B). Complicated skin and skin structure infections, such as those that occur in patients with burns, diabetes mellitus, infected decubitus ulcers and traumatic or surgical wound infections, are more commonly polymicrobial, and can often include gram-negative bacilli such as *Escherichia coli* and *Pseudomonas aeruginosa*. Group A streptococci, *S. aureus*, or *Clostridium* spp., with and without other anaerobes, can cause fulminant soft tissue infection and necrosis, particularly in patients with diabetes mellitus. Necrotizing cellulitis or fasciitis is often caused by group A streptococcus or by methicillin-resistant *S. aureus* (MRSA), an increasingly frequent cause of community-onset infections.[1,2]

Since Infectious Disease Society of America (IDSA) guidelines for management of skin and soft-tissue infections were published in 2005,[3] MRSA has become the predominant cause of suppurative skin infection in many parts of the US.[4] It should be considered if the patient was recently treated with antibiotics, is known to be colonized, has a history of recent hospitalization, or is in a geographic area of high prevalence. In areas with high rates of community-acquired MRSA (CA-MRSA), absence of traditional risk factors does not reliably exclude MRSA.[5]

Vancomycin is the drug of choice for treatment of severe skin and soft tissue infections due to MRSA. Linezolid or daptomycin are reasonable alternatives.[6] Tigecycline can be used, but because it has a very broad spectrum of activity, it is best reserved for patients unable to take other drugs or those with documented polymicrobial coinfection.[7] With less severe infection, many community-acquired strains of MRSA can be treated with clindamycin, trimethoprim/sulfamethoxazole or doxycycline. Fluoroquinolones should not be used empirically to treat MRSA infections because of increasing resistance in both nosocomial and community-associated settings.[8] For small abscesses and less serious CA-MRSA skin or soft tissue infections, drainage or local therapy alone may be effective.

For **uncomplicated** infections unlikely to be due to MRSA, an antistaphylococcal penicillin such as dicloxacillin or a first-generation cephalosporin such as cephalexin would be a reasonable choice. If the patient requires hospitalization, the same classes of drugs (nafcillin, cefazolin) could be given IV. Clindamycin would be a reasonable choice for patients who are allergic to a beta-lactam.

For **complicated** infections that are unlikely to be MRSA, piperacillin/ tazobactam, ticarcillin/clavulanate, imipenem or meropenem would be reasonable empiric monotherapy; in severely ill patients vancomycin or linezolid should be added until MRSA is ruled out. If group A streptococcus or *Clostridium* spp. is the likely cause, a combination of clindamycin and penicillin should be used.[3] Surgical debridement is essential to the management of necrotizing skin and skin structure infections.[9]

BONE AND JOINT — *S. aureus* is the most common cause of **osteomyelitis**. *S. pyogenes* and *S. agalactiae* are less common pathogens. *Salmonella* spp. can cause osteomyelitis in patients with sickle cell disease, as can other gram-negative bacteria *(E. coli, Pseudomonas* spp.)*, particularly in patients who have had orthopedic procedures or have open fractures or vertebral infection. Infections of the feet are common in diabetic patients, involve both bone and soft tissue, and are usually polymicrobial, including both aerobic and anaerobic bacteria.

Septic arthritis may be due to *S. aureus*, *S. pyogenes* or *Streptococcus pneumoniae*,[10] gram-negative bacteria, or in young, sexually active patients, *Neisseria gonorrhoeae*.[11] Coagulase-negative staphylococci and *S. aureus* are the most common causes of prosthetic joint infection.

For empiric treatment of osteomyelitis, IV administration of an antistaphylococcal penicillin such as oxacillin or a first-generation cephalosporin such as cefazolin would be appropriate. Some Medical Letter consultants would use vancomycin until culture results are available. Ceftriaxone would be a reasonable first choice for empiric treatment of a joint infection to include coverage for *S. aureus* and *N. gonorrhoeae*. For both bone and joint infections, IV penicillin or ceftriaxone can be used to treat *Streptococcus* spp. If MRSA or coagulase-negative staphylococcus is the pathogen, vancomycin or linezolid (if the patient cannot take vancomycin) should be used. Ceftriaxone, ceftazidime or ciprofloxacin would be a good option for empiric treatment of bone and joint infections due to gram-negative bacteria.

Chronic osteomyelitis, common in complicated diabetic foot infection, usually requires surgical debridement of involved bone followed by 4-8 weeks of antibacterial therapy. Well absorbed oral antibacterials, such as trimethoprim/sulfamethoxazole, metronidazole, linezolid and the fluoro-quinolones can be used for chronic osteomyelitis depending on the susceptibility of the pathogen(s). Reversible bone marrow suppression has occurred with linezolid, especially with therapy for more than two weeks.

For prosthetic joint infections rifampin is often added to antistaphylo-coccal therapy because of its effect on *S. aureus* isolates that are adherent to the prosthesis; surgical intervention/debridement or prosthesis removal is always necessary to achieve microbiological cure.[12,13]

MENINGITIS

The organisms most commonly responsible for community-acquired bacterial meningitis in children and adults are *S. pneumoniae* (pneumo-coccus) and *Neisseria meningitidis*, which cause about 80% of all cases.[14] Meningitis due to *Haemophilus influenzae* type b has decreased markedly in adults and children as a result of childhood immunization, and the incidence of pneumococcal meningitis is also starting to decline due to routine childhood immunization with the 7-valent pneumococcal conjugate vaccine *(Prevnar)*.[15,16] Enteric gram-negative bacteria cause meningitis in neonates, the elderly, and in those who have had recent neurosurgery or are immunosuppressed. Group B streptococcus often causes meningitis in neonates or in the elderly. *Listeria monocytogenes* may be the cause in pregnant women, neonates, patients >50 years old and in immunosuppressed patients.[17,18]

For empiric treatment of meningitis in **adults and children more than two months old** high-dose ceftriaxone or cefotaxime plus vancomycin to cover highly penicillin- or cephalosporin-resistant pneumococci is generally recommended. Ampicillin (sometimes in combination with gentamicin for severely ill patients) is added in patients in whom *L. monocytogenes* is a consideration. Vancomycin in usual doses may not reach effective levels in cerebrospinal fluid and clinical response should be carefully monitored; some Medical Letter consultants have used up to 4 grams per day to treat meningitis. Vancomycin should be stopped if the etiologic agent proves to be susceptible to a third-generation cephalosporin or penicillin.

Neonatal meningitis is most often caused by group B streptococci, gram-negative enteric organisms or *L. monocytogenes*. For meningitis in the first two months of life, while waiting for the results of cultures and susceptibility tests, many Medical Letter consultants use ampicillin plus ceftriaxone or cefotaxime, with or without gentamicin.

For treatment of **nosocomial** meningitis, vancomycin and a cephalosporin with good activity against *Pseudomonas* such as ceftazidime or cefepime are appropriate; if *P. aeruginosa* is confirmed, addition of an aminoglycoside such as tobramycin, gentamicin or amikacin is recommended. In hospitals where gram-negative bacilli that produce extended-spectrum ß-lactamases are common, use of imipenem or meropenem should be considered.

Ceftriaxone or cefotaxime can often be used safely to treat meningitis in **penicillin-allergic** patients, but occassionally such patients could also have an allergic reaction to some cephalosporins. When allergy truly prevents the use of a cephalosporin, chloramphenicol can be given for initial treatment, but may not be effective if the infecting pathogen is an enteric gram-negative bacilli or *L. monocytogenes*, or in some patients with penicillin nonsusceptible pneumococcal meningitis. For coverage of enteric gram-negative bacilli and *P. aeruginosa* in patients with penicillin and cephalosporin allergy, aztreonam or possibly a fluoroquinolone, could be used. Trimethoprim/sulfamethoxazole can be used for treatment of *Listeria* meningitis in patients allergic to penicillin. As with nonallergic patients, vancomycin should be added to cover resistant pneumococci.

A **corticosteroid**, usually parenteral dexamethasone (*Decadron*, and others), given before or at the same time as the first dose of antibiotics, has been reported to decrease the incidence of hearing loss and other neurological complications in children with bacterial meningitis[19] and is now recommended as a treatment for adults with suspected or proven pneumococcal meningitis.[20,21] The basis of this recommendation is a study in 301 adults with bacterial meningitis that found improved outcome and decreased mortality associated with dexamethasone, started 15-20 minutes before the first dose of an antibacterial and continued every 6 hours for four days.[22] The benefits were most pronounced in patients with pneumococcal meningitis; all pneumococcal isolates in this study were susceptible to penicillin. Some Medical Letter consultants would give 4 days of dexamethasone to all adult patients with bacterial meningitis, regardless of microbial etiology.[23] Concerns that steroid use in meningitis can decrease penetration of antibiotics, particularly vancomycin, into the CNS, may not be justified.[24] With adjuvant steroid use, rifampin is sometimes added to the empirical combination of vancomycin and a third-generation cephalosporin, based on a study in animals that found that dexamethasone decreases vancomycin levels in the CSF when used alone, but not when given in combination with rifampin.[25]

INFECTIONS OF THE UPPER RESPIRATORY TRACT

Acute sinusitis in adults is often due to viral infections. When it is bacterial, it is usually caused by pneumococci, *H. influenzae* or *Moraxella catarrhalis* and is generally treated with an oral antibacterial such as amoxicillin or amoxicillin/clavulanate, cefuroxime axetil or cefpodoxime, or a fluoroquinolone with good antipneumococcal activity such as levofloxacin or moxifloxacin. Monotherapy with a macrolide (erythromycin, clarithromycin or azithromycin) is generally not recommended because of increasing pneumococcal resistance. Doxycycline, trimethoprim/sulfamethoxazole, azithromycin or clarithromycin may be considered for patients with mild acute bacterial sinusitis (ABS) who are allergic to penicillins and cephalosporins.[26] In patients with moderate ABS or with risk factors for infection with drug-resistant *S. pneumoniae*, such as recent antibiotic use, high-dose amoxicillin/clavulanate or an antipneumococcal fluoroquinolone could be used.

Acute exacerbation of chronic bronchitis (AECB) is also often viral. When it is bacterial it may be due to *S. pneumoniae*, *H. influenzae* or *M. catarrhalis* and is treated with the same antimicrobials used to treat ABS. The most common bacterial cause of **acute pharyngitis** in adults is group A streptococci. Penicillin, or a macrolide if the patient has a penicillin allergy, is usually used for treatment.[27] Although there have been reports of resistance to macrolides among pharyngeal isolates of group A streptococci, there is no evidence of widespread resistance in the US.[28,29]

PNEUMONIA

The pathogen responsible for **community-acquired bacterial pneumonia (CAP)** is often not confirmed, but *S. pneumoniae* and the "atypical" pathogens *Mycoplasma pneumoniae* and *Chlamydophila pneumoniae* (formerly *Chlamydia pneumoniae*) probably cause most cases. Among **hospitalized patients with community-acquired bacterial pneumonia**, *S. pneumoniae* is probably the most common pathogen. *Legionella* spp., another atypical organism, is less common. Other bacterial pathogens include *H. influenzae, Klebsiella pneumoniae, S. aureus* and occasionally other gram-negative bacilli and anaerobic mouth organisms.

In **ambulatory** patients, an oral macrolide (erythromycin, azithromycin or clarithromycin) or doxycycline is generally used in otherwise healthy adults. Pneumococci may, however, be resistant to macrolides[30] and to doxycycline, especially if they are resistant to penicillin. For older patients or those with comorbid illness, a fluoroquinolone may be a better choice. A fluoroquinolone with good antipneumococcal activity such as levofloxacin or moxifloxacin is generally used for adults with comorbidities or antibiotic exposure during the prior 90 days.[31] Nationally, less than 1% of pneumococcal isolates are resistant to fluoroquinolones, but in some urban centers the percentage is higher.[32,33]

Choice of Antibacterial Drugs

In **community-acquired pneumonia requiring hospitalization,** a beta-lactam (such as ceftriaxone or cefotaxime) plus a macrolide (erythromycin, azithromycin or clarithromycin), or a fluoroquinolone with good activity against *S. pneumoniae* (levofloxacin or moxifloxacin) is recommended pending culture results.[31,34] If aspiration pneumonia is suspected, metronidazole or clindamycin can be added. Moxifloxacin or ampicillin-sulbactam, which also have anaerobic activity, are reasonable alternatives.

In treating pneumococcal pneumonia due to strains with intermediate degrees of penicillin resistance (minimal inhibitory concentration [MIC] ≤ 1 mcg/mL), ceftriaxone, cefotaxime, or high doses of either IV penicillin (12 million units daily for adults) or oral amoxicillin (1-3 g daily) can be used. For highly resistant strains (MIC ≥ 2 mcg/mL), a fluoroquinolone (levofloxacin or moxifloxacin), vancomycin or linezolid may be required, and should be added in severely ill patients (such as those requiring admission to an ICU) and those not responding to a beta-lactam.

Hospital-acquired (HAP) (nosocomial) or ventilator associated pneumonia (VAP) is often caused by gram-negative bacilli, especially *P. aeruginosa, Klebsiella* spp., *E. coli, Enterobacter* spp., *Serratia* spp., and *Acinetobacter* spp.; it can also be caused by *S. aureus*. Many of these bacteria are multidrug resistant (MDR), particularly when disease onset is after a long hospital admission with prior antibacterial therapy, and further resistance can emerge on treatment. Pneumonia with *S. aureus*, particularly methicillin-resistant strains, is also more common in patients with diabetes mellitus, head trauma, or intensive care unit admission. HAP due to *Legionella* species can also occur, usually in immunocompromised patients.[35]

In the absence of risk factors for MDR organisms, initial empiric therapy for HAP can be limited to one antibiotic, such as ceftriaxone, a fluoroquinolone, ampicillin/sulbactam, or a carbapenem. In other patients, however, particularly those who are severely ill or in an ICU, broader-spectrum coverage with an agent with antipseudomonal activity such as piperacillin/tazobactam, cefepime, imipenem or meropenem, combined with either an aminoglycoside (tobramycin, gentamicin or amikacin) or a fluoroquinolone with antipseudomonal activity (ciprofloxacin or levofloxacin) is a reasonable choice. Addition of vancomycin or linezolid should be considered in hospitals where MRSA are common. Some multidrug resistant gram-negative bacteria causing HAP, such as *Acinetobacter* spp; may be susceptible to colistin (polymyxin E) or tigecycline; some *Acinetobacter* strains are also sensitive to sulbactam.

INFECTIONS OF THE GENITOURINARY TRACT

URINARY TRACT INFECTION (UTI) — *E. coli* causes the majority of uncomplicated cystitis. *Staphylococcus saprophyticus* is the second most common pathogen, and the remaining cases are due to *Proteus* spp. and other gram-negative rods.[36] Fluoroquinolones (especially ciprofloxacin) have become the most common class of antibiotic prescribed for UTI.[37] Due to concerns about cost-effectiveness and emerging fluoroquinolone resistance, however, Medical Letter consultants advise against routine use of fluoroquinolones for acute uncomplicated cystitis.[38]

Acute uncomplicated cystitis in women can be effectively and inexpensively treated, before the infecting organism is known, with a three-day course of oral trimethroprim/sulfamethoxazole. In areas where the prevalence of *E. coli* resistant to trimethoprim/sulfamethoxazole exceeds 15% to 20%, or in women with risk factors for resistance, a 3-day course of a fluoroquinolone (ciprofloxacin, norfloxacin or ofloxacin) or a 7-day course of nitrofurantoin could be substituted.[39] Other alternatives include a single dose of fosfomycin. Based on the results of susceptibility testing, nitrofurantoin, amoxicillin or a cephalosporin can be given for 7 days to treat UTIs in pregnant women[40], but nitrofurantoin should not be given near term or during labor or delivery because it can cause hemolytic anemia in the newborn.

Choice of Antibacterial Drugs

Acute uncomplicated pyelonephritis can often be managed with a 7-day course of an oral fluoroquinolone.[41]

Complicated UTIs that recur after treatment, occur in patients with indwelling urinary catheters, or are acquired in hospitals or nursing homes, are more likely to be due to antibiotic-resistant gram-negative bacilli, *S. aureus* or enterococci. A fluoroquinolone, oral amoxicillin/clavulanate or an oral third-generation cephalosporin such as cefpodoxime, cefdinir, ceftibuten or cefixime can be useful in treating such infections in outpatients. In hospitalized patients with complicated UTIs, treatment with a third-generation cephalosporin, a fluoroquinolone, ticarcillin/clavulanate, piperacillin/tazobactam, imipenem or meropenem is recommended, sometimes together with an aminoglycoside such as gentamicin, especially in patients with sepsis syndromes.

PROSTATITIS — Acute bacterial prostatitis may be due to enteric gram-negative bacteria, especially *E. coli* and *Klebsiella* spp., or to *P. aeruginosa* or *Enterococcus* spp.,[42] but a bacterial pathogen is often not identified. Occasionally, a sexually transmitted organism such as *N. gonorrhoeae*, *Chlamydia trachomatis* or *Ureaplasma urealyticum* is responsible. Chronic bacterial prostatitis, although often idiopathic, may be caused by the same bacteria as acute prostatitis, or by *S. aureus* or coagulase-negative staphylococci. Chronic bacterial prostatitis is the most frequent cause of recurrent UTI in young and middle-aged men.[43,44]

An oral fluoroquinolone with activity against *P. aeruginosa* (ciprofloxacin or levofloxacin) is a reasonable choice for initial treatment of acute bacterial prostatitis in a patient who does not require hospitalization. Trimethoprim/sulfamethoxazole could be used as an alternative. Fluoroquinolones are no longer recommended for treatment of *N. gonorrhoeae*; if gonorrhea is suspected IV ceftriaxone is recommended.[45]

For more severe prostatitis, an IV fluoroquinolone or third-generation cephalosporin, either with or without an aminoglycoside, may be used.

Prostatic abscesses may require drainage in addition to antimicrobial treatment. Chronic bacterial prostatitis is generally treated with a long (4- to 12-week) course of an oral fluoroquinolone or trimethoprim/sulfamethoxazole.

INTRA-ABDOMINAL INFECTIONS

Most intra-abdominal infections, such as **cholangitis** and **diverticulitis,** are due to enteric gram-negative organisms, most commonly *E. coli,* but also *Klebsiella* or *Proteus* spp. Enterococci and anaerobes, particularly *Bacteroides fragilis*, are also common. Changes in bowel flora, such as occur in hospitalized patients treated with antibiotics, lead to an increased risk of infections due to *Pseudomonas* and *Candida* spp. Many intra-abdominal infections, particularly abscesses, are polymicrobial.

Empiric therapy should cover both enteric gram-negative organisms and *B. fragilis*. Monotherapy with piperacillin/tazobactam, ticarcillin/clavulanate, ampicillin/sulbactam or a carbapenem would be a reasonable first choice.[46] Cefoxitin, which has been used in the past, no longer has reliable coverage against *B. fragilis* and cefotetan *(Cefotan)*, once an alternative, is no longer manufactured. A fluoroquinolone (ciprofloxacin, levofloxacin, moxifloxacin) plus metronidazole for anaerobic coverage, or tigecycline alone[7] can be used in patients allergic to beta-lactams. For bacteremia thought to be from the biliary tract, some clinicians would use piperacillin/tazobactam or ampicillin/sulbactam, each with or without an aminoglycoside. In severely ill patients and those with prolonged hospitalization, treatment should include coverage for *Pseudomonas*. Reasonable choices would include an antipseudomonal penicilllin (piperacillin/tazobactam); or a carbapenem (imipenem or meropenem); or ceftazidime, cefepime, aztreonam or ciprofloxacin, each plus metronidazole for *B. fragilis* coverage. An aminoglycoside could be added to any of these regimens.

Choice of Antibacterial Drugs

Clostridium difficile is the most common identifiable cause of antibiotic-associated diarrhea. In recent years, a more toxic epidemic strain has emerged, possibly related to widespread use of fluoroquinolones,[47] causing an increase in the incidence and severity of *C. difficile*–**associated disease** (CDAD).[48-50] Oral metronidazole can be used to treat mild or moderate CDAD. Patients with severe disease and those with delayed response to metronidazole should be treated with oral vancomycin. First recurrences of CDAD can be treated with either metronidazole or vancomycin,[51] but for multiple recurrences, longer courses of oral vancomycin with slow tapering or pulsed doses should be used.[52]

SEPSIS SYNDROME

For treatment of sepsis syndromes, the choice of drugs should be based on the probable source of infection, gram-stained smears of appropriate clinical specimens, and the immune status of the patient. The choice should also reflect local patterns of bacterial resistance.

A third- or fourth-generation cephalosporin (cefotaxime, ceftizoxime, ceftriaxone, ceftazidime or cefepime), piperacillin/tazobactam, ticarcillin/clavulanate, imipenem, meropenem, or aztreonam can be used to treat sepsis caused by most strains of gram-negative bacilli. Ceftazidime has less activity against gram-positive cocci. Cephalosporins other than ceftazidime and cefepime have limited activity against *P. aeruginosa*. Piperacillin/tazobactam, imipenem and meropenem are active against most strains of *P. aeruginosa* and are active against anaerobes. Aztreonam is active against many strains of *P. aeruginosa* but has no activity against gram-positive bacteria or anaerobes.

For initial treatment of life-threatening sepsis in adults, Medical Letter consultants recommend a third- or fourth-generation cephalosporin (cefotaxime, ceftriaxone, ceftazidime or cefepime), piperacillin/tazobactam, imipenem or meropenem, plus vancomycin and perhaps an aminoglycoside (gentamicin, tobramycin or amikacin). However, a recent meta-analysis found no additional benefit from addition of an aminoglycoside.[53]

When **bacterial endocarditis** is suspected and therapy must be started before the pathogen is identified, a combination of ceftriaxone and vancomycin can be used; some Medical Letter consultants would also add low-dose gentamicin.

Recombinant human activated protein C *(Xigris)* is occasionally used in combination with standard therapy for treatment of severe sepsis, but it has many exclusion criteria that limit its use and has serious side effects such as bleeding, particularly intracranial hemorrhage. Most Medical Letter consultants would use it only for the most severely ill patients with no bleeding risk.[54] Recent analyses question its ultimate cost-effectiveness as a therapeutic measure and its use in children.[55,56]

FEVER AND NEUTROPENIA — For empiric treatment of fever in patients with neutropenia, ceftazidime, imipenem, meropenem or cefepime, each alone or, in more seriously ill patients, with an aminoglycoside (gentamicin, tobramycin or amikacin), would be reasonable first choices.[57,58] Piperacillin/ tazobactam combined with amikacin may be equally effective. Addition of vancomycin may be necessary for treatment of neutropenic patients who remain febrile despite antibiotics or who have bacteremia caused by methicillin-resistant staphylococci or penicillin-resistant viridans streptococci. Studies in low-risk hospitalized adults show that when neutropenia is expected to last less than 10 days, high-dose oral ciprofloxacin with amoxicillin/clavulanate is as effective as intravenous ceftazidime or ceftriaxone plus amikacin.[59]

ANTIBACTERIAL RESISTANCE

MULTIPLE-ANTIBIOTIC-RESISTANT ENTEROCOCCI — Many *Enterococcus* spp., particularly *E. faecium,* are now resistant to penicillin and ampicillin, to gentamicin or streptomycin or both, and to vancomycin.

Choice of Antibacterial Drugs

Some of these strains are susceptible *in vitro* to chloramphenicol, doxycycline, or rarely to fluoroquinolones, but clinical results with these drugs have been variable. Linezolid, daptomycin and tigecycline are active against many gram-positive organisms, including both *E. faecium* and *E. faecalis*[7]; resistance to these drugs has been rare.[4,60] Quinupristin/dalfopristin is active against most strains of vancomycin-resistant *E. faecium,* but not *E. faecalis.*[61] Polymicrobial surgical infections that include antibiotic-resistant enterococci may respond to antibiotics aimed at the other organisms. When antibiotic-resistant enterococci cause endocarditis, surgical replacement of the infected valve may be required. UTIs caused by resistant enterococci may respond nevertheless to ampicillin or amoxicillin, which reach very high concentrations in urine; nitrofurantoin, fosfomycin or doxycycline can also be used.

***STAPHYLOCOCCUS AUREUS* WITH REDUCED SUSCEPTIBILITY TO VANCOMYCIN** — *S. aureus* isolates that are resistant to vancomycin due to possession of the *vanA* gene, which encodes for vancomycin resistance in enterococci,[62,63] remain uncommon. Vancomycin-intermediate (VISA) strains were first identified in 1997 and have been reported worldwide, usually in patients requiring long courses of vancomycin.[64] Treatment should be based on results of susceptibility testing.

COMMUNITY-ACQUIRED MRSA (CA-MRSA) — CA-MRSA usually causes skin and soft tissue infections, often associated with furunculosis and abscesses. In part because strains of CA-MRSA, unlike hospital-associated strains, frequently carry a gene encoding the Panton-Valentine leukocidin (PVL) toxin which causes necrosis, some of these infections such as necrotizing fasciitis or pneumonia or sepsis can be severe.[2] Outbreaks have been reported in children, men who have sex with men, prisoners, injection drug users and athletes involved in contact sports, such as wrestlers and football players.[65,66]

Community-acquired strains often are susceptible to trimethoprim/sulfamethoxazole and clindamycin; nosocomial strains often are not. Treatment should be guided by the severity of infection and susceptibility tests. Patients with serious CA-MRSA infections should be treated with IV vancomycin, linezolid or (except for CA-MRSA pneumonia) daptomycin. For small abscesses and less serious CA-MRSA skin or soft tissue infections, drainage or local therapy alone may be effective. When it is not, oral trimethoprim/sulfamethaxazole, minocycline, doxycycline, clindamycin or linezolid could be tried.[67]

ANTIBIOTIC-RESISTANT GRAM-NEGATIVE BACILLI — In many hospitals, gram-negative bacilli have become increasingly resistant to one or more classes of antibiotics, including aminoglycosides, third-generation cephalosporins, cefepime, beta-lactam/beta-lactamase inhibitors (ticarcillin/clavulanate, piperacillin/tazobactam), the carbapenems (imipenem, meropenem, ertapenem), aztreonam and trimethoprim/sulfamethaxazole. Of particular concern are MDR strains of *Pseudomonas*, *Acinetobacter* and *Klebsiella*.[68,69] Treatment options for these serious infections are extremely limited, which has led to a revival in use of the polymyxin class of antibiotics (polymyxin B and colistin) in this setting.[70] Resistance is also increasing in some community-acquired organisms such as *N. gonorrhoeae*, *Campylobacter*, *Salmonella* and *Shigella* spp. Susceptibility testing and resistance patterns within a region, as reported by public health laboratories, should be used to guide therapy.

TABLES BEGIN ON PAGE 56.

1. LG Miller et al. Necrotizing fasciitis caused by community-associated methicillin-resistant *Staphylococcus aureus* in Los Angeles. N Engl J Med 2005; 352:1445.
2. JS Francis et al. Severe community-onset pneumonia in healthy adults caused by methicillin-resistant *Staphylococcus aureus* carrying the Panton-Valentine leukocidin genes. Clin Infect Dis 2005; 40:100.
3. DL Stevens et al. Practice guidelines for the diagnosis and management of skin and soft-tissue infections. Clin Infect Dis 2005; 41:1373.

Choice of Antibacterial Drugs

4. GJ Moran et al. Methicillin-resistant *S. aureus* infections among patients in the emergency department. N Engl J Med 2006; 355:666.
5. LG Miller et al. Clinical and epidemiologic characteristics cannot distinguish community-associated methicillin-resistant *Staphylococcus aureus* infection from methicillin-susceptible *S. aureus* infection: a prospective investigation. Clin Infect Dis 2007; 44:471.
6. Daptomycin *(Cubicin)* for skin and soft tissue infections. Med Lett Drugs Ther 2004; 46:11.
7. Tigecycline *(Tygacil)*. Med Lett Drugs Ther 2005; 47:73.
8. ME Levison and S Fung. Community-associated methicillin-resistant Staphylococcus aureus: reconsideration of therapeutic options. Curr Infect Dis Reports 2006; 8:23.
9. MJ DiNubile and BA Lipsky. Complicated infections of skin and skin structures: when the infection is more than skin deep. J Antimicrob Chemother 2004; 53 suppl 2:37.
10. JJ Ross et al. Pneumococcal septic arthritis: review of 190 cases. Clin Infect Dis 2003; 36:319.
11. I Garcia-De La Torre. Advances in the management of septic arthritis. Rheum Dis Clin North Am 2003; 29:61.
12. W Zimmerli et al. Infection and musculoskeletal conditions: Prosthetic-joint-associated infections. Best Pract Res Clin Rheumatol 2006; 20:1045.
13. W Zimmerli et al. Prosthetic-joint infections. N Engl J Med 2004; 351:1645.
14. MT Fitch and D van de Beek. Emergency diagnosis and treatment of adult meningitis. Lancet Infect Dis 2007; 7:191.
15. MH Kyaw et al. Effect of introduction of the pneumococcal conjugate vaccine on drug-resistant *Streptococcus pneumoniae*. N Engl J Med 2006; 354:1455.
16. D van de Beek et al. Clinical features and prognostic factors in adults with bacterial meningitis. N Engl J Med 2004; 351:1849.
17. X Saez-Lorens and GH McCracken Jr. Bacterial meningitis in children. Lancet 2003; 361:2139.
18. JK Varma et al. Listeria monocytogenes infection from foods prepared in a commercial establishment: a case-control study of potential sources of sporadic illness in the United States. Clin Infect Dis 2007; 44:521.
19. AR Tunkel et al. Practice guidelines for the management of bacterial meningitis. Clin Infect Dis 2004; 39:1267.
20. D van de Beek and J de Gans. Adjunctive corticosteroids in adults with bacterial meningitis. Drugs 2006; 66:415.
21. D van de Beek et al. Corticosteroids for acute bacterial meningitis (Review). Cochrane Database Syst Rev 2007; 1:CD004405.
22. J de Gans et al. Dexamethasone in adults with bacterial meningitis. N Engl J Med 2002; 347:1549.
23. D van de Beek et al. Community-acquired bacterial meningitis in adults. N Engl J Med 2006; 354:44.
24. J-D Ricard et al. Levels of vancomycin in cerebrospinal fluid of adult patients receiving adjunctive corticosteroids to treat pneumococcal meningitis: a prospective multicenter observational study. Clin Infect Dis 2007; 44:250.

25. J Martinez-LaCasa et al. Experimental study of the efficacy of vancomycin, rifampicin and dexamethasone in the therapy of pneumococcal meningitis. J Antimicrob Chemother 2002; 49:507.

26. B Anon et al. Antimicrobial treatment guidelines for acute bacterial rhinosinusitis. Otolaryngol Head Neck Surg 2004; 130 suppl:1.

27. AL Bisno. Acute pharyngitis. New Engl J Med 2001; 344:205.

28. M Green et al. Reemergence of macrolide resistance in pharyngeal isolates of group a streptococci in southwestern Pennsylvania. Antimicrob Agent Chemother 2004; 48:473.

29. RR Tanz. Community-based surveillance in the united states of macrolide-resistant pediatric pharyngeal group A streptococci during 3 respiratory disease seasons. Clin Infect Dis 2004; 39:1794.

30. JR Lonks et al. Implications of antimicrobial resistance in the empirical treatment of community-acquired respiratory tract infections: the case of macrolides. J Antimicrob Chemother 2002; 50 suppl 2:87.

31. LA Mandell et al. Infectious Diseases Society of America/American Thoracic Society consensus guidelines on the management of community-acquired pneumonia in adults. Clin Infect Dis 2007; 44 Suppl 2: S27.

32. AM Ferrara. New fluoroquinolones in lower respiratory tract infections and emerging patterns of pneumococcal resistance. Infection 2005; 33:106.

33. MJ Rybak. Increased bacterial resistance: PROTEKT US—an update. Ann Pharmacother 2004; 38:S8.

34. RB Brown et al. Impact of initial antibiotic choice on clinical outcomes in community-acquired pneumonia: analysis of a hospital claims-made database. Chest 2003; 123:1503.

35. American Thoracic Society and The Infectious Diseases Society of America. Guidelines for the management of adults with hospital-acquired, ventilator-associated, and health-care-associated pneumonia. AM J Respir Crit Care Med 2005; 171:388.

36. EA Katchman et al. Three-day vs longer duration of antibiotic treatment for cystitis in women: systematic review and meta-analysis. Am J Med 2005; 118:1196.

37. AJ Kallen et al. Current antibiotic therapy for isolated urinary tract infections in women. Arch Intern Med 2006; 166:635.

38. TM Hooton et al. Acute uncomplicated cystitis in an era of increasing antibiotic resistance: a proposed approach to empirical therapy. Clin Infect Dis 2004; 39:75.

39. K Gupta et al. Increasing antimicrobial resistance and the management of uncomplicated community-acquired urinary tract infections. Ann Intern Med 2001; 135:41.

40. AM Macejko and AJ Schaeffer. Asymptomatic bacteriuria and symptomatic urinary tract infections during pregnancy. Urol Clin North Am 2007; 34:35.

41. BP Brown. Antimicrobial selection in the treatment of pyelonephritis. Curr Infect Dis Reports 2004; 6:457.

42. HS Gurunadha Rao Tunuguntla and CP Evans. Management of prostatitis. Prostate Cancer Prostatic Dis 2002; 5:172.

43. FME Wagenlehner and KG Naber. Fluoroquinolone antimicrobial agents in the treatment of prostatitis and recurrent urinary tract infections in men. Curr Infect Dis Reports 2005; 7:9.

44. JN Krieger et al. Chronic prostatitis: epidemiology and role of infection. Urology 2002; 60 suppl 6A:8.

45. Centers for Disease Control and Prevention (CDC). Update to CDC's sexually transmitted diseases treatment guidelines, 2006: fluoroquinolones no longer recommended for treatment of gonococcal infections. MMWR Morbid Mortal Wkly Rep 2007; 56:332.

46. JS Solomkin et al. Guidelines for the selection of anti-infective agents for complicated intra-abdominal infections. Clin Infect Dis 2003; 37:997.

47. J Pepin et al. Emergence of fluoroquinolones as the predominant risk factor for *Clostridium difficile*-associated diarrhea: a cohort study during an epidemic in Quebec. Clin Infect Dis 2005; 41:1254.

48. LC McDonald et al. An epidemic, toxin gene-variant strain of *Clostridium difficile*. N Engl J Med 2005; 353:2433.

49. VG Loo et al. A predominantly clonal multi-institutional outbreak of *Clostridium difficile*-associated diarrhea with high morbidity and mortality. N Engl J Med 2005; 353:2442.

50. LC McDonald et al. *Clostridium difficile* infection in patients discharged from US short-stay hospitals, 1996-2003. Emerg Infect Dis 2006; 12:409.

51. J Pepin et al. Management of outcomes of a first recurrence of *Clostridium difficile*–associated dosease in Quebec, Canada. Clin Infect Dis 2006; 42:758.

52. Treatment of *Clostridium difficile*-associated disease (CDAD). Med Lett Drugs Ther 2006; 48:89.

53. M Paul et al. Beta lactam monotherapy versus beta lactam-aminoglycoside combination therapy for sepsis in immunocompetent patients: systematic review and meta-analysis of randomised trials. BMJ 2004.

54. Activated protein C *(Xigris)* for severe sepsis. Med Lett Drugs Ther 2002; 44:17.

55. M Haley et al. Activated protein C in sepsis: emerging insights regarding its mechanism of action and clinical effectiveness. Curr Opin Infect Dis 2004; 17:205.

56. SM Opal. Can we RESOLVE the treatment of sepsis? Lancet 2007; 369:803.

57. H Link et al. Antimicrobial therapy of unexplained fever in neutropenic patients — guidelines of the Infectious Diseases Working Party (AGIHO) of the German Society of Hematology and Oncology (DGHO), Study Group Interventional Therapy of Unexplained Fever, Arbeitsgemeinschaft Supportivmassnahmen in der Onkologie (ASO) of the Deutsche Krebsgesellschaft (DKG-German Cancer Society). Ann Hematol 2003; suppl 2:S105.

58. WT Hughes et al. 2002 guidelines for the use of antimicrobial agents in neutropenic patients with cancer. Clin Infect Dis 2002; 34:730.

59. A Koh and PA Pizzo. Empirical oral antibiotic therapy for low risk febrile cancer patients with neutropenia. Cancer Invest 2002; 20:420.

60. VG Meka and HS Gold. Antimicrobial resistance to linezolid. Clin Infect Dis 2004; 39:1010.

61. DJ Winston et al. Quinupristin/Dalfopristin therapy for infections due to vancomycin-resistant *Enterococcus faecium*. Clin Infect Dis 2000; 30:790.

62. S Chang et al. Infection with vancomycin-resistant *Staphylococcus aureus* containing the *vanA* resistance gene. N Engl J Med 2003; 348:1342.

63. Centers for Disease Control and Prevention (CDC). Vancomycin-resistant *Staphylococcus aureus* — Pennsylvania, 2002. MMWR Morb Mortal Wkly Rep 2002 51:902.

64. PC Appelbaum. The emergence of vancomycin-intermediate and vancomycin-resistant *Staphylococcus aureus*. Clin Microbiol Infect 2006; 12 Suppl 1:16.

65. SV Kazakova et al. A clone of methicillin-resistant *Staphylococcus aureus* among professional football players. N Engl J Med 2005; 352:468.

66. Centers for Disease Control and Prevention (CDC). Methicillin-resistant *Staphylococcus aureus* infections in correctional facilities—-Georgia, California, and Texas, 2001-2003. MMWR Morb Mortal Wkly Rep 2003; 52:992.

67. Treatment of community-associated MRSA infections. Med Lett Drugs Ther 2006; 48:13.

68. J Quale et al. Molecular epidemiology and mechanisms of carbapenem resistance in *Acinetobacter baumannii* endemic in New York City. Clin Infect Dis 2003; 37:214.

69. EP Hyle et al. Risk factors for increasing multidrug resistance among extended-spectrum beta-lactamase-producing *Escherichia coli* and *Klebsiella* species. Clin Infect Dis 2005; 40:1317.

70. ME Falagas and SK Kasiakou. Colistin: the revival of polymyxins for the management of multidrug-resistant gram-negative bacterial infections. Clin Infect Dis 2005; 40:1333.

CHOICE OF ANTIBACTERIAL DRUGS[†]

Drug of First Choice	Alternative Drugs
GRAM-POSITIVE COCCI	
Enterococcus spp.[1]	
endocarditis or other severe infection:	
penicillin G or ampicillin + gentamicin or streptomycin[2]	vancomycin + gentamicin or streptomycin[2]; linezolid[3]; daptomycin[4]; quinupristin/ dalfopristin[5]
uncomplicated urinary tract infection:	
ampicillin or amoxicillin	nitrofurantoin; a fluoroquinolone[6]; fosfomycin

† Brand names are listed on page 82. * Resistance may be a problem; susceptibility tests should be used to guide therapy.
1. Disk sensitivity testing may not provide adequate information; β-lactamase assays, "E" tests and dilution tests for susceptibility should be used in serious infections.
2. Aminoglycoside resistance is increasingly common among enterococci; treatment options include ampicillin 2 g IV q4h, continuous infusion of ampicillin, a combination of ampicillin plus a fluoro-quinolone, or a combination of ampicillin, imipenem and vancomycin.
3. Reversible bone marrow suppression has occurred, especially with therapy for more than two weeks. Linezolid is an MAO inhibitor and can interact with serotonergic and adrenergic drugs and with tyramine-containing foods (JJ Taylor et al, Clin Infect Dis 2006; 43:180).
4. Daptomycin should not be used to treat pneumonia.
5. Quinupristin/dalfopristin is not active against *Enterococcus faecalis*.
6. Among the fluoroquinolones, levofloxacin, gemifloxacin and moxifloxacin have excellent *in vitro* activity against most *S. pneumoniae*, including penicillin- and cephalosporin-resistant strains. Levofloxacin, gemifloxacin and moxifloxacin also have good activity against many strains of *S. aureus*, but resistance has become frequent among methicillin-resistant strains. Gemifloxacin is associated with a high rate of rash; other fluoroquinolones are preferred. Ciprofloxacin has the greatest activity against *Pseudomonas aeruginosa*. For urinary tract infections, norfloxacin can be used. For tuberculosis, levofloxacin, ofloxacin, ciprofloxacin or moxifloxacin could be used (Treat Guidel Med Lett 2007; 5:15). Ciprofloxacin, ofloxacin, levofloxacin and moxifloxacin are available for IV use. None of these agents is recommended for children or pregnant women.

Continued on next page.

CHOICE OF ANTIBACTERIAL DRUGS[†] (continued)

Drug of First Choice	Alternative Drugs

GRAM-POSITIVE COCCI (continued)

*Staphylococcus aureus or epidermidis

methicillin-susceptible

    a penicillinase-resistant penicillin[7] — a cephalosporin[8,9]; vancomycin; imipenem or meropenem; clindamycin; linezolid[3]; daptomycin[4]; a fluoroquinolone[6]

methicillin-resistant[10]

    vancomycin ± gentamicin ± rifampin — linezolid[3]; daptomycin[4]; tigecycline[11]; a fluoroquinolone[6]; trimethoprim/ sulfamethoxazole; quinupristin/ dalfopristin; doxycycline[11]

[†] Brand names are listed on page 82. * Resistance may be a problem; susceptibility tests should be used to guide therapy.

7. For oral use against staphylococci, cloxacillin or dicloxacillin is preferred; for severe infections, a parenteral formulation (nafcillin or oxacillin) should be used. Ampicillin, amoxicillin, carbenicillin, ticarcillin and piperacillin are not effective against penicillinase-producing staphylococci. The combinations of clavulanate with amoxicillin or ticarcillin, sulbactam with ampicillin, and tazobactam with piperacillin may be active against these organisms.

8. Cephalosporins have been used as alternatives to penicillins in patients allergic to penicillins, but such patients may also have allergic reactions to cephalosporins.

9. For parenteral treatment of staphylococcal or non-enterococcal streptococcal infections, a first-generation cephalosporin such as cefazolin can be used. For oral therapy, cephalexin or cephradine can be used. The second-generation cephalosporins cefamandole, cefprozil, cefuroxime, cefotetan, cefoxitin and loracarbef are more active than the first-generation drugs against gram-negative bacteria. Cefotetan and cefamandole are no longer available. Cefuroxime is active against ampicillin-resistant strains of *H. influenzae*. Cefoxitin is the most active of the cephalosporins against *B. fragilis*. The third-generation cephalosporins cefotaxime, cefoperazone, ceftizoxime, ceftriaxone and ceftazidime and the fourth-generation cefepime have greater activity than the second-generation drugs against enteric gram-negative bacilli. Ceftazidime has poor activity against many gram-positive cocci and anaerobes, and ceftizoxime has poor activity against penicillin-resistant *S. pneumoniae*. Cefepime has *in vitro* activity against gram-positive cocci similar to cefotaxime and ceftriaxone and somewhat greater activity against enteric gram-negative bacilli. The activity of cefepime against *P. aeruginosa* is similar to that of ceftazidime. Cefixime, cefpodoxime, cefdinir, ceftibuten and cefditoren are oral cephalosporins with more activity than second-generation cephalosporins against facultative gram-negative bacilli; they have no useful activity against anaerobes or *P. aeruginosa*, and cefixime and ceftibuten have no useful activity against staphylococci. With the exception of cefoperazone (which can cause bleeding), ceftazidime and cefepime, the activity of all currently available cephalosporins against *P. aeruginosa* is poor or inconsistent.

10. Many strains of coagulase-positive and coagulase-negative staphylococci are resistant to penicillinase-resistant penicillins; these strains are also resistant to cephalosporins and carbapenems and are often resistant to fluoroquinolones, trimethoprim/sulfamethoxazole and clindamycin. Community-acquired MRSA often is susceptible to clindamycin and trimethoprim/sulfamethoxazole.

11. Tetracyclines and tigecycline, a derivative of minocycline, are generally not recommended for pregnant women or children less than 8 years old.

Continued on next page.

CHOICE OF ANTIBACTERIAL DRUGS† (continued)

Drug of First Choice	Alternative Drugs
GRAM-POSITIVE COCCI (continued)	
Streptococcus pyogenes (group A[12]) and groups C and G	
penicillin G or V[13]	clindamycin; erythromycin; a cephalosporin[8,9]; vancomycin; clarithromycin[14]; azithromycin; linezolid[3]; daptomycin[4]
Streptococcus, group B	
penicillin G or ampicillin	a cephalosporin[8,9]; vancomycin; daptomycin[4]; erythromycin
Streptococcus, viridans group[1]	
penicillin G ± gentamicin	a cephalosporin[8,9]; vancomycin
Streptococcus bovis	
penicillin G	a cephalosporin[8,9]; vancomycin
Streptococcus, anaerobic or *Peptostreptococcus*	
penicillin G	clindamycin; a cephalosporin[8,9]; vancomycin

† **Brand names are listed on page 82. * Resistance may be a problem; susceptibility tests should be used to guide therapy.**

12. For serious soft-tissue infection due to group A streptococci, clindamycin may be more effective than penicillin. group A streptococci may, however, be resistant to clindamycin; therefore, some Medical Letter consultants suggest using both clindamycin and penicillin, with or without IV immune globulin, to treat serious soft-tissue infections. Surgical debridement is usually needed for necrotizing soft tissue infections due to group A streptococci. Group A streptococci may also be resistant to erythromycin, azithromycin and clarithromycin.

13. Penicillin V (or amoxicillin) is preferred for oral treatment of infections caused by non-penicillinase-producing streptococci. For initial therapy of severe infections, penicillin G, administered parenterally, is the first choice. For somewhat longer action in less severe infections due to group A streptococci, pneumococci or *Treponema pallidum*, procaine penicillin G, an IM formulation, can be given once or twice daily, but is seldom used now. Benzathine penicillin G, a slowly absorbed preparation, is usually given in a single monthly injection for prophylaxis of rheumatic fever, once for treatment of group A streptococcal pharyngitis and once or more for treatment of syphilis.

14. Not recommended for use in pregnancy.

Continued on next page.

CHOICE OF ANTIBACTERIAL DRUGS† (continued)

Drug of First Choice	Alternative Drugs

GRAM-POSITIVE COCCI (continued)

*Streptococcus pneumoniae[15] (pneumococcus)

penicillin-susceptible (MIC <0.1 mcg/mL)

penicillin G or V[13]; amoxicillin	a cephalosporin[8,9]; erythromycin; azithromycin; clarithromycin[14]; levofloxacin, gemifloxacin or moxifloxacin[6]; meropenem, imipenem or ertapenem; trimethoprim/ sulfamethoxazole; clindamycin; a tetracycline[11]; vancomycin

penicillin-intermediate resistance (MIC 0.1 – 1 mcg/mL)

penicillin G IV (12 million units/day for adults); ceftriaxone or cefotaxime	levofloxacin, gemifloxacin or moxifloxacin[6]; vancomycin; clindamycin

penicillin-high-level resistance (MIC ≥2 mcg/mL)

meningitis:

vancomycin +
ceftriaxone or cefotaxime, ±
rifampin

other infections:

vancomycin + ceftriaxone or cefotaxime; levofloxacin, gemifloxacin or moxifloxacin[6]	linezolid[3]; quinupristin/ dalfopristin

† Brand names are listed on page 82. * **Resistance may be a problem; susceptibility tests should be used to guide therapy.**
15. Some strains of *S. pneumoniae* are resistant to erythromycin, clindamycin, trimethoprim/sulfamethoxazole, clarithromycin, azithromycin and chloramphenicol, and resistance to the newer fluoroquinolones is rare but increasing. Nearly all strains tested so far are susceptible to linezolid and quinupristin/dalfopristin *in vitro*.

Continued on next page.

CHOICE OF ANTIBACTERIAL DRUGS[†] (continued)

Drug of First Choice	Alternative Drugs
GRAM-NEGATIVE COCCI	
Moraxella (Branhamella) catarrhalis	
cefuroxime[8]; a fluoroquinolone[6]	trimethoprim/sulfamethoxazole; amoxicillin/clavulanate; erythromycin; clarithromycin[14]; azithromycin; doxycycline[11]; cefotaxime[8]; ceftizoxime[8]; ceftriaxone[8]; cefpodoxime[8]
*Neisseria gonorrhoeae (gonococcus)[16]	
ceftriaxone[8]	cefixime[8]; cefotaxime[8]; penicillin G
Neisseria meningitidis[17] (meningococcus)	
penicillin G	cefotaxime[8]; ceftizoxime[8]; ceftriaxone[8]; chloramphenicol[18]; a sulfonamide[19]; a fluoroquinolone[6]
GRAM-POSITIVE BACILLI	
*Bacillus anthracis [20] (anthrax)	
ciprofloxacin[6]; a tetracycline[11]	penicillin G; amoxicillin; erythromycin; imipenem; clindamycin; levofloxacin[6]
Bacillus cereus, subtilis	
vancomycin	imipenem or meropenem; clindamycin

† Brand names are listed on page 82. * Resistance may be a problem; susceptibility tests should be used to guide therapy.

16. Patients with gonorrhea should be treated presumptively for co-infection with *C. trachomatis* with azithromycin or doxycycline. Fluoroquinolones are no longer recommended for treatment (Centers for Disease Control and Prevention (CDC). MMWR Morbid Mortal Wkly Rep 2007; 56:332).

17. Rare strains of *N. meningitidis* are resistant or relatively resistant to penicillin. A fluoroquinolone or rifampin is generally recommended for prophylaxis after close contact with infected patients, but fluoroquinolone-resistant strains have been reported. A single dose of azithromycin is another alternative (Centers for Disease Control and Prevention (CDC). MMWR Morbid Mortal Wkly Rep 2008; 57:173).

18. Because of the possibility of serious adverse effects, this drug should be used only for severe infections when less hazardous drugs are ineffective.

19. Sulfonamide-resistant strains are frequent in the US; sulfonamides should be used only when susceptibility is established by susceptibility tests.

20. For post-exposure prophylaxis, ciprofloxacin for 4 weeks if given with vaccination, and 60 days if not given with vaccination, might prevent disease; if the strain is susceptible, doxycycline is an alternative (JG Bartlett et al, Clin Infect Dis 2002; 35:851).

Continued on next page.

CHOICE OF ANTIBACTERIAL DRUGS† (continued)

Drug of First Choice	Alternative Drugs
GRAM-POSITIVE BACILLI (continued)	
Clostridium perfringens [21]	
penicillin G; clindamycin	metronidazole; imipenem, meropenem or ertapenem; chloramphenicol[18]
Clostridium tetani [22]	
metronidazole	penicillin G; doxycycline[11]
Clostridium difficile [23]	
metronidazole (oral)	vancomycin (oral)
Corynebacterium diphtheriae[24]	
erythromycin	penicillin G
Corynebacterium, jeikeium	
vancomycin	penicillin G + gentamicin; erythromycin
*Erysipelothrix rhusiopathiae	
penicillin G	erythromycin; a cephalosporin[8,9]; a fluoroquinolone[6]
Listeria monocytogenes	
ampicillin ± gentamicin	trimethoprim/sulfamethoxazole

† **Brand names are listed on page 82. * Resistance may be a problem; susceptibility tests should be used to guide therapy.**
21. Debridement is primary. Large doses of penicillin G are required. Hyperbaric oxygen therapy may be a useful adjunct to surgical debridement in management of the spreading, necrotizing type of infection.
22. For prophylaxis, a tetanus toxoid booster and, for some patients, tetanus immune globulin (human) are required.
23. In order to decrease the emergence of vancomycin-resistant enterococci in hospitals and to reduce costs, most clinicians now recommend use of metronidazole first in treatment of patients with *C. difficile* associated diarrhea, with oral vancomycin used only for seriously ill patients or those who do not respond to metronidazole. Patients who are unable to take oral medications can be treated with IV metronidazole.
24. Antitoxin is primary; antimicrobials are used only to halt further toxin production and to prevent the carrier state.

Continued on next page.

CHOICE OF ANTIBACTERIAL DRUGS[†] (continued)

Drug of First Choice	Alternative Drugs
ENTERIC GRAM-NEGATIVE BACILLI	
Campylobacter fetus	
a third-generation cephalosporin[9]; gentamicin	ampicillin; imipenem or meropenem
Campylobacter jejuni	
erythromycin or azithromycin	a fluoroquinolone[6]; a tetracycline[11]; gentamicin
Citrobacter freundi	
imipenem or meropenem[25]	a fluoroquinolone[6]; ertapenem; amikacin; doxycycline[11]; trimethoprim/sulfamethoxazole; cefotaxime[8,25], ceftizoxime[8,25], ceftriaxone[8,25], cefepime[8,25], or ceftazidime[8,25]
Enterobacter spp.	
imipenem or meropenem[25]; cefepime[8,25]	gentamicin, tobramycin or amikacin; trimethoprim-sulfamethoxazole; ciprofloxacin[6]; ticarcillin/clavulanate[26] or piperacillin/tazobactam[26]; aztreonam[25]; cefotaxime, ceftizoxime, ceftriaxone, or ceftazidime[8,25]; tigecycline[11]

† Brand names are listed on page 82. * Resistance may be a problem; susceptibility tests should be used to guide therapy.
25. In severely ill patients, most Medical Letter consultants would add gentamicin, tobramycin or amikacin.
26. In severely ill patients, most Medical Letter consultants would add gentamicin, tobramycin or amikacin (but see footnote 39).

Continued on next page.

CHOICE OF ANTIBACTERIAL DRUGS† (continued)

Drug of First Choice	Alternative Drugs
ENTERIC GRAM-NEGATIVE BACILLI (continued)	
Escherichia coli [27]	
cefotaxime, ceftriaxone, cefepime or ceftazidime[8,25]	ampicillin ± gentamicin, tobramycin or amikacin; gentamicin, tobramycin or amikacin; amoxicillin/ clavulanate; ticarcillin/ clavulanate[26]; piperacillin/ tazobactam[26]; ampicillin/ sulbactam[25]; trimethoprim/ sulfamethoxazole; imipenem, meropenem or ertapenem[25]; aztreonam[25]; a fluoroquinolone[6]; another cephalosporin[8,9]; tigecycline[11]
Klebsiella pneumoniae [27]	
cefotaxime, ceftriaxone, cefepime or ceftazidime[8,25]	imipenem, meropenem or ertapenem[25]; gentamicin, tobramycin or amikacin; amoxicillin/clavulanate; ticarcillin/clavulanate[26]; piperacillin/tazobactam[26]; ampicillin/sulbactam[25]; trimethoprim/ sulfamethoxazole; aztreonam[25]; a fluoro-quinolone[6]; another cephalosporin[8,9]; tigecycline[11]

† **Brand names are listed on page 82. * Resistance may be a problem; susceptibility tests should be used to guide therapy.**

27. For an acute, uncomplicated urinary tract infection, before the infecting organism is known, the drug of first choice is trimethoprim/sulfamethoxazole. Antibacterial treatment of gastroenteritis due to *E. coli* O157:H7 may increase toxin release and risk of hemolytic uremic syndrome and is not recommended (Centers for Disease Control and Prevention CDC). Morbid Mortal Wkly Rep, MMWR 2006; 55:1045).

Continued on next page.

CHOICE OF ANTIBACTERIAL DRUGS[†] (continued)

Drug of First Choice	Alternative Drugs

ENTERIC GRAM-NEGATIVE BACILLI (continued)

Proteus mirabilis[27]

ampicillin[28]	a cephalosporin[8,9,25]; ticarcillin/clavulanate or piperacillin/tazobactam[26]; gentamicin, tobramycin or amikacin; trimethoprim/sulfamethoxazole; imipenem, meropenem or ertapenem[25]; aztreonam[25]; a fluoroquinolone[6]; chloramphenicol[18]

Proteus, indole-positive (including *Providencia rettgeri, Morganella morganii,* and *Proteus vulgaris*)

cefotaxime, ceftriaxone, cefepime or ceftazidime[8,25]	imipenem, meropenem or ertapenem[25]; gentamicin, tobramycin or amikacin; amoxicillin/clavulanate; ticarcillin/clavulanate[26]; piperacillin/tazobactam[26]; ampicillin/sulbactam[25]; aztreonam[25]; trimethoprim-sulfamethoxazole; a fluoroquinolone[6]

Providencia stuartii

cefotaxime, ceftriaxone, cefepime or ceftazidime[8,25]	imipenem, meropenem or ertapenem[25]; ticarcillin/clavulanate[26]; piperacillin/tazobactam[26]; gentamicin, tobramycin or amikacin; aztreonam[25]; trimethoprim/sulfamethoxazole; a fluoroquinolone[6]

[†] **Brand names are listed on page 82. * Resistance may be a problem; susceptibility tests should be used to guide therapy.**
28. Large doses (6 grams or more daily) are usually necessary for systemic infections. In severely ill patients, some Medical Letter consultants would add gentamicin, tobramycin or amikacin.

Continued on next page.

CHOICE OF ANTIBACTERIAL DRUGS[†] (continued)

Drug of First Choice	Alternative Drugs
ENTERIC GRAM-NEGATIVE BACILLI (continued)	
Salmonella typhi (typhoid fever)[29]	
a fluoroquinolone[6] or ceftriaxone[8]	chloramphenicol[18]; trimethoprim/ sulfamethoxazole; ampicillin; amoxicillin; azithromycin[30]
Other Salmonella spp. [31]	
cefotaxime[8] or ceftriaxone[8] or a fluoroquinolone[6]	ampicillin or amoxicillin; trimethoprim/sulfamethoxazole; chloramphenicol[18]
Serratia spp.	
imipenem or meropenem[25]	gentamicin or amikacin; cefotaxime, ceftizoxime, ceftriaxone, cefepime or ceftazidime[8,25]; aztreonam[25]; trimethoprim/sulfamethoxazole; a fluoroquinolone[6]
Shigella spp.	
a fluoroquinolone[6]	azithromycin; trimethoprim/ sulfamethoxazole; ampicillin; ceftriaxone[8]
Yersinia enterocolitica	
trimethoprim/sulfamethoxazole	a fluoroquinolone[6]; gentamicin, tobramycin or amikacin; cefotaxime[8]

† **Brand names are listed on page 82. * Resistance may be a problem; susceptibility tests should be used to guide therapy.**
29. A fluoroquinolone or amoxicillin is the drug of choice for *S. typhi* carriers (CM Parry et al, N Engl J Med 2002; 347:1770).
30. RW Frenck Jr, et al, Clin Infect Dis 2000; 31:1134.
31. Most cases of *Salmonella* gastroenteritis subside spontaneously without antimicrobial therapy. Immunosuppressed patients, young children and the elderly may benefit the most from antibacterials.

Continued on next page.

CHOICE OF ANTIBACTERIAL DRUGS[†] (continued)

Drug of First Choice	Alternative Drugs
OTHER GRAM-NEGATIVE BACILLI	
Acinetobacter	
imipenem or meropenem[25]	an aminoglycoside; cipro-floxacin[6]; trimethoprim sulfamethoxazole; ticarcillin/clavulanate[26] or piperacillin/tazobactam[26]; ceftazidime[25]; doxycycline[11]; sulbactam[32]; colistin[18]
Aeromonas	
trimethoprim/sulfamethoxazole	gentamicin or tobramycin; imipenem; a fluoroquinolone[6]
Bacteroides	
metronidazole	imipenem, meropenem or ertapenem; amoxicillin/clavulanate, ticarcillin/clavulanate, piperacillin/tazobactam or ampicillin/sulbactam; chloramphenicol[18]
Bartonella henselae or *quintana* (bacillary angiomatosis, trench fever)	
erythromycin	azithromycin; doxycycline[11]
Bartonella henselae [33] (cat scratch bacillus)	
azithromycin	erythromycin; ciprofloxacin[6]; trimethoprim/sulfamethoxazole; gentamicin; rifampin
Bordetella pertussis (whooping cough)	
azithromycin; erythromycin; clarithromycin[14]	trimethoprim/sulfamethoxazole

† **Brand names are listed on page 82.** * **Resistance may be a problem; susceptibility tests should be used to guide therapy.**
32. Sulbactam may be useful to treat multi-drug resistant *Acinetobacter*. It is only available in combination with ampicillin as *Unasyn*. Medical Letter consultants recommend 3 g IV q4h.
33. Role of antibiotics is not clear (DA Conrad, Curr Opin Pediatr 2001; 13:56).

Continued on next page.

CHOICE OF ANTIBACTERIAL DRUGS† (continued)

Drug of First Choice	Alternative Drugs
OTHER GRAM-NEGATIVE BACILLI (continued)	
Brucella spp.	
a tetracycline[11] + rifampin	a tetracycline[11] + streptomycin or gentamicin; chloramphenicol[18] ± streptomycin; trimethoprim-sulfamethoxazole ± gentamicin; ciprofloxacin[6] + rifampin
Burkholderia cepacia	
trimethoprim/sulfamethoxazole	ceftazidime[8]; chloramphenicol[18]; imipenem
Burkholderia (Pseudomonas) mallei (glanders)	
streptomycin + a tetracycline[11]	streptomycin + chloramphenicol[18]; imipenem
Burkholderia (Pseudomonas) pseudomallei (melioidosis)	
imipenem; ceftazidime[8]	meropenem; chloramphenicol[18] + doxycycline[11] + trimethoprim/sulfamethoxazole; amoxicillin/clavulanate
Calymmatobacterium granulomatis (granuloma inguinale)	
trimethoprim/sulfamethoxazole	doxycycline[11] or ciprofloxacin[6] ± gentamicin
Capnocytophaga canimorsus [34]	
penicillin G	cefotaxime, ceftizoxime or ceftriaxone[8]; imipenem or meropenem; vancomycin; a fluoroquinolone[6]; clindamycin

† Brand names are listed on page 82. * Resistance may be a problem; susceptibility tests should be used to guide therapy.
34. C Pers et al, Clin Infect Dis 1996; 23:71.

Continued on next page.

CHOICE OF ANTIBACTERIAL DRUGS† (continued)

Drug of First Choice	Alternative Drugs
OTHER GRAM-NEGATIVE BACILLI (continued)	
Eikenella corrodens	
ampicillin	erythromycin; azithromycin; clarithromycin[14]; doxycycline[11]; amoxicillin/clavulanate; ampicillin/sulbactam; ceftriaxone[8]
Francisella tularensis (tularemia)[35]	
gentamicin (or streptomycin) + a tetracycline[11]	chloramphenicol[18]; ciprofloxacin[6]
Fusobacterium	
penicillin G; metronidazole	clindamycin; cefoxitin[8]; chloramphenicol[18]
Gardnerella vaginalis (bacterial vaginosis)	
oral metronidazole[36]	topical clindamycin or metronidazole; oral clindamycin
Haemophilus ducreyi (chancroid)	
azithromycin or ceftriaxone	ciprofloxacin[6] or erythromycin

† **Brand names are listed on page 82. * Resistance may be a problem; susceptibility tests should be used to guide therapy.**

35. For post-exposure prophylaxis, doxycycline or ciprofloxacin begun during the incubation period and continued for 14 days might prevent disease (Med Lett Drugs Ther 2001; 43:87).

36. Metronidazole is effective for bacterial vaginosis even though it is not usually active *in vitro* against *Gardnerella*.

Continued on next page.

CHOICE OF ANTIBACTERIAL DRUGS† (continued)

Drug of First Choice	Alternative Drugs

OTHER GRAM-NEGATIVE BACILLI (continued)

Haemophilus influenzae

meningitis, epiglottitis, arthritis and other serious infections:

cefotaxime or ceftriaxone[8] — cefuroxime[8] (not for meningitis); chloramphenicol[18]; meropenem

upper respiratory infections and bronchitis:

trimethoprim/sulfamethoxazole — cefuroxime[8]; amoxicillin/clavulanate; cefuroxime axetil[8]; cefpodoxime[8]; cefaclor[8]; cefotaxime[8]; ceftizoxime[8]; ceftriaxone[8]; cefixime[8]; doxycycline[11]; clarithromycin[14]; azithromycin; a fluoroquinolone[6]; ampicillin or amoxicillin

Helicobacter pylori [37]

proton pump inhibitor[38] + clarithromycin[14] + either amoxicillin or metronidazole — bismuth subsalicylate + metronidazole + tetracycline HCl[11] + either a proton pump inhibitor[38] or H_2-blocker[38]

Legionella species

azithromycin or a fluoroquinolone[6] ± rifampin — doxycycline[11] ± rifampin; trimethoprim-sulfamethoxazole; erythromycin

Leptotrichia buccalis

penicillin G — doxycycline[11]; clindamycin; erythromycin

---

† Brand names are listed on page 82. * Resistance may be a problem; susceptibility tests should be used to guide therapy.

37. Eradication of *H. pylori* with various antibacterial combinations, given concurrently with a proton pump inhibitor or H_2-blocker, has led to rapid healing of active peptic ulcers and low recurrence rates.

38. Proton pump inhibitors available in the US are omeprazole (*Prilosec*, and others), lansoprazole (*Prevacid*), pantoprazole (*Protonix*), esomeprazole (*Nexium*) and rabeprazole (*Aciphex*). Available H_2-blockers include cimetidine (*Tagamet*, and others), famotidine (*Pepcid*, and others), nizatidine (*Axid*, and others) and ranitidine (*Zantac*, and others).

Continued on next page.

CHOICE OF ANTIBACTERIAL DRUGS[†] (continued)

Drug of First Choice	Alternative Drugs

OTHER GRAM-NEGATIVE BACILLI (continued)

Pasteurella multocida
    penicillin G — doxycycline[11]; a second- or third-generation cephalosporin[8,9]; amoxicillin/ clavulanate; ampicillin/ sulbactam

*Pseudomonas aeruginosa
urinary tract infection:
    ciprofloxacin[6] — levofloxacin[6]; piperacillin/tazobactam; ceftazidime[8]; cefepime[8]; imipenem or meropenem; aztreonam; tobramycin, gentamicin or amikacin

other infections:
    piperacillin/tazobactam or ticarcillin/clavulanate, — ceftazidime[8]; ciprofloxacin[6]; imipenem or meropenem; aztreonam; cefepime[8]

    plus/minus tobramycin, gentamicin or amikacin[39] — **plus/minus** tobramycin, gentamicin or amikacin

Spirillum minus (rat bite fever)
    penicillin G — doxycycline[11]; streptomycin[18]

*Stenotrophomonas maltophilia
    trimethoprim/sulfamethoxazole — ticarcillin/clavulanate[26]; minocycline[11]; a fluoroquinolone[6]; tigecycline[11]

Streptobacillus moniliformis (rat bite fever; Haverhill fever)
    penicillin G — doxycycline[11]; streptomycin[18]

† **Brand names are listed on page 82. * Resistance may be a problem; susceptibility tests should be used to guide therapy.**
39. Neither gentamicin, tobramycin, netilmicin or amikacin should be mixed in the same bottle with car-benicillin, ticarcillin, mezlocillin or piperacillin for IV administration. When used in high doses or in patients with renal impairment, these penicillins may inactivate the aminoglycosides.

Continued on next page.

CHOICE OF ANTIBACTERIAL DRUGS[†] (continued)

Drug of First Choice	Alternative Drugs
OTHER GRAM-NEGATIVE BACILLI (continued)	
Vibrio cholerae (cholera)[40]	
a tetracycline[11]	a fluoroquinolone[6]; trimethoprim/sulfamethoxazole
Vibrio vulnificus	
a tetracycline[11]	cefotaxime[8]; ciprofloxacin[14]
Yersinia pestis (plague)	
streptomycin ± a tetracycline[11]	chloramphenicol[18]; gentamicin; trimethoprimsulfamethoxazole; ciprofloxacin[14]
MYCOBACTERIA	
*Mycobacterium tuberculosis[41]	
isoniazid + rifampin + pyrazinamide ± ethambutol or streptomycin[18]	a fluoroquinolone[6]; cycloserine[18]; capreomycin[18] or kanamycin[18] or amikacin[18]; ethionamide[18]; paraaminosalicylic acid[18]
*Mycobacterium kansasii[41]	
isoniazid + rifampin ± ethambutol or streptomycin[18]	clarithromycin[14] or azithromycin; ethionamide[18]; cycloserine[18]
*Mycobacterium avium complex[41]	
treatment:	
clarithromycin[14] or azithromycin, plus ethambutol ± rifabutin	ciprofloxacin[6]; amikacin[18]
prophylaxis	
clarithromycin[14] or azithromycin ± rifabutin	

† Brand names are listed on page 82. * Resistance may be a problem; susceptibility tests should be used to guide therapy.
40. Antibiotic therapy is an adjunct to and not a substitute for prompt fluid and electrolyte replacement.
41. Multidrug regimens are necessary for successful treatment. Drugs listed as alternatives are subsitutions for primary regimens and are meant to be used in combination. For additional treatment recommendations for tuberculosis, see Treat Guidel Med Lett 2007; 5:15.

Continued on next page.

CHOICE OF ANTIBACTERIAL DRUGS† (continued)

Drug of First Choice	Alternative Drugs
MYCOBACTERIA (continued)	
Mycobacterium fortuitum/chelonae[41] complex	
amikacin + clarithromycin[14]	cefoxitin[8]; rifampin; a sulfonamide; doxycycline[11]; ethambutol; linezolid[3]
Mycobacterium marinum (balnei)[42]	
minocycline[11]	trimethoprim/sulfamethoxazole; rifampin; clarithromycin[14]; doxycycline[11]
Mycobacterium leprae (leprosy)[41]	
dapsone + rifampin ± clofazimine	minocycline[11]; ofloxacin[6]; clarithromycin[14]
ACTINOMYCETES	
Actinomyces israelii (actinomycosis)	
penicillin G	doxycycline[11]; erythromycin; clindamycin
Nocardia	
trimethoprim/sulfamethoxazole	sulfisoxazole; amikacin[18]; a tetracycline[11]; ceftriaxone; imipenem or meropenem; cycloserine[18]; linezolid[3]
Rhodococcus equi	
vancomycin ± a fluoroquinolone[6], rifampin, imipenem or meropenem; amikacin	erythromycin
Tropheryma whippeli[43] (Whipple's disease)	
trimethoprim/sulfamethoxazole	penicillin G; a tetracycline[11]; ceftriaxone

† Brand names are listed on page 82. * Resistance may be a problem; susceptibility tests should be used to guide therapy.
42. Most infections are self-limited without drug treatment.
43. F Fenollar et al, N Engl J Med 2007; 356:55.

Continued on next page.

CHOICE OF ANTIBACTERIAL DRUGS[†] (continued)

Drug of First Choice	Alternative Drugs
CHLAMYDIAE	
Chlamydia trachomatis	
trachoma:	
azithromycin	doxycycline[11]; a sulfonamide (topical plus oral)
inclusion conjunctivitis:	
erythromycin (oral or IV)	a sulfonamide
pneumonia:	
erythromycin	a sulfonamide
urethritis, cervicitis:	
azithromycin or doxycycline[11]	erythromycin; ofloxacin[6]; amoxicillin
lymphogranuloma venereum:	
a tetracycline[11]	erythromycin
Chlamydophila (formerly *Chlamydia*) *pneumoniae*	
erythromycin; a tetracycline[11]; clarithromycin[14] or azithromycin	a fluoroquinolone[6]
Chlamydophila (formerly *Chlamydia*) *psittaci* (psittacosis; ornithosis)	
a tetracycline[11]	chloramphenicol[18]
EHRLICHIA	
Anaplasma phagocytophilum (formerly *Ehrlichia phagocytophila*)	
doxycycline[11]	rifampin
Ehrlichia chaffeensis	
doxycycline[11]	chloramphenicol[18]
Ehrlichia ewingii	
doxycycline[11]	

† Brand names are listed on page 82. * Resistance may be a problem; susceptibility tests should be used to guide therapy.

Continued on next page.

CHOICE OF ANTIBACTERIAL DRUGS[†] (continued)

Drug of First Choice	Alternative Drugs
MYCOPLASMA	
Mycoplasma pneumoniae	
erythromycin; a tetracycline[11]; clarithromycin[14] or azithromycin	a fluoroquinolone[6]
Ureaplasma urealyticum	
azithromycin	erythromycin; a tetracycline[11]; clarithromycin[14]; ofloxacin[6]
RICKETTSIOSES	
Rickettsia rickettsii (Rocky Mountain spotted fever)	
doxycycline[11]	a fluoroquinolone[6]; chloramphenicol[18]
Rickettsia typhi (endemic typhus-murine)	
doxycycline[11]	a fluoroquinolone[6]; chloramphenicol[18]
Rickettsia prowazekii (epidemic typhus-louseborne)	
doxycycline[11]	a fluoroquinolone[6]; chloramphenicol[18]
Orientia tsutsugamushi (scrub typhus)	
doxycycline[11]	a fluoroquinolone[6]; chloramphenicol[18]
Coxiella burnetii (Q fever)	
doxycycline[11]	a fluoroquinolone[6]; chloramphenicol[18]
SPIROCHETES	
Borrelia burgdorferi (Lyme disease)[44]	
doxycycline[11]; amoxicillin; cefuroxime axetil[8]	ceftriaxone[8]; cefotaxime[8]; penicillin G; azithromycin; clarithromycin[14]

† Brand names are listed on page 82. * Resistance may be a problem; susceptibility tests should be used to guide therapy.
44. For treatment of erythema migrans, uncomplicated facial nerve palsy, mild cardiac disease and arthritis, oral therapy is satisfactory; for other neurologic or more serious cardiac disease, parenteral therapy with ceftriaxone, cefotaxime or penicillin G is recommended. For recurrent arthritis after an oral regimen, another course of oral therapy or a parenteral drug may be given (Med Lett Drugs Ther 2005; 47:41).

Continued on next page.

CHOICE OF ANTIBACTERIAL DRUGS† (continued)

Drug of First Choice	Alternative Drugs
SPIROCHETES (continued)	
Borrelia recurrentis (relapsing fever)	
a tetracycline[11]	penicillin G; erythromycin
Leptospira	
penicillin G	doxycycline[11]; ceftriaxone[8,45]
Treponema pallidum (syphilis)	
penicillin G[13]	doxycycline[11]; ceftriaxone[8]
Treponema pertenue (yaws)	
penicillin G	doxycycline[11]

† Brand names are listed on page 82. * Resistance may be a problem; susceptibility tests should be used to guide therapy.
45. JM Vinetz, Clin Infect Dis 2003; 36:1514; T Panaphot et al, Clin Infect Dis 2003; 36:1507.

COST OF ORAL ANTIBACTERIAL DRUGS

Drug	Formulations
AZITHROMYCIN – generic	250, 500, 600 mg tabs; susp; inj
Zithromax	
ZMax	2 g ER susp
CEPHALOSPORINS	
Cefaclor – generic	250, 500 mg caps; susp
Ceclor	
extended-release – generic	350, 500 mg ER tabs
Ceclor CD	
Cefadroxil – generic	500 mg caps; 1 g tabs; susp
Duricef	
Cefdinir – *Omnicef*	300 mg caps; susp
Cefditoren – *Spectracef*	200 mg tabs
Cefpodoxime – generic	100, 200 mg tabs; susp
Vantin	
Cefprozil – generic	250, 500 mg tabs; susp
Cefzil	
Ceftibuten – *Cedax*	400 mg caps; susp
Cefuroxime axetil – generic	125, 250, 500 mg tabs; inj
Ceftin	
Cephalexin – generic	250, 500 mg caps; susp
Keflex	
Cephradine – generic	250, 500 mg caps; susp
Velosef	
Loracarbef – *Lorabid*	200 mg caps; susp
CLARITHROMYCIN – generic	250, 500 mg tabs; susp
Biaxin	
extended-release – generic	500 mg ER tabs
Biaxin XL	
CLINDAMYCIN – generic	75, 150, 300 mg caps; susp; inj
Cleocin	

Usual Adult Dosage	Usual Pediatric Dosage	Cost[1]
500 mg day 1, then	5-12 mg/kg q24h	$39.06
250 mg days 2-5		55.02
2 g single dose		55.20
500 mg q8h	6.6-13.3 mg/kg q8h	88.20
		135.60
500 mg q12h		88.40
		88.40
1 gram daily	15 mg/kg q12h	69.70
		181.30
300 mg q12h	7 mg/kg q12h or 14 mg/kg q24h	103.00
400 mg q12h		103.20
200 mg q12h	10 mg/kg q24h or 5 mg/kg q12h	98.80
		134.20
500 mg q12h	15 mg/kg q12h	154.60
		187.60
400 mg daily	9 mg/kg q24h	102.60
500 mg bid	10-15 mg/kg q12h	123.20
		283.00
500 mg q6h	6.25-25 mg/kg q6h	44.00
		162.00
500 mg q6h	6.25-25 mg/kg q6h or 12.5-50 mg/kg q12h	42.00
		77.60
400 mg q12h	7.5-15 mg/kg q12h	124.10
500 mg q12h	7.5 mg/kg q12h	70.40
		107.00
1000 mg q24h		93.60
		112.40
300 mg q6h	2-8 mg/kg q6-8h	123.20
		255.20

Continued on next page.

COST OF ORAL ANTIBACTERIAL DRUGS (continued)

Drug	Formulations
ERYTHROMYCIN	
base, delayed-release capsules	250 mg caps
generic	
ERYC	
base, enteric-coated tablets	
E-Mycin	250, 333 mg tabs
Ery-tab	250, 333, 500 mg tabs
FLUOROQUINOLONES	
Ciprofloxacin – generic	250, 500, 750 mg tabs; susp
Cipro	
Cipro XR	500, 1000 ER tabs
Gemifloxacin – *Factive*	320 mg tabs
Levofloxacin – *Levaquin*	250, 500, 750 mg tabs; susp; inj
Moxifloxacin – *Avelox*	400 mg tabs; inj
Norfloxacin – *Noroxin*	400 mg tabs
Ofloxacin – generic	200, 300, 400 mg tabs
Floxin	
FOSFOMYCIN – *Monurol*	3 g powder
LINEZOLID – *Zyvox*	400, 600 mg tabs; susp; inj
KETOLIDE	
Telithromycin – *Ketek*	400 mg tabs
METRONIDAZOLE	
generic	250, 500 mg tabs, 375 mg caps; inj
Flagyl	
generic	750 mg ER tabs
Flagyl ER	
NITROFURANTOIN	
macrocrystals – generic	25, 50, 100 mg caps
Macrodantin	
monohydrate-macrocrystals–	100 mg caps
generic	
Macrobid	

Usual Adult Dosage	Usual Pediatric Dosage	Cost[1]
500 mg q6h	7.5-12.5 mg/kg q6h	
		19.20
		58.40
500 mg q6h	7.5-12.5 mg/kg q6h	11.20
		22.40
		17.20
500 mg q12h	see footnote 2	103.20
		118.60
1000 mg q24h		118.70
320 mg daily		223.30
500 mg daily		121.10
400 mg daily		116.10
400 mg bid		75.20
400 mg q12h		117.20
		120.60
3 grams once		41.00
600 mg q12h	10 mg/kg q8h[3]	1480.20
800 mg daily		115.20
500 mg tid	30 mg/kg/d divided q6h	18.00
		153.60
750 mg once/day		60.90
		105.80
100 mg q6h	1.25-1.75 mg/kg q6h	63.60
		94.40
100 mg q12h		
		33.40
		52.20

Continued on next page.

COST OF ORAL ANTIBACTERIAL DRUGS (continued)

Drug	Formulations
PENICILLINS	
Penicillin V[4] – generic	250, 500 mg tabs; susp
Veetids	
Amoxicillin – generic	250, 500 mg caps; chewable tabs; susp
Amoxil	
Amoxicillin/clavulanate[5]	250/125, 500/125, 875/125 tabs; chewable
Augmentin	tabs; susp
Augmentin XR [6]	1000/62.5 mg ER tabs
Ampicillin – generic	250, 500 mg caps; susp
Principen	
Cloxacillin – generic	250, 500 mg caps; susp
Dicloxacillin – generic	250, 500 mg caps; susp
TETRACYCLINES	
Doxycycline –	50, 100 mg caps
generic (capsules)	
Vibramycin	
generic (tablets)	
Vibra-tabs	
Minocycline – generic	50, 75, 100 mg caps; inj
Minocin	
Tetracycline HCl – generic	250, 500 mg caps, tabs; susp
Sumycin	
TRIMETHOPRIM/SULFAMETHOXAZOLE	
generic –	400/80 mg tabs; susp
Bactrim	
Septra	
double strength (DS) –	800/160 mg tabs
generic	
Bactrim DS	
Septra DS	

Usual Adult Dosage	Usual Pediatric Dosage	Cost[1]
500 mg q6h	6.25-12.5 mg/kg q6h	11.20
		14.80
500 mg q8h	6.6-13.3 mg/kg q8h or 15 mg/kg q12h	10.50
		3.90
875 mg q12h	6.6-13.3 mg/kg q8h or 15 mg/kg q12h	
		144.80
2000 mg q12h		134.80
500 mg q6h	12.5-25 mg/kg q6h	15.60
		15.60
500 mg q6h	12.5-25 mg/kg q6h	30.40
500 mg q6h	3.125-12.5 mg/kg q6h	47.60
100 mg bid	2.2 mg/kg q12-24h[7]	
		21.80
		104.00
		12.20
		106.80
200 mg once, then		54.60
100 mg bid		197.19
500 mg q6h	6.25-12.5 mg/kg q6h[7]	3.60
		9.20
1 tablet q6h	4-5 mg/kg (TMP) q6h	23.60
		41.60
		50.00
1 DS tablet q12h		
		16.40
		39.40
		40.20

Continued on next page.

Choice of Antibacterial Drugs

COST OF ORAL ANTIBACTERIAL DRUGS (continued)

Drug	Formulations
VANCOMYCIN	
Vancocin	125, 250 mg caps

1. Cost for 10 days' treatment (5 days with azithromycin and 1 day with fosfomycin and *Zmax*), for an adult, based on the most recent data (February 2007) from retail pharmacies nationwide available from Wolters Kluwer Health.
2. Pediatric dose for post-exposure prophylaxis for anthrax is 10-15 mg/kg bid.
3. For children ≤11 years of age. Usual dose for children ≥12 years old is 600 mg q12h.
4. One mg is equal to 1600 units.
5. Dosage based on amoxicillin content. For doses of 500 or 875 mg, 500-mg or 875-mg tablets should be used, because multiple smaller tablets would contain too much clavulanate. The 875-mg, 500-mg and 250-mg tablets each contain 125 mg clavulanate. 125-mg chewable tablets and 125 mg/5 mL oral suspension both contain 31.25 mg clavulanate; 250-mg chewable tablets and 250-mg/5 mL oral suspension both contain 62.5 mg clavulanate.

LIST OF SOME GENERIC AND BRAND NAMES

* Amikacin – *Amikin*
* *Amikin* – Amikacin
* Aminosalicylic acid – *Paser*
* Amoxicillin/clavulanate – *Augmentin*
* Ampicillin – *Principen*
* *Ancef* – Cefazolin
* *Augmentin* – Amoxicillin/clavulanate
  Avelox – Moxifloxacin
  Azactam – Aztreonam
  Azithromycin – *Zithromax*
  Aztreonam – *Azactam*
* *Bactrim* – Trimethoprim/sulfamethoxazole
  Biaxin – Clarithromycin
* *Ceclor* – Cefaclor
  Cedax – Ceftibuten
* Cefadroxil – *Duricef*

* Cefazolin – *Ancef; Kefzol*
  Cefdinir – *Omnicef*
  Cefepime – *Maxipime*
  Cefixime – *Suprax*
  Cefizox – Ceftizoxime
  Cefobid – Cefoperazone
  Cefoperazone – *Cefobid*
  Cefotan – Cefotetan
  Cefotaxime – *Claforan*
  Cefotetan – *Cefotan*
* Cefoxitin – *Mefoxin*
* Cefpodoxime – *Vantin*
* Cefprozil – *Cefzil*
  Ceftazidime – *Fortaz; Tazicef; Tazidime*
  Ceftibuten – *Cedax*
  Ceftin – Cefuroxime axetil
  Ceftizoxime – *Cefizox*
  Ceftriaxone – *Rocephin*

Continued on next page.

Usual Adult Dosage	Usual Pediatric Dosage	Cost[1]
125 mg q6h	40 mg/kg/d divided q6-8h	666.80

6. Dosage based on amoxicillin content.
7. Not recommended for children <8 years old.

LIST OF SOME GENERIC AND BRAND NAMES (continued)

Cefuroxime – *Zinacef*
Cefuroxime axetil – *Ceftin*
* *Cefzil* – Cefprozil
* Cephalexin – *Keflex*
* Cephalothin – *Keflin*
* Cephradine – *Velosef*
* Chloramphenicol – *Chloromycetin*
* *Chloromycetin* – Chloramphenicol
* *Cipro* – Ciprofloxacin
* Ciprofloxacin – *Cipro*
  Claforan – Cefotaxime
  Clarithromycin – *Biaxin*
* *Cleocin* – Clindamycin
* Clindamycin – *Cleocin*
  Clofazimine – *Lamprene*
  Cubicin – Daptomycin
* Cycloserine – *Seromycin*
* Dapsone – generics
  Daptomycin – *Cubicin*

* Dicloxacillin – generics
* Doxycycline – *Vibramycin*, *Vibra-Tabs*
* *Duricef* – Cefadroxil
* *E-Mycin* – Erythromycin
  Enoxacin – *Penetrex*
  Ertapenem – *Invanz*
* *ERYC* – Erythromycin
* *Ery-Tab* – Erythromycin
* Erythromycin – *E-Mycin*; *Ery-Tab*
* Ethambutol – *Myambutol*
  Ethionamide – *Trecator-SC*
  Factive – Gemifloxacin
* *Flagyl* – Metronidazole
* *Floxin* – Ofloxacin
  Fortaz – Ceftazidime
  Fosfomycin – *Monurol*
* *Gantrisin* – Sulfisoxazole
* *Garamycin* – Gentamicin

Continued on next page.

LIST OF SOME GENERIC AND BRAND NAMES (continued)

Gemifloxacin – *Factive*
* Gentamicin – *Garamycin*
Imipenem – *Primaxin*
* *INH* – Isoniazid
Invanz – Ertapenem
* Isoniazid – *INH*
* Kanamycin – *Kantrex; Keflin*
* *Kantrex* – Kanamycin
* *Keflex* – Cephalexin
* *Keflin* – Cephalothin
* *Kefzol* – Cefazolin
Ketek – Telithromycin
Lamprene – Clofazimine
Levaquin – Levofloxacin
Levofloxacin – *Levaquin*
Linezolid – Zyvox
Lorabid – Loracarbef
Loracarbef – *Lorabid*
* *Macrobid* – Nitrofurantoin
* *Macrodantin* – Nitrofurantoin
Maxipime – Cefepime
* *Mefoxin* – Cefoxitin
Meropenem – *Merrem*
Merrem – Meropenem
* Metronidazole – *Flagyl*
* *Minocin* – Minocycline
* Minocycline – *Minocin*
Monurol – Fosfomycin
Moxifloxacin – *Avelox*
* *Myambutol* – Ethambutol
Mycobutin – Rifabutin
* Nafcillin – *Nallpen*
* *Nallpen* – Nafcillin
* *Nebcin* – Tobramycin
* Nitrofurantoin – *Macrobid*;
  Macrodantin
Norfloxacin – *Noroxin*
Noroxin – Norfloxacin

* Ofloxacin – *Floxin*
Omnicef – Cefdinir
* Oxacillin – generics
Para-aminosalicylic acid – *Paser*
Paser – Para-aminosalicylic acid
Penetrex – Enoxacin
* Penicillin G – generics
* Penicillin V – *Pen-Vee K; Veetids*
* *Pen-Vee K* – Penicillin V
Piperacillin/tazobactam – *Zosyn*
Primaxin – Imipenem
* *Principen* – Ampicillin
Pyrazinamide – *PZA*
PZA – Pyrazinamide
Quinupristin/dalfopristin – *Synercid*
Rifabutin – Mycobutin
Rifadin – Rifampin
Rifampin – *Rifadin*
Rifaxamin – *Xifaxan*
Rocephin – Ceftriaxone
* *Septra* – Trimethoprim/
  sulfamethoxazole
* *Seromycin* – Cycloserine
* Streptomycin – generics
* Sulfisoxazole – *Gantrisin*
* *Sumycin* – Tetracycline
* *Suprax* – Cefixime
Synercid – Quinupristin/dalfopristin
Tazicef – Ceftazidime
Tazidime – Ceftazidime
Telithromycin – *Ketek*
* Tetracycline – *Sumycin*
Ticar – Ticarcillin
Ticarcillin – *Ticar*
Ticarcillin/clavulanate – *Timentin*
Tigecycline – *Tygacil*
Timentin – Ticarcillin/clavulanate
* Tobramycin – *Nebcin*

Continued on next page.

LIST OF SOME GENERIC AND BRAND NAMES (continued)

Trecator-SC – Ethionamide
* Trimethoprim – *Trimpex*
* Trimethoprim/sulfamethoxazole –
   Bactrim; *Septra*
* *Trimpex* – Trimethoprim
  Tygacil – Tigecycline
* *Vancocin* – Vancomycin
* Vancomycin – *Vancocin*
* *Vantin* – Cefpodoxime
* *Veetids* – Penicillin V

* *Velosef* – Cephradine
* *Vibramycin* – Doxycycline
* *Vibra-Tabs* – Doxycycline
  Xifaxan – Rifaxamin
  Zinacef – Cefuroxime
  Zithromax – Azithromycin
  Zmax – Azithromycin
  Zosyn – Piperacillin/tazobactam
  Zyvox – Linezolid

* Also available generically.

Treatment of *Clostridium difficile*–Associated Disease (CDAD)

Originally published in The Medical Letter – November 2006; 48:89

The gram-positive anaerobic bacillus *Clostridium difficile* is the most common identifiable cause of antibiotic-associated diarrhea. The antibiotics most often implicated have been ampicillin, second- and third-generation cephalosporins, clindamycin and fluoroquinolones.[1] The emergence in recent years of a new, more toxic epidemic strain (BI/NAP1), possibly related to widespread use of fluoroquinolones,[2] has caused a marked increase in the incidence and severity of *C. difficile*–associated disease (CDAD).[3-5]

STANDARD TREATMENT — In the past, mild *C. difficile* diarrhea often responded within 2-3 days simply to discontinuation of antibiotics. For patients with persistent symptoms, oral metronidazole and oral vancomycin have been the drugs of choice for many years. Oral administration of vancomycin results in very high concentrations in the intestinal lumen, and little or no systemic absorption. Metronidazole can be given intravenously for patients who cannot take oral drugs.

Recently, observational studies of CDAD caused by the new epidemic strain have suggested a reduced primary response to metronidazole and higher rates of recurrent disease in patients treated with the drug.[6-8] There is no evidence that the decreased response rates are due to bacterial resistance to metronidazole. Data on failure rates with vancomycin in patients infected with epidemic strains are still limited.

Initial Treatment – Since the emergence of the current epidemic strain, which has been associated with rapid clinical deterioration in some patients, prompt treatment has become common practice. Most patients with mild to moderate illness will respond to oral metronidazole 500 mg three times a day for 10 days, but some may need to be treated longer.

Treatment of Clostridium difficile–Associated Disease (CDAD)

Because of the recent increase in metronidazole failures, patients should be reassessed frequently during treatment.

Patients whose symptoms have not responded to metronidazole within 7 days, or who have deteriorating clinical signs and symptoms during treatment, should be treated with oral vancomycin, initially 125 mg four times a day.

In order to prevent emergence of vancomycin-resistant enterococci and staphylococci in hospitals, the Centers for Disease Control and Prevention has discouraged use of vancomycin as first-line therapy. Since it may, however, be more effective than metronidazole for CDAD,[9] many experts now use vancomycin as initial treatment for patients who appear seriously ill, particularly if they have a white blood cell (WBC) count >20,000/mm^3.

Treatment of Recurrences – With either metronidazole or vancomycin, about 20-25% of patients will have a recurrence of symptoms when treatment is discontinued.[10] Patients with a first recurrence typically respond to a second course of treatment with the same drug. Regardless of which drug was used initially, no significant difference has been found in the response of patients treated with metronidazole vs. vancomycin for a first recurrence, but there has been a trend toward a better outcome with vancomycin.[11]

Patients with first recurrences of CDAD have had a high rate of second recurrences (33% in one study).[11] For patients with multiple recurrences, no therapy has been proven to reduce the number of further recurrences; the most common approach has been prolonged tapering or pulsed doses of oral vancomycin, such as one week each of vancomycin (125 mg orally) 4 times daily, twice daily, daily, and every other day, followed by treatment every 3 days for 2 weeks.

Treatment of Clostridium difficile–Associated Disease (CDAD)

SOME DRUGS FOR CDAD

Drug	Dosage	Cost[1]
Metronidazole[2] – generic	500 mg PO 3x/d	$18.00
Flagyl (Pfizer)		146.70
Vancomycin – Vancocin[3]	125-500 mg PO 4x/d	610.80
(Viropharma)		

1. Cost of 10 days' treatment at lowest dose based on the most recent data (September 30, 2006) from retail pharmacies nationwide available from Wolters Kluwer Health.
2. Not approved by the FDA for this indication.
3. Oral vancomycin is not available generically.

Treatment of Fulminant CDAD – Patients who develop fulminant CDAD (rapidly progressive severe disease including toxic megacolon, shock, acute abdomen and colonic perforation) have a mortality rate of >50%. Metronidazole, which is excreted enterohepatically, can be given intravenously. Vancomycin can be given orally, via nasogastric tube, and by rectal instillation via enemas but is not effective for CDAD when given intravenously. In some patients, the two drugs have been used together. In severely ill patients refractory to other treatment, colectomy can be life-saving.[12]

OTHER OPTIONS — Intravenous immunoglobulin (IVIG) has been helpful in a small number of patients, presumably by providing antibodies against *C. difficile* toxins.[13,14]

Tolevamer, an oral investigational nonantibiotic, toxin-binding polymer, has been shown to be non-inferior to vancomycin for treatment of mild to moderate CDAD.[15]

Rifaximin *(Xifaxan)*, a non-absorbed oral antibiotic approved for use in travelers' diarrhea,[16] was effective in 9 of 10 patients in one study.[17,18]

Nitazoxanide *(Alinia)*, an antiparasitic drug,[19] was at least as effective as metronidazole in a prospective randomized trial,[20] and might be an alternative for patients not responding to metronidazole or vancomycin.

Fecal transplantation has been used successfully to treat CDAD recurrences by reconstituting the normal colonic flora, but is aesthetically unappealing and potentially could transfer other pathogens.[21]

Probiotic agents such as *Lactobacillus* spp. and *Bifidobacterium* spp. (found in most yogurt) have been used to treat or prevent CDAD, but with the possible exception of the yeast *Saccharomyces boulardii* (*Florastor* – Biocodex) in combination with high-dose vancomycin for multiple recurrences,[22] there is no convincing evidence that these agents are efficacious.[23]

The **resins** cholestyramine (*Questran*, and others) and colestipol *(Colestril)*, which bind *C. difficile* toxin, have been used to treat recurrent infection, sometimes in combination with vancomycin, but controlled trials demonstrating their efficacy are lacking, and these agents can also bind vancomycin.

PREVENTION — Unnecessary use of antibiotics, especially clindamycin, cephalosporins and fluoroquinolones, should, of course, be avoided. Healthcare workers caring for patients with *C. difficile* infection should follow contact isolation precautions, especially use of gloves and hand washing with soap and water after glove removal. Alcohol-based products such as hand sanitizers will not eradicate *C. difficile* spores.[24]

CONCLUSION — An epidemic strain of *Clostridium difficile* is causing an increase in the incidence and severity of *C. difficile*–associated disease (CDAD) that is sometimes refractory to standard treatment. Oral metronidazole can be used for patients with mild or moderate CDAD. Patients with severe disease should probably be treated initially with oral vancomycin. First recurrences of CDAD can be treated with either metronidazole or vancomycin, but for multiple recurrences, vancomycin should be used in tapering or pulsed doses. No current treatment reliably prevents further recurrences.

1. S Aslam and DM Musher. An update on diagnosis, treatment and prevention of *Clostridium difficile*–associated disease. Gastroenterol Clin N Am 2006; 35:315.
2. J Pepin et al. Emergence of fluoroquinolones as the predominant risk factor for *Clostridium difficile*–associated diarrhea: a cohort study during an epidemic in Quebec. Clin Infect Dis 2005; 41:1254.
3. LC McDonald et al. An epidemic, toxin gene–variant strain of *Clostridium difficile*. N Engl J Med 2005; 353:2433.
4. VG Loo et al. A predominantly clonal multi-institutional outbreak of *Clostridium difficile*–associated diarrhea with high morbidity and mortality. N Engl J Med 2005; 353:2442.
5. LC McDonald et al. *Clostridium difficile* infection in patients discharged from US short-stay hospitals, 1996-2003. Emerg Infect Dis 2006; 12:409.
6. DM Musher et al. Relatively poor outcome after treatment of *Clostridium difficile* colitis with metronidazole. Clin Infect Dis 2005; 40:1586.
7. J Pepin et al. Increasing risk of relapse after treatment of *Clostridium difficile* colitis in Quebec, Canada. Clin Infect Dis 2005; 40:1591.
8. DN Gerding. Metronidazole for *Clostridium difficile*–associated disease: Is it okay for Mom? Clin Infect Dis 2005; 40:1598.
9. FA Zar et al. Vancomycin (V) is superior to metronidazole (M) in the treatment of severe *Clostridium difficile*-associated diarrhea (CDAD). 44th Annual Meeting of IDSA in Toronto, Canada, October 12-15, 2006; page 60, abstract 686.
10. JG Bartlett. New drugs for *Clostridium difficile* infection. Clin Infect Dis 2006; 43:428.
11. J Pepin et al. Management and outcomes of a first recurrence of *Clostridium difficile*–associated disease in Quebec, Canada. Clin Infect Dis 2006: 42:758.
12. K Koss et al. The outcome of surgery in fulminant *Clostridium difficile* colitis. Colorectal Dis 2006; 8:149.
13. MH Wilcox. Descriptive study of intravenous immunoglobulin for the treatment of recurrent *Clostridium difficile* diarrhoea. J Antimicrob Chemother 2004; 53:882.
14. S McPherson et al. Intravenous immunoglobulin for the treatment of severe, refractory, and recurrent *Clostridium difficile* diarrhea. Dis Colon Rectum 2006; 49:640.
15. TJ Louie et al for the Tolevamer Study Investigator Group. Tolevamer, a novel nonantibiotic polymer, compared with vancomycin in the treatment of mild to moderately severe *Clostridium difficile*–associated diarrhea. Clin Infect Dis 2006; 43:411.
16. Rifaximin *(Xifaxan)* for travelers' diarrhea. Med Lett Drugs Ther 2004; 46:74.
17. M Boero et al. Treatment for colitis caused by *Clostridium difficile*: results of a randomized, open-label study of rifaximin vs. vancomycin [Italian]. Microbiol Medica 1990; 5:74.
18. L Gerard et al. Rifaximin: a nonabsorbable rifamycin antibiotic for use in nonsystemic gastrointestinal infections. Expert Rev Anti Infect Ther 2005; 3:201.
19. Nitazoxanide *(Alinia)*—a new anti-protozoal agent. Med Lett Drugs Ther 2003; 45:29.

20. DM Musher et al. Nitazoxanide for the treatment of *Clostridium difficile* colitis. Clin Infect Dis 2006; 43:421.
21. J Aas et al. Recurrent *Clostridium difficile* colitis: case series involving 18 patients threated with donor stool administered via a nasogastric tube. Clin Infect Dis 2003; 36:580.
22. CM Surawicz et al. The search for a better treatment for recurrent *Clostridium difficile* disease: use of high-dose vancomycin combined with *Saccharomyces boulardii*. Clin Infect Dis 2000; 31:1012.
23. N Dendukuri et al. Probiotic therapy for the prevention and treatment of *Clostridium difficile*–associated diarrhea: a systematic review. CMAJ 2005; 173:167.
24. M Wullt et al. Activity of three disinfectants and acidified nitrite against *Clostridium difficile* spores. Infect Control Hosp Epidemiol 2003; 24:765.

Drugs for Community-Acquired Bacterial Pneumonia

Originally published in The Medical Letter – July 2007; 49:62

Most patients with community-acquired pneumonia (CAP) are treated empirically. New guidelines published jointly by the Infectious Diseases Society of America and the American Thoracic Society have recently become available.[1]

PATHOGENS — The pathogens responsible for CAP are usually not identified, but *Streptococcus pneumoniae*, *Haemophilus influenzae*, the "atypical" pathogens *Mycoplasma pneumoniae* and *Chlamydophila pneumoniae* (formerly *Chlamydia pneumoniae*), and viruses such as influenza probably cause most cases. *M. pneumoniae* is most common in otherwise healthy people <50 years old and *S. pneumoniae* is the most common pathogen in older patients or those with comorbidities. *H. influenzae* is also more common in patients with other illnesses, particularly chronic obstructive pulmonary disease (COPD).

Among patients with CAP requiring hospitalization, *S. pneumoniae* is probably the most common pathogen. Other possible bacterial pathogens include *Moraxella catarrhalis*, *Klebsiella pneumoniae*, *Staphylococcus aureus* and occasionally other gram-negative bacilli or anaerobic mouth organisms. *Legionella* spp., another atypical organism, is less common, but like *S. pneumoniae*, *S. aureus* and gram-negative bacilli, should be considered in severely ill patients requiring ICU admission. Nonambulatory residents of nursing homes and other long-term care facilities are often infected with organisms commonly associated with hospital-acquired pneumonia, such as *Enterobacteriaceae* spp., *Pseudomonas aeruginosa* and methicillin-resistant *S. aureus*.[2]

EMPIRIC THERAPY — Ambulatory CAP – In otherwise healthy ambulatory young adults with CAP, an oral macrolide or doxycycline is generally prescribed empirically. Pneumococci may, however, be resistant to macrolides and doxycycline, especially if they are resistant to peni-

SOME ORAL ANTIBIOTICS FOR CAP[1]

Drug	Usual Adult Dosage	Cost[2]
CEPHALOSPORINS		
Cefpodoxime proxetil – generic	200 mg q12h	$56.20
Vantin (Pfizer)		68.20
Cefuroxime axetil – generic	500 mg q12h	76.20
Ceftin (GlaxoSmithKline)		143.80
MACROLIDES		
Azithromycin – generic	500 mg on day 1, then	39.06
Zithromax (Pfizer)	250 mg/day on days 2-5	55.20
Clarithromycin – generic	250-500 mg q12h	36.20
Biaxin (Abbott)		53.30
Biaxin XL	1000 mg q24h	55.50
Erythromycin base	250-500 mg q6h	
enteric-coated tabs – generic		9.60
E-mycin (Knoll)		11.60
FLUOROQUINOLONES		
Gemifloxacin – *Factive* (Oscient)	320 mg q24h	112.30
Levofloxacin – *Levaquin*	750 mg q24h	113.60
(Ortho-McNeil)		
Moxifloxacin – *Avelox* (Bayer)	400 mg q24h	60.50
TETRACYCLINES		
Doxycycline – generic	100 mg q12h	11.00
Vibramycin (Pfizer)		55.80
PENICILLINS		
Amoxicillin – generic	1 g q8h	9.00
Amoxil (GlaxoSmithKline)		11.00
Amoxicillin/clavulanate –		
Augmentin XR	2 g q12h[3]	67.80

1. Patients with a normally functioning gastrointestinal tract who are able to ingest oral medication should be switched from IV to PO therapy when hemodynamically stable and clinically improving.
2. Cost for 5 days' treatment at the lowest adult dosage, according to the most recent data (June 30, 2007) from retail pharmacies nationwide provided by Wolters Kluwer Health.
3. Dosage based on amoxicillin content. Multiple smaller tablets of amoxicillin/clavulanate (*Augmentin*, and others) would contain too much clavulanate.

SOME IV DRUGS FOR CAP[1]

Drug	Usual Adult Dosage	Cost[2]
CEPHALOSPORINS		
Cefotaxime – generic	1 g q8h	$89.40
Claforan (Aventis)		93.75
Ceftriaxone – generic	1 g q24h	130.05
Rocephin (Roche)		240.10
MACROLIDES		
Azithromycin – generic	500 mg q24h	112.90
Zithromax (Pfizer)		148.30
Erythromycin – generic	1 g q6h	334.40[3]
FLUOROQUINOLONES		
Levofloxacin – *Levaquin* (Ortho-McNeil)	750 mg q24h	303.00
Moxifloxacin – *Avelox* (Bayer)	400 mg q24h	212.50
TETRACYCLINES		
Doxycycline – generic	100 mg q12h	141.80
PENICILLINS		
Ampicillin – generic	1-2 g q6h	147.60
Ampicillin/sulbactam – generic		280.40
Unasyn (Pfizer)	3 g q6h[4]	347.20

1. Patients with a normally functioning gastrointestinal tract who are able to ingest oral medication should be switched from IV to PO therapy when hemodynamically stable and clinically improving.
2. Cost for 5 days' treatment at the lowest adult dosage, according to the most recent data (June 30, 2007) from retail pharmacies nationwide provided by Wolters Kluwer Health.
3. Price based on AWP listings in *Red Book* 2007.
4. A 3 g vial contains ampicillin 2 g and sulbactam 1 g.

cillin. For patients at risk of infection with drug-resistant *S. pneumoniae*, such as older patients (>65 years), those with comorbid illness, or those with antibiotic exposure during the previous 90 days, a fluoroquinolone with good antipneumococcal activity or a beta-lactam (a cephalosporin or a penicillin) plus a macrolide, is preferred.[3] Nationally, less than 1% of pneumococcal isolates are resistant to fluoroquinolones, but in some

EMPIRIC THERAPY FOR AMBULATORY CAP[1]

Young and otherwise healthy:
An oral macrolide (azithromycin, clarithromycin, erythromycin)

OR

Oral doxycycline

At risk for drug-resistant *S. pneumoniae*[2]:
Monotherapy with an oral respiratory fluoroquinolone (levofloxacin, moxifloxacin, gemifloxacin[3])

OR

An oral beta-lactam (amoxicillin, amoxicillin-clavulanate, cefpodoxime, cefuroxime)

plus

An oral macrolide (azithromycin, clarithromycin, erythromycin)[4]

---

1. See Tables on page 2 and 3 for CAP-specific dosage recommendations.
2. Because of age >65 years, comorbid illness or recent antibiotic use.
3. Gemifloxacin has a high rate of rash; Medical Letter consultants prefer levofloxacin or moxifloxacin.
4. Doxycycline is an alternative for patients who cannot tolerate a macrolide.

urban centers the percentage is higher.[4,5] These strains are more common among patients previously treated with a fluoroquinolone.

Hospitalized CAP — In patients with CAP requiring hospitalization, the combination of an intravenous (IV) beta-lactam plus a macrolide or monotherapy with a fluoroquinolone with good activity against *S. pneumoniae* is recommended pending culture results. Anaerobic coverage is seldom needed; when it is, ampicillin-sulbactam or moxifloxacin could be used.

Empiric treatment of patients with severe CAP who are admitted to the ICU should include an IV beta-lactam plus either a fluoroquinolone or azithromycin. An antipseudomonal, antipneumococcal beta-lactam, such as piperacillin/tazobactam *(Zosyn)*, plus either ciprofloxacin or lev-

EMPIRIC THERAPY FOR HOSPITALIZED CAP[1]

Non-ICU:
An IV or oral respiratory fluoroquinolone (levofloxacin, moxifloxacin, gemifloxacin[2])

OR

An IV beta-lactam (ceftriaxone, cefotaxime, ampicillin)

plus

An IV macrolide (azithromycin, erythromycin)[3]

ICU:
An IV beta-lactam (ceftriaxone, cefotaxime, ampicillin-sulbactam)

plus

An IV fluoroquinolone (levofloxacin, moxifloxacin) or IV azithromycin

1. See tables on page 94-95 for CAP-specific dosage recommendations.
2. Gemifloxacin is not available in an IV formulation and has been associated with a high rate of rash; Medical Letter consultants prefer levofloxacin or moxifloxacin.
3. Doxycycline is an alternative for patients who cannot tolerate a macrolide.

ofloxacin, should be used in patients in whom infection with *P. aeruginosa* is strongly suspected.

Drug-resistant *S. pneumoniae* (DRSP) – In treating patients with pneumococcal pneumonia due to strains resistant to penicillin, either ceftriaxone, cefotaxime or a respiratory fluoroquinolone can be used. Telithromycin *(Ketek)*, a ketolide with activity against DRSP, is not recommended because it has been associated with fatal hepatotoxicity. Vancomycin *(Vancocin, and others)* or linezolid *(Zyvox)* could be considered in severely ill patients.

CA-MRSA — Community-acquired strains of methicillin-resistant *S. aureus* (CA-MRSA) are a rare cause of CAP, but have recently been associated with severe, sometimes fatal pneumonia in young, previously healthy adults and children with influenza.[6] MRSA should be suspected in patients with severe pneumonia, particularly during influenza season, in patients with cavitary infiltrates, and in those with a history of MRSA infection. Vancomycin or linezolid should be used in such patients.

CONCLUSION — Atypical organisms such as *Mycoplasma pneumoniae* or *Chlamydophila pneumoniae* and respiratory viruses cause most cases of community-acquired pneumonia in young people with mild disease. Pneumococci are probably the most common cause in patients who need hospitalization. Before the infecting organism is known, it would be reasonable to treat young healthy patients with mild disease with an oral macrolide. For older or sicker patients not requiring hospitalization, an oral fluoroquinolone with good anti-pneumococcal activity, or a beta-lactam plus a macrolide, would be a better choice.

1. LA Mandell et al. Infectious Diseases Society of America/American Thoracic Society Consensus Guidelines on the Management of Community-Acquired Pneumonia in Adults. Clin Infect Dis 2007; 44 suppl 2:S27.
2. Guidelines for the management of adults with hospitalized-acquired, ventilator-associated, and healthcare-associated pneumonia. Am J Respir Crit Care Med 2005; 171:388.
3. JR Lonks et al. Implications of antimicrobial resistance in the empirical treatment of community-acquired respiratory tract infections: the case of macrolides. J Antimicrob Chemother 2002; 50 suppl 2:87.
4. AM Ferrara. New fluoroquinolones in lower respiratory tract infections and emerging patterns of pneumococcal resistance. Infection 2005; 33:106.
5. MJ Rybak. Increased bacterial resistance: PROTEKT US — an update. Ann Pharmacother 2004; 38 suppl:S8.
6. CDC. Severe methicillin-resistant Staphylococcus aureus community-acquired pneumonia associated with influenza-Louisiana and Georgia, December 2006-January 2007. MMWR Morbid Mortal Wkly Rep 2007; 56:325.

Doripenem *(Doribax)*

Doripenem *(Doribax)* — A New Parenteral Carbapenem
Originally published in The Medical Letter – January 2008; 50:75

Doripenem *(Doribax* – Ortho-McNeil Janssen), an intravenous (IV) car-bapenem antibiotic with a spectrum of activity similar to that of imipenem and meropenem, has been approved by the FDA for treatment of complicated intra-abdominal and urinary tract infections. Use of doripenem for treatment of nosocomial pneumonia, including ventilator-associated pneumonia, is still under FDA review.

ANTIBACTERIAL ACTIVITY — Like imipenem and meropenem, doripenem is active against a broad range of gram-positive, gram-nega-tive and anaerobic pathogens.[1] *In vitro*, it is more active than imipenem and meropenem against *Pseudomonas aeruginosa*[2] and is active against some pseudomonal isolates resistant to the other carbapenems[3,4]; the clinical significance of this *in vitro* activity is unknown. Carbapenems have little or no activity against methicillin-resistant *Staphylococcus aureus* (MRSA), *Enterococcus faecium, Stenotrophomonas maltophilia* or *Burkholderia cepacia*.

STANDARD TREATMENT — **Complicated intra-abdominal infec-tions** are often polymicrobial and are commonly due to enteric gram-negative organisms, enterococci, anaerobes and sometimes, in severely ill or hospitalized patients, *P. aeruginosa*. Empiric monotherapy with piperacillin/tazobactam or a carbapenem would be a reasonable first choice.[5] A fluoroquinolone (ciprofloxacin, levofloxacin, moxifloxacin) plus metronidazole for anaerobic coverage or tigecycline[6] alone could be used in patients allergic to beta-lactams.

Complicated urinary tract infections that recur after treatment are likely to be due to antibiotic-resistant gram-negative bacilli, *S. aureus* or enterococci. In hospitalized patients with symptomatic infections, initial empiric treatment with a third-generation cephalosporin such as cef-

PHARMACOLOGY

Drug class	Carbapenem
Mechanism of action	Inhibition of bacterial cell wall synthesis
Formulation	500 mg (on an anhydrous basis) powder; single-use vial
Dosage	500 mg every 8 hours; dosage adjustment needed for renal dysfunction
Administration	IV over 1 hour
Plasma concentrations	C_{max}: 23.0 mcg/mL $AUC_{0-\infty}$: 36.3 mcg·hr/mL
Metabolism	By dehydropeptidase to inactive metabolite
Excretion	Primarily renal; 70% as unchanged drug
Mean plasma half-life	~1 hour

tazidime, a fluoroquinolone, piperacillin/tazobactam or a carbapenem is recommended, sometimes together with an aminoglycoside.[7]

Nosocomial or ventilator-associated pneumonia is often caused by gram-negative bacilli, especially *P. aeruginosa, Klebsiella* spp., *Enterobacter* spp., *Serratia* spp. and *Acinetobacter* spp.; it can also be caused by *S. aureus*. Many of these bacteria are multi-drug resistant (MDR). Nosocomial pneumonia is usually treated with broad-spectrum drugs such as piperacillin/tazobactam, cefepime, a carbapenem or a fluoroquinolone; addition of an aminoglycoside or a fluoroquinolone with anti-pseudomonal activity (in patients who are not already taking one) is reasonable. Addition of vancomycin or linezolid should be considered in hospitals where MRSA are common.[7]

CLINICAL STUDIES — FDA approval of doripenem was entirely based on unpublished clinical trials available only as abstracts.

Complicated intra-abdominal infection – Two prospective, randomized, double-blind studies compared doripenem with meropenem for the

Doripenem *(Doribax)*

SOME PARENTERAL ANTIBIOTICS

Drug	Daily Dosage[1]	Cost[2]
Ampicillin/sulbactam – generic	1.5-3 g q6h	$26.96
Unasyn (Pfizer)	35.64	
Aztreonam – *Azactam* (Elan)	1-2 g q6-8h	94.44
Cefepime – *Maxipime* (Elan)	1-2 g q8-12h	43.40
Ciprofloxacin – generic	200-400 mg q8-12h	15.40[3]
Cipro (Schering)		31.20[3]
Doripenem – *Doribax* (Ortho-McNeil)	500 mg q8h	138.00[3]
Ertapenem – *Invanz* (Merck)	1 g q24h	60.00
Imipenem/cilastatin – *Primaxin* (Merck)	250 mg-1 g q6-8h	146.68[4]
Levofloxacin – *Levaquin* (Ortho-McNeil)	250-750 mg q24h	22.50
Meropenem – *Merrem* (Astrazeneca)	1-2 g q8h	188.43
Metronidazole – generic	500 mg q8h	45.00
Moxifloxacin – *Avelox* (Schering)	400 mg q24h	37.50
Piperacillin/tazobactam – *Zosyn* (Wyeth)	3.375 g q4-6h	71.12
	or 4.5 g q6-8h	
Ticarcillin/clavulanic acid – *Timentin* (GSK)	3.1 g q4-6h	62.84
Tigecycline – *Tygacil* (Wyeth)	100 mg x 1, then 50 mg q12	116.98

1. Dosage adjustment may be necessary in patients with renal or hepatic dysfunction.
2. Cost of one day's treatment for the drug alone with the lowest daily dosage, according to the most recent data (December 31, 2007) from retail pharmacies nationwide, provided by Wolter's Kluwer Health.
3. Price based on AWP listings in *Red Book* 2007 or January 2008 *Update*.
4. Cost of four, 500-mg vials.

treatment of patients with complicated appendicitis, bowel perforation, cholecystitis, intra-abdominal or solid organ abscess, or generalized peritonitis. The clinical cure rates for doripenem were similar to that of meropenem among all microbiologically evaluable patients in both trials: 83.3% (135/162) for doripenem and 83.0% (127/153) for meropenem in the first trial,[8] and 85.9% (140/163) for doripenem and 85.3% (133/156) for meropenem in the second trial.[9]

Complicated urinary tract infection – One double-blind study compared the efficacy of doripenem to IV levofloxacin. Microbiological cure rates were similar in both treatment arms: 82.1% (230/280) for doripenem and 83.4% (221/265) for levofloxacin.[10]

Nosocomial pneumonia, including ventilator-associated pneumonia – In an open-label study comparing doripenem to piperacillin/tazobactam, the clinical cure rates among microbiologically evaluable patients were similar: 82.1% (69/84) for doripenem and 78.3% (65/83) for piperacillin/tazobactam.[11] In a second study comparing doripenem to imipenem, the clinical cure rates among microbiologically evaluable patients were also similar: 69.0% (80/116) for doripenem and 64.5% (71/110) for imipenem.[12,13]

ADVERSE EFFECTS — Doripenem is generally well tolerated. It can cause serious allergic reactions in patients allergic to beta-lactams. Headache, nausea, diarrhea, rash and injection site phlebitis have occurred. Unlike the other carbapenems, doripenem has not demonstrated any epileptogenic potential in animal studies.[14]

DRUG INTERACTIONS — Carbapenems can reduce serum concentrations of valproic acid (*Depakene*, and others), leading to loss of seizure control. Probenecid interferes with tubular secretion of doripenem, increasing serum concentrations of the drug.

CONCLUSION — Doripenem *(Doribax)* is a broad-spectrum parenteral antibiotic similar to meropenem and imipenem. Like the other carbapenems, it should be reserved for use in seriously ill and/or hospitalized patients in whom polymicrobial infections or infections with *Pseudomonas* or multi-drug resistant gram-negatives are a concern.

1. PD Lister. Carbapenems in the USA: focus on doripenem. Expert Rev Anti Infect Ther. 2007; 5:793.
2. GG Zhanel et al. Comparative review of the carbapenems. Drugs 2007; 67:1027.

Doripenem *(Doribax)*

3. RN Jones et al. Activities of doripenem (S-4661) against drug-resistant pathogens. Antimicrob Agents Chemother 2004; 48: 3136.

4. S Mushtaq et al. Doripenem versus Pseudomonas aeruginosa in vitro: activity against characterized isolates, mutants, and transconjugants and resistance selection potential. Antimicrob Agents Chemother 2004; 48:3086.

5. JS Solomkin et al. Guidelines for the selection of anti-infective agents for complicated intra-abdominal infections. Clin Infect Dis 2003; 37:997.

6. Tigecycline (Tygacil). Med Lett Drugs Ther 2005; 47:73.

7. Choice of antibacterial drugs. Treat Guidel Med Lett 2007; 5:33.

8. O Malafaia et al. Doripenem versus meropenem for the treatment of complicated intra-abdominal infections. 46th Interscience Conference on Antimicrobial Agents and Chemotherapy; San Francisco, CA; September 17-20, 2006. Abstract L-1654b.

9. C Lucasti et al. Treatment of complicated intra-abdominal infections: doripenem versus meropenem. Clin Microbiol Infect 2007; 13 (suppl 1): S212. Poster P834.

10. K Naber et al. Intravenous therapy with doripenem versus levofloxacin with an option for oral step-down therapy in the treatment of complicated urinary tract infection and pyelonephritis. Clin Microbiol Infect 2007; 13 (suppl 1): S212. Poster P833.

11. A Rea-Neto, et al. Efficacy and safety of intravenous doripenem vs. piperacillin/tazobactam in nosocomial pneumonia. 47th Annual Interscience Conference on Antimicrobial Agents and Chemotherapy; Chicago, IL; September 17-20, 2007. Presentation L-731

12. J Chastre et al. Efficacy and safety of doripenem versus imipenem for ventilator-associated pneumonia. 47th Annual Interscience Conference on Antimicrobial Agents and Chemotherapy; Chicago, IL; September 17-20, 2007. Presentation L-486.

13. M Clavel et al. Efficacy of doripenem versus imipenem in patients with ventilator-associated pneumonia and high disease severity. 45th Annual Meeting of the Infectious Diseases Society of America; San Diego, CA; October 4-7, 2007. Abstract 1081.

14. M Horiuchi et al. Absence of convulsive liability of doripenem, a new carbapenem antibiotic, in comparision with B-lactam antibiotics. Toxicology 2006; 222:114.

DRUGS FOR
Tuberculosis

Original publication date – March 2007

Even though the incidence continues to decline, tuberculosis (TB) is still a problem in the United States.[1] Treatment of TB can be divided into treatment of latent infection and treatment of active disease. A table listing the first-line drugs used for treatment of TB with their doses and adverse effects can be found on page 106. Other guidelines with more detailed management recommendations are available.[2,3]

DIRECTLY OBSERVED THERAPY

Poor adherence to TB therapy is the most common cause of treatment failure and is associated with emergence of drug resistance. Medical Letter consultants recommend that almost all patients, including those with disease due to susceptible strains, take drugs for active TB disease under direct observation. Compared to self-administered regimens, directly observed therapy (DOT) has been shown to decrease drug resistance, relapse and mortality rates, and to improve cure rates.[4,5] Due to the complexity and duration of TB treatment regimens, DOT is particularly important for treatment of patients with drug-resistant infections and for those on intermittent regimens because these are more susceptible to failure. Patients with latent infection who are at high risk for developing active TB or are taking an intermittent regimen should also be considered for DOT. DOT services are available through most local and state health departments.

LATENT TB INFECTION

The risk of patients with latent TB infection developing active TB disease is extremely high in those who are co-infected with HIV or are receiving immunosuppressive therapy. It is also high in children, in close contacts of patients with recent pulmonary TB, in previously untreated patients with radiographic evidence of prior TB, during the first 2 years after development of a positive tuberculin test, and in immigrants from countries with a high incidence of TB.[6,7]

The risk of serious disease, including miliary TB and tuberculous meningitis, is highest in infants, the elderly, and in patients with HIV infection or other causes of severe immunosuppression. Recent reports also indicate high risk for development of active TB disease in persons with latent TB infection who are treated with the TNF-alpha inhibitors infliximab *(Remicade)*, etanercept *(Enbrel)*, and adalimumab *(Humira)* for rheumatoid arthritis or some other condition. These reports include cases of extrapulmonary and disseminated disease, and deaths. Before beginning therapy with these drugs, testing for latent TB infection is recommended.[8,9]

Diagnosis – The tuberculin skin test (purified protein derivative, PPD) has been in clinical use for over a century. Recently, interferon-gamma release assays (IGRAs) that measure host cell-mediated immune response to *Mycobacterium tuberculosis* have become available for diagnosis of latent TB infection. Unlike PPD skin testing, IGRA results are not affected by prior immunization with Bacille Calmette-Guérin (BCG) or exposure to most nontuberculous mycobacteria, which gives them higher specificity than skin testing.

Currently, the only FDA-approved IGRA is the QuantiFERON-TB Gold (QFT-G) assay.[10] QFT-G detects the immune response to two *M. tuberculosis* antigens that are absent from all BCG vaccine preparations and most nontuberculous mycobacteria (exceptions are *M. kansasii, M. mar-*

inum and *M. szulgai*). It has not been well studied in high-risk groups such as children, healthcare workers, and HIV-infected and other immunocompromised persons. An enzyme-linked immunospot IGRA assay, T-SPOT. *TB*, is available in Europe.[11]

Treatment – Isoniazid (INH) is the drug of choice for treatment of latent TB infection presumed to be due to susceptible strains. It should be given daily or intermittently for 9 months.[12] Monthly follow-up visits, patient education, and identification of barriers to adherence can all promote completion of therapy for latent TB. Directly observed therapy (DOT) should be considered for high-risk patients such as children or patients co-infected with HIV and for all patients taking intermittent regimens.

An alternative regimen for treatment of latent TB, particularly for persons intolerant to isoniazid or those found to be tuberculin-positive after exposure to patients with organisms resistant to isoniazid, is daily rifampin alone for 4 months (6 months in children).[13,14] One meta-analysis found short-course therapy with 3 months of isoniazid plus rifampin equivalent to the standard 9 months of isoniazid.[15] The combination of rifampin and pyrazinamide for 2 months, which formerly was used as an alternative to isoniazid treatment of latent infection, is no longer recommended because of its association with potentially lethal hepatotoxicity.[16,17]

Drug-Resistant Latent TB Infection – There are no data-based recommendations for treatment of latent TB infection in high-risk patients with known exposure to multi-drug resistant TB (MDRTB), defined as isolates with resistance to at least isoniazid and rifampin. Regimens with two drugs to which the organism is susceptible (e.g., pyrazinamide plus either ethambutol or a fluoroquinolone for 9-12 months) have been used, but are poorly tolerated, can be hepatotoxic and are of uncertain efficacy.[18,19]

Extensively drug-resistant TB (XDRTB), now defined as isolates with resistance not only to isoniazid and rifampin but also to any fluoro-

FIRST-LINE DRUGS

Drug/formulation	Adult dosage	
	Daily	Intermittent[1]
Isoniazid (INH)[2] 100, 300 mg tabs, 50 mg/5mL syrup, 100 mg/mL inj	5 mg/kg (max 300 mg) PO, IM or IV	15 mg/kg (max 900 mg) 2-3x/wk
Rifampin *(Rifadin, Rimactane)* 150, 300 mg caps, 600 mg inj powder	10 mg/kg (max 600 mg) PO or IV	10 mg/kg (max 600 mg) 2-3x/wk
Rifabutin[3] *(Mycobutin)* 150 mg caps	5 mg/kg (max 300 mg) PO	5 mg/kg (max 300 mg) 2-3x/wk
Rifapentine *(Priftin)* 150 mg tabs	—	10-15 mg/kg/wk (max 600-900 mg) PO
Pyrazinamide 500 mg tabs	20-25 mg/kg PO (max 2 g)	30-50 mg/kg 2x/wk (max 3 g); 3x/wk (max 4 g)
Ethambutol[4] *(Myambutol)* 100, 400 mg tabs	15-25 mg/kg PO (max 1.6 g)	25-50 mg/kg 2x/wk (max 2.4 g); 3x/wk (max 4 g)

1. Intermittent therapy is usually begun after a few weeks or months of treatment with a daily regimen.
2. Pyridoxine 25-50 mg should be given to prevent neuropathy in malnourished or pregnant patients and those with HIV infection, alcoholism or diabetes.
3. For use with amprenavir, fosamprenavir, nelfinavir or indinavir, the rifabutin dose is 150 mg/day or 300 mg 3 times a week. For use with atazanavir, ritonavir alone or ritonavir combined with other protease inhibitors, and lopinavir/ritonavir *(Kaletra)*, the rifabutin dose is further decreased to 150 mg every other day or 3 times weekly. For use with efavirenz, the rifabutin dose is increased to 450 mg/day or 600 mg 2-3 times weekly. Not recommended with saquinavir alone or delavirdine.

quinolone and either capreomycin, kanamycin or amikacin (see table on page 110), is an increasing problem worldwide; there are no data-based recommendations for treatment of latent TB following exposure to XDRTB.[20-22]

	Pediatric dosage	Main
Daily	Intermittent[1]	adverse effects
10-20 mg/kg (max 300 mg)	20-30 mg/kg (max 900 mg) 2x/wk	Hepatic toxicity, rash, peripheral neuropathy
10-20 mg/kg (max 600 mg)	10-20 mg/kg (max 600 mg) 2x/wk	Hepatic toxicity, rash, flu-like syndrome, pruritis, drug interactions
10-20 mg/kg (max 300 mg)	No data available	Hepatic toxicity, flu-like syndrome, uveitis, neutropenia, drug interactions
No data available	No data available	Similar to rifampin
15-30 mg/kg (max 2 g)	50 mg/kg (max 2 g) 2x/wk	Arthralgias, hepatic toxicity, pruritis, rash, hyperuricemia, GI upset
15-25 mg/kg (max 1 g)	50 mg/kg (max 2.5 g) 2x/wk	Decreased red-green color discrimination, decreased visual acuity

4. Usually not recommended for children when visual acuity cannot be monitored. Some clinicians use 25 mg/kg/day during first one or two months or longer if organism is isoniazid-resistant. Decrease dosage if renal function is diminished.

Medical Letter consultants recommend that treatment of patients with drug-resistant latent TB be provided by or in collaboration with a clinician experienced in treatment of these infections. Whatever treatment is chosen, such patients should be observed for up to 2 years following exposure.

ACTIVE TB DISEASE

All initial isolates of *M. tuberculosis* should be tested for antimicrobial susceptibility, but results generally do not become available for at least 2-4 weeks.[23] Standard treatment of active TB includes a 2-month initial phase and a continuation phase of either 4 or 7 months, depending on the presence or absence of cavitary disease at the time of diagnosis and the results of sputum cultures taken at 2 months (see table). Patients should be monitored monthly to assess for adverse reactions, adherence and response to treatment. Medical Letter consultants recommend that patients on self-administered therapy receive no more than a 1-month supply of medication at each visit.

Initial Therapy – Until susceptibility results are available, empiric initial treatment should consist of a 4-drug regimen of isoniazid, rifampin, pyrazinamide and ethambutol.[24] Patients in areas with low rates of drug-resistant TB who cannot take pyrazinamide, such as those who have severe liver disease or gout, should receive empiric initial therapy with isoniazid, rifampin and ethambutol.

When TB disease proves to be caused by a fully susceptible strain, the initial phase of treatment should consist of isoniazid, rifampin and pyrazinamide for 2 months.

Continuation Therapy – Two factors increase the risk of treatment failure and relapse: cavitary disease at presentation and a positive sputum culture taken at 2 months. For patients with one or no risk factors, the continuation phase of treatment should be with isoniazid and rifampin for 4 months. For patients with both risk factors, and for those who could not take pyrazinamide as part of the initial regimen, the continuation phase is extended to 7 months.

For selected patients with neither cavitary disease nor a positive smear after 2 months of therapy, the long-acting rifamycin rifapentine, given

DURATION OF CONTINUATION THERAPY[1]

Cavity on Chest X-ray	Drugs	Sputum culture taken at 2 mos	Duration (months)[2]
No	INH/RIF	Negative	4
	or INH/RPT[3]		4
No	INH/RIF	Positive[4]	4
	or INH/RPT[3]		7
Yes	INH/RIF	Negative	4
Yes	INH/RIF	Positive	7

INH = Isoniazid; RIF = rifampin; RPT = rifapentine
1. For treatment of drug-susceptible disease after two months of initial therapy.
2. Always 7 months for patients who could not take pyrazinamide as part of the initial regimen. Can be shortened to 2 months in non-HIV patients with culture-negative pulmonary TB.
3. RPT is a treatment option only for non-pregnant, HIV-negative adults without cavitary or extrapulmonary disease who are smear-negative at 2 months.
4. If the culture is positive and the patient is taking INH/RPT, some Medical Letter consultants would switch to INH/RIF.

once-weekly by DOT is an additional option for continuation therapy.[24] Rifapentine should not be used if the patient has extrapulmonary TB or co-infection with HIV, is younger than 12 years of age or pregnant, or if drug susceptibility is unknown. If the culture taken at 2 months proves to be positive and rifapentine is being used, some Medical Letter consultants would switch to rifampin.

If sputum cultures remain positive after 4 months of treatment, nonadherence to treatment or infection with drug-resistant TB must be considered. Only after these are excluded should other causes (e.g., malabsorption) be considered as possible explanations of poor response. Treatment duration should be prolonged in such patients.

SOME SECOND-LINE DRUGS

Drug	Daily adult dosage
Streptomycin[1]	15 mg/kg IM (max 1 g)
Capreomycin (Capastat)	15 mg/kg IM (max 1 g)
Kanamycin (Kantrex, and others)	15 mg/kg IM or IV (max 1 g)
Amikacin (Amikin)	15 mg/kg IM or IV (max 1 g)
Cycloserine[2] (Seromycin)	10-15 mg/kg in 2 doses (max 500 mg bid) PO
Ethionamide (Trecator-SC)	15-20 mg/kg in 2 doses (max 500 mg bid) PO
Levofloxacin (Levaquin)	500-1000 mg PO or IV
Moxifloxacin (Avelox)	400 mg PO or IV
Aminosalicylic acid (PAS; Paser)	8-12 g in 2-3 doses PO

1. Streptomycin is generally given 5-7 times per week (15 mg/kg, or a maximum of 1 g per dose) for an initial 2 to 12 week period, and then (if needed) 2 to 3 times per week (20 to 30 mg/kg, or a maximum of 1.5 g per dose). For patients >59 years old, dosage is reduced to 10 mg/kg/d (max 750 mg/d). Dosage should be decreased if renal function is diminished.
2. Some authorities recommend pyridoxine 50 mg for every 250 mg of cycloserine to decrease the incidence of adverse neurological effects.

TB osteomyelitis is usually treated for 6-9 months. Tuberculous meningitis is usually treated for a total of 9-12 months. Addition of a corticosteroid for 1-2 months is recommended for tuberculous pericarditis or meningitis.[25]

Culture-Negative TB – Patients with pulmonary disease who have no positive cultures for *M. tuberculosis* before treatment and after 2 months of therapy have "culture-negative TB"; in these patients, the continuation phase with isoniazid and rifampin can generally be shortened to 2 months. Exceptions are patients with extrapulmonary TB or those co-infected with HIV, who should be treated for 6 months or longer.

Daily pediatric dosage	Main adverse effects
20-40 mg/kg	Vestibular and auditory toxicity, renal damage
15-30 mg/kg	Auditory and vestibular toxicity, renal damage
15-30 mg/kg	Auditory toxicity, renal damage
15-30 mg/kg	Auditory toxicity, renal damage
10-15 mg/kg	Psychiatric symptoms, seizures
15-20 mg/kg	GI and hepatic toxicity, hypothyroidism
See footnote 3	GI toxicity, CNS effects, rash, dysglycemia
See footnote 3	GI toxicity, CNS effects, rash, dysglycemia
200-300 mg/kg, in 2-4 doses	GI disturbance

3. According to the American Academy of Pediatrics, although fluoroquinolones are generally contraindicated in children <18 years old, their use may be justified in special circumstances. Medical
Letter consultants would use these drugs to treat children with MDRTB.

Drug Intolerance – For patients who cannot tolerate rifamycins, alternative regimens include 9-12 months of isoniazid, ethambutol and pyrazinamide, with or without a fluoroquinolone (levofloxacin or moxifloxacin). Levofloxacin has been safe for long-term use in patients with drug-resistant TB or those intolerant to isoniazid or a rifamycin. Moxifloxacin is currently in clinical trials for use in TB treatment and may be more active than levofloxacin against *M. tuberculosis*, but clinical data are limited.

Isoniazid plus ethambutol for 18 months has also been used for patients intolerant of rifamycins. Rifabutin has been substituted for rifampin in standard regimens for some patients who could not take rifampin

COMBINATION DRUGS

Drug	Daily adult dosage
Rifamate[1] (isoniazid 150 mg, rifampin 300 mg)	2 capsules
Rifater[1] (isoniazid 50 mg, rifampin 120 mg, pyrazinamide 300 mg)	≤44 kg: 4 tablets 45-54 kg: 5 tablets 55-90 kg: 6 tablets >90 kg: 6 tablets plus additional pyrazinamide[2]

1. Pyridoxine 25-50 mg should be given to prevent neuropathy in malnourished or pregnant patients and those with HIV infection, alcoholism or diabetes.
2. Six tablets provide 1800 mg of pyrazinamide. Patients should take additional pyrazinamide tablets to achieve a total dose of 20-25 mg/kg/d.

because of drug interactions (such as HIV co-infected patients on a pro-tease inhibitor). Patients who cannot take pyrazinamide in the initial phase of treatment should receive continuation therapy with isoniazid and rifampin for 7 months (a total course of 9 months).

Intermittent Treatment – Intermittent 4-drug regimens with 2 or 3 doses per week are also effective for treatment of TB, but must be given by DOT. Intermittent therapy is most commonly used in the continuation phase, after at least 2 months of daily (or 5x/wk) therapy during the initiation phase. It should never be used for treatment of drug-resistant TB. A once-weekly continuation-therapy regimen of isoniazid plus rifapentine (instead of rifampin), started after 2 months of standard initial therapy, is also effective for susceptible TB in selected patients.[2,24] This regimen has, however, been associated with development of rifamycin resistance in HIV-infected patients and should not be used in these individuals.[26-28]

Twice-weekly intermittent regimens have also been associated with rifamycin resistance in HIV co-infected patients with low CD4 counts; such patients should receive daily or 3x/wk therapy.

Fixed-Dose Combinations – A combination formulation of rifampin, isoniazid and pyrazinamide *(Rifater)* is approved by the FDA for the initial 2 months of daily anti-tuberculosis therapy. A combination of rifampin and isoniazid *(Rifamate)* has been available in the US since 1975. Fixed-dose combinations may be particularly useful for patients self-administering their therapy.[29]

DRUG-RESISTANT TB DISEASE

Resistance to Isoniazid – TB that is resistant to isoniazid can be treated with rifampin, pyrazinamide and ethambutol for 6-9 months. If the organism is susceptible, streptomycin is an alternative to ethambutol. Patients who cannot tolerate pyrazinamide can take rifampin and ethambutol for 12 months. A fluoroquinolone or an injectable drug (capreomycin, amikacin, kanamycin or streptomycin) is sometimes added, especially if the patient cannot tolerate pyrazinamide or if there is extensive disease.

Multidrug Resistance – Recommendations for treatment of MDRTB and XDRTB are based on limited data and should be undertaken in collaboration with someone familiar with the management of these conditions. MDRTB and XDRTB should be treated with ≥4 drugs to which the organism is susceptible. When MDRTB is likely, or in patients with a history of treatment for TB, some experienced clinicians start with combinations of 5-7 drugs before laboratory susceptibility data become available. Typically, empiric therapy for suspected MDRTB includes isoniazid, rifampin, ethambutol, pyrazinamide, an aminoglycoside (streptomycin, kanamycin or amikacin) or capreomycin, a fluoroquinolone and either cycloserine, ethionamide or aminosalicylic acid (PAS).[30-32] Drug selection is based on a hierarchy of drugs to which the isolate is susceptible. This involves inclusion of all active first-line drugs (pyrazinamide, ethambutol), a fluoroquinolone and one injectable drug.

Monthly bacteriologic results (AFB smear and culture) should be monitored and treatment continued for 18-24 months, or 12-18 months after the culture becomes negative. The parenteral drug should be continued for 6 months after culture conversion. Surgical resection has improved outcome in some patients and should be considered if cultures fail to convert to negative after 3-4 months of appropriate treatment.[33]

HIV-INFECTED PATIENTS

Testing for HIV infection is recommended for all patients with active TB. Persons with HIV, once infected, are at markedly increased risk of developing active TB disease. HIV-infected patients with a history of prior untreated or inadequately treated TB disease should be re-evaluated for active disease regardless of age or results of tests for latent TB infection. If active TB disease is ruled out, patients should receive treatment for latent TB infection. HIV-infected persons who have had recent close contact with a patient with active TB disease should receive empiric treatment for latent infection regardless of age, results of tests for TB infection, or history of previous treatment.

To minimize the emergence of drug-resistant TB, co-infected patients in the continuation phase of TB treatment should take medication once daily or three times weekly.[34] Twice-weekly regimens have been associated with acquisition of rifamycin resistance in patients with CD4 cell counts <100 cells/mm^3.[35] Once-weekly rifapentine is not recommended for TB treatment in HIV-infected patients because it has been associated with development of rifamycin resistance.[28]

Patients Not on HAART – For HIV-infected patients requiring TB treatment who are not currently being treated with highly active antiretroviral therapy (HAART), it may be prudent to delay HAART for 2-3 months in order to avoid a paradoxical worsening of TB due to immune reconstitution, decrease the risk of overlapping drug adverse effects and interactions, reduce pill burden, and enhance adherence to both drug regimens,[36-38] but the optimal timing for initiating HAART in patients with newly diagnosed TB is not known.

Patients on HAART – Rifamycins induce hepatic CYP enzymes, especially CYP3A4, and can accelerate metabolism of protease inhibitors and some non-nucleoside reverse transcriptase inhibitors (NNRTIs), decreasing their serum concentrations, possibly to ineffective levels. The degree to which each drug induces CYP3A4 differs: rifampin is the most potent and rifabutin the least. In addition, rifabutin is a substrate for CYP3A4; protease inhibitors decrease its metabolism, increasing serum concentrations and possibly toxicity.

Standard 4-drug treatment regimens including rifampin can be given to HIV-infected patients with active TB who are simultaneously receiving HAART if the HAART regimen consists of efavirenz *(Sustiva)* and two nucleoside reverse transcriptase inhibitors (NRTIs). Standard doses of rifampin can also be used in patients taking ritonavir *(Norvir)* as the only protease inhibitor, combined with 2 NRTIs.[39]

Two alternative TB/HAART regimens are based on **rifabutin**, which appears to be as effective as rifampin against TB and has less effect on protease inhibitor concentrations. The first substitutes low-dose rifabutin (150 mg once/day or 300 mg 3x/week) for rifampin in the standard TB regimen (i.e., isoniazid, rifabutin, pyrazinamide and ethambutol) and uses higher-than-usual doses of indinavir *(Crixivan)* or nelfinavir *(Viracept)*, or standard doses of amprenavir *(Agenerase)* or fosamprenavir *(Lexiva)* as the HIV protease inhibitor. The second decreases the rifabutin dose further to 150 mg every other day or 3 times weekly and the HAART regimen includes standard doses of atazanavir *(Reyataz)*, ritonavir/lopinavir *(Kaletra)* or ritonavir alone or combined with other protease inhibitors. Saquinavir *(Invirase)* alone should not be used. Higher rifabutin doses (450 mg daily or 600 mg 2-3 times per week) are needed if the HAART regimen contains efavirenz.

TB IN PREGNANCY

Active TB disease during pregnancy requires treatment. The treatment of **latent TB infection** during pregnancy is more controversial because of the risk of isoniazid hepatotoxicity. In general, it is recommended that treatment of latent TB be delayed until 2 or 3 months after delivery. However, for women who are HIV-positive or have been infected with TB recently, initiation of therapy should not be delayed because of pregnancy.

Treatment of **active TB** disease should be initiated in pregnancy when there is moderate to high suspicion of disease because the risk to the fetus is much greater than the risk of adverse drug effects. The initial regimen should include isoniazid, rifampin and ethambutol. Each of these drugs crosses the placenta, but none is teratogenic. Pyrazinamide has not been extensively studied in pregnancy, but some Medical Letter consultants would use it in addition to isoniazid, rifampin and ethambutol.[40] If pyrazinamide is not used, treatment should be continued for a total of at least 9 months. Pyrazinamide is always recommended as part of the initial regimen in pregnant women who are HIV co-infected or when drug resistance is suspected.

Limited data are available on the treatment of MDRTB in pregnancy. Regimens using various combinations of amikacin, ethionamide, PAS, cycloserine, capreomycin and fluoroquinolones have been successful without causing fetal adverse effects, even though these drugs are generally not considered safe in pregnancy.[41-43]

ADVERSE EFFECTS

Isoniazid – Serum aminotransferase activity increases in 10-20% of patients taking isoniazid, especially in the early weeks of treatment, but often returns to normal even when the drug is continued. Severe liver damage due to isoniazid is less common than previously thought. It is more likely to occur in patients more than 35 years old. Clinical monitoring should occur monthly; monitoring of serum transaminases is not routinely recommended except for patients with pre-existing liver disease and those at increased risk for isoniazid hepatotoxicity, such as those patients who drink alcohol regularly. Medical Letter consultants recommend stopping isoniazid when serum aminotransferase activity reaches five times the upper limit of normal or if the patient has symptoms of hepatitis. In patients with active TB disease it can sometimes be restarted later. Rechallenge with isoniazid is not recommended for patients with latent TB infection.

Peripheral neuropathy occurs rarely and can usually be prevented by supplementation with pyridoxine (vitamin B6, 25-50 mg/day), which is recommended for patients with chronic alcohol use, diabetes, chronic renal failure or HIV infection, and for those who are pregnant, breast-feeding or malnourished. Some Medical Letter consultants routinely use pyridoxine for all patients taking isoniazid. Pyridoxine does not need to be given to a nursing infant unless the baby is also being given isoniazid.

Rifamycins – Rifampin, like isoniazid, is potentially hepatotoxic, and gastrointestinal disturbances, morbilliform rash and thrombocytopenic purpura can occur. Whenever possible, rifampin should be continued despite minor adverse reactions such as pruritus and gastrointestinal upset. When taken erratically, the drug can cause a febrile "flu-like" syndrome and, very rarely, shortness of breath, hemolytic anemia, shock and acute renal failure. Patients should be warned that rifampin may turn urine, tears and other body fluids reddish-orange and can permanently stain contact lenses and lens implants.

Rifampin is an inducer of CYP isozymes 3A4, 2C9, 2C19, 2D6, 2B6, and 2C8. It can increase the metabolism and decrease the effect of many other drugs, including hormonal contraceptives (patients should be advised to use another method of contraception), sulfonylureas such as glyburide (*Diabeta*, and others), corticosteroids, warfarin (*Coumadin*, and others), quinidine, methadone (*Dolophine*, and others), delavirdine (*Rescriptor*), clarithromycin (*Biaxin*, and others), ketoconazole (*Nizoral*, and others), itraconazole (*Sporanox*, and others) and fluconazole (*Diflucan*, and others), as well as protease inhibitors and most statins (such as atorvastatin and simvastatin).[44]

Rifabutin and **rifapentine** have adverse effects similar to those of rifampin. Rifabutin can also cause uveitis, skin hyperpigmentation and neutropenia, but is less likely than rifampin to interact with other drugs.

Other Drugs – **Pyrazinamide** can cause gastrointestinal disturbances, hepatotoxicity, morbilliform rash, arthralgias and asymptomatic hyper-uricemia, and can block the hypouricemic action of allopurinol (*Zyloprim*, and others). **Ethambutol** can cause optic neuritis, but only very rarely when using a dosage of 15 mg/kg daily. Testing of visual acuity and color perception should be performed at the start of therapy, and monthly thereafter. The decision to use ethambutol in children too young to have visual acuity monitored must take into consideration the risk/benefit for each particular patient.[45]

Streptomycin causes ototoxicity (usually vestibular disturbance) and, less frequently, renal toxicity. **Amikacin** and **kanamycin** can cause tinnitus and high-frequency hearing loss. These drugs and **capreomycin** can also cause renal and vestibular toxicity. **Cycloserine** can cause psychiatric symptoms and seizures. **Ethionamide** has been associated with gastrointestinal, hepatic and thyroid toxicity. A delayed-release granular formulation of **aminosalicylic acid** (PAS) has better gastrointestinal tolerability than older formulations. **Fluoroquinolones** are usually well-tolerated, but can cause gastrointestinal and CNS disturbances, and dysglycemia can occur, particularly in the elderly and in patients with diabetes.

CONCLUSION

All initial isolates of *M. tuberculosis* should be tested for antimicrobial susceptibility. Initial therapy for most patients with active TB should include at least isoniazid, rifampin, pyrazinamide and ethambutol until susceptibility is known. Directly observed therapy (DOT) by a health-care worker is the standard of care and should be offered to all patients with active TB to minimize failure rates, relapse and the emergence of drug resistance. Confirmed multidrug-resistant tuberculosis (MDRTB) should be treated with DOT in collaboration with a clinician familiar with the management of the disease. Regimens for MDRTB must include at least 4 drugs to which the organism is susceptible; the duration of therapy usually should be 18-24 months.

1. Centers for Disease Control and Prevention (CDC). Trends in tuberculosis — United States, 2005. MMWR Morb Mortal Wkly Rep 2006; 55:305.
2. American Thoracic Society; CDC; Infectious Diseases Society of America. Treatment of tuberculosis. MMWR Recomm Rep 2003; 52 (RR-11):1.
3. PC Hopewell et al. International standards for tuberculosis care. Lancet Infect Dis 2006; 6:710.
4. TR Frieden and SS Munsiff. The DOTS strategy for controlling the global tuberculosis epidemic. Clin Chest Med 2005; 26:197.
5. K DeRiemer et al. Does DOTS work in populations with drug-resistant tuberculosis? Lancet 2005; 365:1239.
6. CR Horsburgh Jr. Priorities for the treatment of latent tuberbulosis infection in the United States. N Engl J Med 2004; 350:2060.
7. KP Cain et al. Tuberculosis among foreign-born persons in the United States: achieving tuberculosis elimination. Am J Respir Crit Care Med 2007; 175:75.
8. Centers for Disease Control and Prevention (CDC). Tuberculosis associated with blocking agents against tumor necrosis factor-alpha—California, 2002-2003. MMWR Morb Mortal Wkly Rep 2004; 53:683.
9. KL Winthrop. Risk and prevention of tuberculosis and other serious opportunistic infections associated with the inhibition of tumor necrosis factor. Nat Clin Pract Rheumatol 2006; 2:602.
10. Centers for Disease Control and Prevention (CDC). Guidelines for using the QuantiFERON®-TB Gold test for detecting *Mycobacterium tuberculosis* infection, United States. MMWR Recomm Rep 2005;54 (RR-15):49.
11. M Pai et al. New tools and emerging technologies for the diagnosis of tuberculosis: part I. Latent tuberculosis. Expert Rev Mol Diagn 2006; 6:413.
12. Centers for Disease Control and Prevention (CDC). Targeted tuberculin testing and treatment of latent tuberculosis infection. MMWR Recomm Rep 2000; 49 (RR-6):1.
13. KR Page et al. Improved adherence and less toxicity with rifampin vs isoniazid for treatment of latent tuberculosis: a retrospective study. Arch Intern Med 2006; 166:1863.
14. A Lardizabal et al. Enhancement of treatment completion for latent tuberculosis infection with 4 months of rifampin. Chest 2006; 130:1712.
15. J Ena and V Valls. Short-course therapy with rifampin plus isoniazid, compared with standard therapy with isoniazid, for latent tuberculosis infection: a meta-analysis. Clin Infect Dis 2005; 40:670.
16. Centers for Disease Control and Prevention (CDC); American Thoracic Society. Update: Adverse event data and revised American Thoracic Society/CDC recommendations against the use of rifampin and pyrazinamide for treatment of latent tuberculosis infection – United States, 2003. MMWR Morb Mortal Wkly Rep 2003; 52:735.

17. PD McElroy et al. National survey to measure rates of liver injury, hospitalization, and death associated with rifampin and pyrazinamide for latent tuberculosis infection. Clin Infect Dis 2005; 41:1125.

18. T Papastavros et al. Adverse events associated with pyrazinamide and levofloxacin in the treatment of latent multidrug-resistant tuberculosis. CMAJ 2002; 167:131.

19. R Ridzon et al. Asymptomatic hepatitis in persons who received alternative preventive therapy with pyrazinamide and ofloxacin. Clin Infect Dis 1997; 24:1264.

20. Centers for Disease Control and Prevention (CDC). Emergence of *Mycobacterium tuberculosis* with extensive resistance to second-line drugs — worldwide, 2000-2004. MMWR Morb Mortal Wkly Rep 2006; 55:301.

21. Centers for Disease Control and Prevention (CDC). Revised definition of extensively drug-resistant tuberculosis. MMWR Morb Mortal Wkly Rep 2006; 55:1176.

22. NR Gandhi et al. Extensively drug-resistant tuberculosis as a cause of death in patients co-infected with tuberculosis and HIV in a rural area of South Africa. Lancet 2006; 368:1575.

23. GL Woods. The mycobacteriology laboratory and new diagnostic techniques. Infect Dis Clin North Am 2002; 16:127.

24. H Blumberg et al. Update on the treatment of tuberculosis and latent tuberculosis infection. JAMA 2005; 293:2776.

25. GE Thwaites et al. Dexamethasone for the treatment of tuberculous meningitis in adolescents and adults. N Engl J Med 2004; 351:1741.

26. M Weiner et al. Pharmacokinetics of rifapentine at 600, 900, and 1,200 mg during once-weekly tuberculosis therapy. Am J Respir Crit Care Med 2004; 169:1191.

27. FM Gordin. Rifapentine for the treatment of tuberculosis: is it all it can be? Am J Respir Crit Care Med 2004; 169:1176.

28. A Vernon et al. Acquired rifamycin monoresistance in patients with HIV-related tuberculosis treated with once-weekly rifapentine and isoniazid. Tuberculosis Trials Consortium. Lancet 1999; 353:1843.

29. B Blomberg and B Fourie. Fixed-dose combination drugs for tuberculosis: application in standardised treatment regimens. Drugs 2003; 63:535.

30. JA Caminero. Treatment of multidrug-resistant tuberculosis: evidence and controversies. Int J Tuberc Lung Dis 2006; 10:829.

31. JB Nachega and RE Chaisson. Tuberculosis drug resistance: a global threat. Clin Infect Dis 2003; 36 suppl 1:S24.

32. JS Mukherjee et al. Programmes and principles in treatment of multidrug-resistant tuberculosis. Lancet 2004; 363:474.

33. ED Chan et al. Treatment and outcome analysis of 205 patients with multidrug-resistant tuberculosis. Am J Respir Crit Care Med 2004; 169:1103.

34. Centers for Disease Control and Prevention (CDC). Acquired rifamycin resistance in persons with advanced HIV disease being treated for active tuberculosis with intermittent rifamycin-based regimens. MMWR Morb Mortal Wkly Rep 2002; 51:214.

35. RE Nettles et al. Risk factors for relapse and acquired rifamycin resistance after directly observed tuberculosis treatment: a comparison by HIV serostatus and rifamycin use. Clin Infect Dis 2004; 38:731.

36. W Manosuthi et al. Immune reconstitution inflammatory syndrome of tuberculosis among HIV-infected patients receiving antituberculous and antiretroviral therapy. J Infect 2006; 53:357.

37. SA Shelburne et al. Incidence and risk factors for immune reconstitution inflammatory syndrome during highly active antiretroviral therapy. AIDS 2005; 14:399.

38. G Breton et al. Determinants of immune reconstitution inflammatory syndrome in HIV type 1-infected patients with tuberculosis after initiation of antiretroviral therapy. Clin Infect Dis 2004; 39:1709.

39. Centers for Disease Control and Prevention (CDC). Updated guidelines for the use of rifamycins for the treatment of tuberculosis among HIV-infected patients taking protease inhibitors or nonnucleoside reverse transcriptase inhibitors. Available at www.cdc.gov/nchstp/tb/ tb_hiv_drugs/toc.htm. Accessed February 13, 2007.

40. G Bothamley. Drug treatment for tuberculosis during pregnancy: safety considerations. Drug Saf 2001; 24:553.

41. S Shin et al. Treatment of multidrug-resistant tuberculosis during pregnancy: a report of 7 cases. Clin Infect Dis 2003; 36:996.

42. KD Lessnau and S Qarah. Multidrug-resistant tuberculosis in pregnancy: case report and review of the literature. Chest 2003; 123:953.

43. PC Drobac et al. Treatment of multidrug-resistant tuberculosis during pregnancy: long-term follow-up of 6 children with intrauterine exposure to second-line agents. Clin Infect Dis 2005; 40:1689.

44. Medical Letter Adverse Drug Interactions Program.

45. World Health Organization. Ethambutol efficacy and toxicity: literature review and recommendations for daily and intermittent dosage in children. Available at http://whqlibdoc.who.int/hq/2006/who_htm_ tb_2006.365_eng.pdf, Accessed February 13, 2007.

A Blood Test for Tuberculosis

Originally published in The Medical Letter – October 2007; 49:83

Quantiferon – TB Gold (Cellestis) is a T-cell interferon-gamma release assay approved by the FDA as an alternative to the tuberculin skin test for diagnosis of infection with *Mycobacterium tuberculosis* (TB). An earlier assay *(Quantiferon-TB)*, which is no longer commercially available, was approved by the FDA in 2001. Other interferon-gamma release assays (IGRAs) are available abroad.

THE TEST — *Quantiferon – TB Gold* (QFT-G) and other IGRA blood tests measure the production of a single cytokine, interferon-gamma, by a subset of T-cells. Unlike the tuberculin skin test, they use highly specific *M. tuberculosis* antigens, and the antigenic challenge occurs *ex vivo*. Use of a blood test eliminates the need for a second visit to read a skin test and may reduce the inconsistencies in test administration and interpretation that are common with skin testing.

As with any blood test, IGRAs are susceptible to errors in specimen management and laboratory methods. Current methods require anticoagulation of the blood specimen, storage at room temperature, and initiation of processing in the laboratory within 12 hours of venipuncture. Possible test results include an "indeterminate" category for which optimal interpretation and management have not been determined.

ANTIGENS — The purified protein derivative (PPD) that is used for the tuberculin skin test contains dozens of potential antigens derived from growing *M. tuberculosis* in culture media. To a variable extent, individuals can have false-positive results to PPD due to infection with mycobacteria other than *M. tuberculosis*, such as *M. avium* or *M. kansasii*, or due to vaccination with Bacille Calmette-Guérin (BCG), a live attenuated anti-TB vaccine derived from *M. bovis*.

The 2 antigenic proteins used in QFT-G are present in *M. tuberculosis* but absent from BCG, making QFT-G unlikely to yield a false-positive result due to vaccination with BCG.[1-3] These antigens may also be present in some other pathogenic mycobacteria, including *M. kansasii*, *M. marinum* and *M. szulgai*, but are absent from *M. avium*, which is the most commonly encountered non-TB mycobacterium. The performance of QFT-G relative to infection with these mycobacteria is unknown, but the results of one small study suggest that IGRA results may be negative in patients with *M. avium* disease.[4]

SENSITIVITY/SPECIFICITY — The sensitivity of QFT-G has been similar to that of the skin test in detecting active infection in patients who have confirmed TB disease (about 80%). Its specificity has been higher than that of a skin test, particularly in persons who have been vaccinated with BCG.[5] The IGRA's reliance on fewer antigens theoretically might make it less sensitive than the skin test in detecting latent TB infection.[6,7] Studies comparing the QFT-G with the skin test for use in serial testing or in special populations such as the immunocompromised and children are limited.[8,9]

CURRENT GUIDELINES — The Centers for Disease Control and Prevention (CDC) has stated that QFT-G can be used in all circumstances in which the tuberculin skin test is used.[10] Like the tuberculin skin test, IGRAs do not distinguish between latent infection and active disease. Negative results should be interpreted with caution, particularly in patients with impaired immune function and those at greater risk for severe TB disease, such as young children, the elderly and the immunocompromised. The time between initial *M. tuberculosis* exposure and the development of a positive result has not been determined for QFT-G or other IGRAs. For the moment, the known delay of 8 weeks (maximum) observed with the tuberculin skin test has been extrapolated to QFT-G.

COST — The average cost of one test using QFT-G, including personnel costs, has been estimated to be $35-120, compared to about $13 for each skin test. However, since IGRAs are more specific than skin tests, their use may reduce the cost of follow-up x-rays and laboratory tests, and the cost (and toxicity) of unnecessary TB therapy.

CONCLUSION — *Quantiferon-TB Gold*, an interferon-gamma release assay (IGRA) blood test, offers several advantages over the tuberculin skin test in the diagnosis of tuberculosis. It requires only a single visit, and is less susceptible to false-positive results due to BCG vaccination or infection with non-tuberculous mycobacteria.

1. D Menzies et al. Meta-analysis: new tests for the diagnosis of latent tuberculosis infection: areas of uncertainty and recommendations for research. Ann Intern Med 2007; 146:340.

2. M Farhat et al. False-positive tuberculin skin tests: what is the absolute effect of BCG and non-tuberculous mycobacteria? Int J Tuberc Lung Dis 2006; 10:1192.

3. B Soborg et al. Detecting a low prevalence of latent tuberculosis among health care workers in Denmark detected by M. tuberculosis specific IFN-gamma whole-blood test, Scand J Infect Dis 2007; 39:554.

4. AD Lein et al. Cellular immune responses to ESAT-6 discriminate between patients with pulmonary disease due to Mycobacterium avium complex and those with pulmonary disease due to Mycobacterium tuberculosis. Clin Diagn Lab Immunol 1999; 6:606.

5. T Mori et al. Specific detection of tuberculosis infection: an interferon-gamma-based assay using new antigens. Am J Respir Crit Care Med 2004; 170:59.

6. P Andersen et al. The prognosis of latent tuberculosis: can disease be predicted? Trends Mol Med 2007; 13:175.

7. M Pai et al. Interferon-gamma assays in the immunodiagnosis of tuberculosis: a systematic review. Lancet Infect Dis 2004; 4:761.

8. TG Connell et al. Quantiferon-TB Gold: state of the art for the diagnosis of tuberculosis infection? Expert Rev Mol Diagn 2006; 6:663.

9. M Pai and R O'Brien. Serial testing for tuberculosis: can we make sense of T cell assay conversions and reversions? PLoS Med 2007; 4:e208.

10. GH Mazurek et al. Guidelines for using Quantiferon-TB Gold test for detecting mycobacterium tuberculosis infection, United States. MMWR Recomm Rep 2005; 54 (RR-15):49.

ANTIMICROBIAL PROPHYLAXIS FOR
Surgery

Original publication date – December 2006

Antimicrobial prophylaxis can decrease the incidence of infection, particularly surgical site infection, after certain procedures. Recommendations for prevention of surgical site infection are listed in the table that begins on page 128.

CHOICE OF A PROPHYLACTIC AGENT

An effective prophylactic regimen should be directed against the most likely infecting organisms, but need not eradicate every potential pathogen. For most procedures, the first-generation cephalosporin, **cefazolin** (*Ancef*, and others), which is active against many staphylococci and streptococci, has been effective.

Some Exceptions – For procedures that might involve exposure to bowel anaerobes, including *Bacteroides fragilis*, the second-generation cephalosporin **cefoxitin** (*Mefoxin*, and others), has been recommended because it is more active than cefazolin against these organisms. Cefoxitin availability has been limited, however, due to high demand and cefotetan *(Cefotan)*, an alternative, is available generically.[1] **Cefazolin** plus **metronidazole** (*Flagyl*, and others), or **ampicillin/sulbactam** (*Unasyn*, and others) alone, are other reasonable alternatives.[2]

Cefuroxime (*Zinacef*, and others) is a second-generation cephalosporin with little activity against *B. fragilis*, but it can be used instead of cefazolin in cardiac, non-cardiac thoracic and orthopedic operations.

Ertapenem *(Invanz)* has been approved by the FDA for prophylaxis of elective colorectal procedures, but most Medical Letter consultants would not recommend routine use of such a broad-spectrum drug.

Not Recommended – Third-generation cephalosporins, such as cefotaxime *(Claforan)*, ceftriaxone *(Rocephin)*, cefoperazone *(Cefobid)*, ceftazidime *(Fortaz*, and others), or ceftizoxime *(Cefizox)*, and fourth-generation cephalosporins such as cefepime *(Maxipime)* should not be used for routine surgical prophylaxis because they are expensive, some are less active than cefazolin against staphylococci, and their spectrum of activity includes organisms rarely encountered in elective surgery.

Penicillin Allergy – Cefazolin can often be used for prophylaxis in patients with penicillin allergy, but some may rarely have allergic reactions to cephalosporins.[3] When allergy prevents use of a cephalosporin, vancomycin (*Vancocin*, and others) or clindamycin (*Cleocin*, and others) can be used, but neither is effective against gram-negative bacteria; many Medical Letter consultants would add gentamicin (*Garamycin*, and others), ciprofloxacin (*Cipro*, and others), levofloxacin *(Levaquin)* or aztreonam *(Azactam)*, particularly for colorectal procedures, hysterectomies, and vascular surgery involving groin incisions.

Resistant Organisms – Long preoperative hospitalizations are associated with increased risk of infection with an antibiotic-resistant organism; local resistance patterns should be taken into account. In institutions where surgical site infections are frequently due to methicillin-resistant *Staphylococcus aureus* (MRSA) or methicillin-resistant coagulase-negative staphylococci, vancomycin can be used for prophylaxis, but routine use should be discouraged because vancomycin does not appear to be any more effective than cefazolin in these settings.[4,5] Preoperative administration of intranasal mupirocin (*Bactroban*, and others) may decrease the rate of post-operative infections with MRSA in some patients undergoing cardiac surgery who are known to be colonized with the organism preoperatively[6]; use of this approach is increasing, but it is controversial and the need for preoperative evaluation of colonization also makes it difficult.

TIMING AND NUMBER OF DOSES

It has been common practice to give antibiotics at the time of anesthesia induction, which results in adequate serum and tissue levels; there is no consensus on whether the infusion must be completed by the time of incision. For procedures lasting less than 4 hours, Medical Letter consultants recommend a **single intravenous dose of an antimicrobial** started within 60 minutes before the initial skin incision, which should provide adequate tissue concentrations throughout the procedure. If vancomycin or a fluoroquinolone is used, the infusion should begin 60-120 minutes before the incision is made in order to minimize the risk of antibiotic-associated reactions around the time of anesthesia induction and ensure adequate tissue levels of the drug at the time of the initial incision.

Additional Doses – If the procedure is prolonged (>4 hours) or major blood loss occurs, redosing every 1-2 half-lives of the drug (in patients with normal renal function) should provide adequate antimicrobial concentrations during the procedure (ampicillin/sulbactam q2-4 hours, cefazolin q2-5 hours, cefuroxime q3-4 hours, cefoxitin q2-3 hours, clindamycin q3-6 hours, vancomycin q6-12 hours, and metronidazole q6-8 hours).[7] Published studies of antimicrobial prophylaxis often use one or two doses postoperatively in addition to one dose just before surgery. Most Medical Letter consultants believe, however, that postoperative doses are unnecessary after wound closure and can increase the risk of antimicrobial resistance.

ANTIMICROBIAL PROPHYLAXIS FOR SURGERY

Nature of operation	Common pathogens
CARDIAC	*Staphylococcus aureus, S. epidermidis*
GASTROINTESTINAL	
Esophageal, gastroduodenal	Enteric gram-negative bacilli, gram-positive cocci
Biliary tract	Enteric gram-negative bacilli, enterococci, clostridia
Colorectal	Enteric gram-negative bacilli, anaerobes, enterococci
Appendectomy, non-perforated[8]	Enteric gram-negative bacilli, anaerobes, enterococci
GENITOURINARY	Enteric gram-negative bacilli, enterococci
GYNECOLOGIC AND OBSTETRIC	
Vaginal, abdominal or laparoscopic hysterectomy	Enteric gram-negative bacilli, anaerobes, Gp B strep, enterococci
Cesarean section	same as for hysterectomy
Abortion	same as for hysterectomy

	Recommended Antimicrobials	Adult dosage before surgery[1]
	cefazolin or	1-2 g IV[2]
	cefuroxime	1.5 g IV[2]
OR	vancomycin[3]	1 g IV
	High risk[4] only: cefazolin[7]	1-2 g IV
	High risk[5] only: cefazolin[7]	1-2 g IV
	Oral: neomycin + erythromycin base[6]	
OR	metronidazole[6]	
	Parenteral:	
	cefoxitin[7]	1-2 g IV
OR	cefazolin	1-2 g IV
	+ metronidazole[7]	0.5 g IV
OR	ampicillin/sulbactam	3 g IV
	cefoxitin[7]	1-2 g IV
OR	cefazolin	1-2 g IV
	+ metronidazole[7]	0.5 g IV
OR	ampicillin/sulbactam[7]	3 g IV
	High risk[9] only:	
	ciprofloxacin	500 mg PO or 400 mg IV
	cefoxitin[7] or cefazolin[7]	1-2 g IV
OR	ampicillin/sulbactam[7]	3 g IV
	cefazolin[7]	1-2 g IV after cord clamping
	First trimester, high risk[10]:	
	aqueous penicillin G	2 mill units IV
OR	doxycycline	300 mg PO[11]
	Second trimester:	
	cefazolin[7]	1-2 g IV

Continued on next page.

ANTIMICROBIAL PROPHYLAXIS FOR SURGERY (continued)

Nature of operation	Common pathogens
HEAD AND NECK SURGERY Incisions through oral or pharyngeal mucosa	Anaerobes, enteric gram-negative bacilli, *S. aureus*
NEUROSURGERY	*S. aureus, S. epidermidis*
OPHTHALMIC	*S. epidermidis, S. aureus*, streptococci, enteric gram-negative bacilli, *Pseudomonas spp.*
ORTHOPEDIC	*S. aureus, S. epidermidis*
THORACIC (NON-CARDIAC)	*S. aureus, S. epidermidis*, streptococci, enteric gram-negative bacilli
VASCULAR Arterial surgery involving a prosthesis, the abdominal aorta, or a groin incision	*S. aureus, S. epidermidis*, enteric gram-negative bacilli
Lower extremity amputation for ischemia	*S. aureus, S. epidermidis*, enteric gram-negative bacilli, clostridia

	Recommended Antimicrobials	Adult dosage before surgery[1]
	clindamycin	600-900 mg IV
	+ gentamicin	1.5 mg/kg IV
OR	cefazolin	1-2 g IV
	cefazolin	1-2 g IV
OR	vancomycin[3]	1 g IV
	gentamicin, tobramycin, ciprofloxacin, gatifloxacin levofloxacin, moxifloxacin, ofloxacin or neomycin-gramicidin-polymyxin B	multiple drops topically over 2 to 24 hours
	cefazolin	100 mg subconjunctivally
	cefazolin[12]	1-2 g IV
	or cefuroxime[12]	1.5 g IV
OR	vancomycin[3,12]	1 g IV
	cefazolin or	1-2 g IV
	cefuroxime	1.5 g IV
OR	vancomycin[3]	1 g IV
	cefazolin	1-2 g IV
OR	vancomycin[3]	1 g IV
	cefazolin	1-2 g IV
OR	vancomycin[3]	1 g IV

Continued on next page.

ANTIMICROBIAL PROPHYLAXIS FOR SURGERY (continued)

1. Parenteral prophylactic antimicrobials can be given as a single IV dose begun 60 minutes or less before the operation. For prolonged operations (>4 hours), or those with major blood loss, additional intraoperative doses should be given at intervals 1-2 times the half-life of the drug for the duration of the procedure in patients with normal renal function. If vancomycin or a fluoroquinolone is used, the infusion should be started 60-120 minutes before the initial incision in order to minimize the possibility of an infusion reaction close to the time of induction of anesthesia and to have adequate tissue levels at the time of incision.
2. Some consultants recommend an additional dose when patients are removed from bypass during open-heart surgery.
3. Vancomycin is used in hospitals in which methicillin-resistant *S. aureus* and *S. epidermidis* are a frequent cause of postoperative wound infection, for patients previously colonized with MRSA, or for those who are allergic to penicillins or cephalosporins. Rapid IV administration may cause hypotension, which could be especially dangerous during induction of anesthesia. Even when the drug is given over 60 minutes, hypotension may occur; treatment with diphenhydramine (*Benadryl*, and others) and further slowing of the infusion rate may be helpful. Some experts would give 15 mg/kg of vancomycin to patients weighing more than 75 kg, up to a maximum of 1.5 g, with a slower infusion rate (90 minutes for 1.5 g). To provide coverage against gram-negative bacteria, most Medical Letter consultants would also include cefazolin or cefuroxime in the prophylaxis regimen for patients not allergic to cephalosporins; ciprofloxacin, levofloxacin, gentamicin, or aztreonam, each one in combination with vancomycin, can be used in patients who cannot tolerate a cephalosporin.

INDICATIONS

Cardiac Surgery – Prophylactic antibiotics can decrease the incidence of infection after cardiac surgery, and intraoperative redosing has been associated with a decreased risk of postoperative infection in procedures lasting >400 minutes.[8] Antimicrobial prophylaxis for prevention of **device-related infections** has not been rigorously studied, but is generally used before placement of electrophysiologic devices, ventricular assist devices, ventriculoatrial shunts and arterial patches.[9] Studies of antimicrobial prophylaxis for implantation of **permanent pacemakers** have shown a significant reduction in the incidence of wound infection, inflammation and skin erosion.[10]

Gastrointestinal Surgery – Antimicrobial prophylaxis is recommended for **esophageal** surgery in the presence of obstruction, which increases the risk of infection. After **gastroduodenal** surgery the risk of infection is high when gastric acidity and gastrointestinal motility are diminished by obstruction, hemorrhage, gastric ulcer or malignancy, or

4. Morbid obesity, esophageal obstruction, decreased gastric acidity or gastrointestinal motility.
5. Age >70 years, acute cholecystitis, non-functioning gall bladder, obstructive jaundice or common duct stones.
6. After appropriate diet and catharsis, 1 g of neomycin plus 1 g of erythromycin at 1 PM, 2 PM and 11 PM or 2 g of neomycin plus 2 g of metronidazole at 7 PM and 11 PM the day before an 8 AM operation.
7. For patients allergic to penicillins and cephalosporins, clindamycin with either gentamicin, ciprofloxacin, levofloxacin or aztreonam is a reasonable alternative.
8. For a ruptured viscus, therapy is often continued for about five days. Ruptured viscus in postoperative setting (dehiscence) requires antibacterials to include coverage of nosocomial pathogens.
9. Urine culture positive or unavailable, preoperative catheter, transrectal prostatic biopsy, placement of prosthetic material.
10. Patients with previous pelvic inflammatory disease, previous gonorrhea or multiple sex partners.
11. Divided into 100 mg one hour before the abortion and 200 mg one half hour after.
12. If a tourniquet is to be used in the procedure, the entire dose of antibiotic must be infused prior to its inflation.

by therapy with an H_2-blocker or proton pump inhibitor, and is also high in patients with morbid obesity.[11] A dose of cefazolin before surgery can decrease the incidence of postoperative infection in these circumstances. Prophylaxis is not indicated for routine gastroesophageal endoscopy, but most clinicians use it before placement of a percutaneous gastrostomy.[12,13]

Antimicrobial prophylaxis is recommended before **biliary tract** surgery for patients with a high risk of infection, such as those more than 70 years old and those with acute cholecystitis, a non-functioning gallbladder, obstructive jaundice or common duct stones. Many clinicians follow similar guidelines for antibiotic prophylaxis of endoscopic retrograde cholangiopancreatography (ERCP).[14] Prophylactic antibiotics are generally not necessary for low-risk patients undergoing elective laparoscopic cholecystectomy.[15,16]

Preoperative antibiotics can decrease the incidence of infection after **colorectal** surgery; for elective operations, an oral regimen of neomycin (not available in Canada) plus either erythromycin or metronidazole appears to be as effective as parenteral drugs. Many surgeons in the US use a combination of oral and parenteral agents. Whether such combinations are more effective than just one or the other is controversial.[17]

Preoperative antimicrobials can decrease the incidence of infection after surgery for acute appendicitis.[18] If **perforation** has occurred, antibiotics are often used therapeutically rather than prophylactically and are continued for 5-7 days. In studies of penetrating abdominal and intestinal injuries, however, a short course (12-24 hours) was as effective as 5 days of therapy.[19-21]

Genitourinary Surgery – Medical Letter consultants do not recommend antimicrobial prophylaxis before most urological surgical procedures in patients with sterile urine. When the urine culture is positive or unavailable, or the patient has a preoperative urinary catheter, patients should be treated to sterilize the urine before surgery or receive a single preoperative dose of an agent active against the likely microrganisms.

Antimicrobial prophylaxis decreases the incidence of postoperative bacteriuria and septicemia in patients with sterile preoperative urine undergoing **transurethral prostatectomy**.[22] Prophylaxis is recommended before **transrectal prostatic biopsies** because urosepsis can occur.[23] Surgical prophylaxis is generally used if a **urologic prosthesis** (penile implant, artificial sphincter, synthetic pubovaginal sling, bone anchors for pelvic floor reconstruction) will be placed.[24]

Gynecology and Obstetrics – Antimicrobial prophylaxis decreases the incidence of infection after vaginal and abdominal **hysterectomy**.[25] Prophylaxis is also used for laparoscopic hysterectomies. Antimicrobials, usually given after cord clamping, can prevent infection after elective and non-elective **cesarean sections**.[26-28] Antimicrobial prophylaxis can also prevent infection after **elective abortion**.[29]

Head and Neck Surgery – Prophylaxis with antimicrobials has decreased the incidence of surgical site infection after head and neck operations that involve an incision through the oral or pharyngeal mucosa.

Neurosurgery – An antistaphylococcal antibiotic can decrease the incidence of infection after **craniotomy**. In **spinal surgery**, the infection rate after conventional lumbar discectomy is low, but the serious consequences of a surgical site infection have led many surgeons to use perioperative antibiotics. One meta-analysis concluded that antibiotic prophylaxis prevents infection even in low-risk spinal surgery.[30] Infection rates are higher after prolonged spinal surgery or spinal procedures involving fusion or insertion of foreign material, and prophylactic antibiotics are usually used.[31] Studies of antimicrobial prophylaxis for implantation of permanent **cerebrospinal fluid shunts** have produced conflicting results.

Ophthalmology – Data are limited on the effectiveness of antimicrobial prophylaxis for ophthalmic surgery, but postoperative endophthalmitis can be devastating. Most ophthalmologists use antimicrobial eye drops for prophylaxis, and some also give a subconjunctival injection or add antimicrobial drops to the intraocular irrigation solution.[32] There is no consensus supporting a particular choice, route or duration of antimicrobial prophylaxis.[33] Preoperative povidone-iodine applied to the skin and conjunctiva has been associated with a lower incidence of culture-proven endophthalmitis.[34] There is no evidence that prophylactic antibiotics are needed for procedures that do not invade the globe.

Orthopedic Surgery – Prophylactic antistaphylococcal drugs administered preoperatively can decrease the incidence of both early and late infection following joint replacement. One large randomized trial found a single dose of a cephalosporin more effective than placebo in preventing wound infection after surgical repair of **closed fractures**.[35] They also decrease the rate of infection when **hip and other closed fractures** are treated with internal fixation by nails, plates, screws or wires, and in compound or open fractures.[36] In such cases antibiotics may be used therapeutically and continued for a number of days; the optimal duration is unknown.[37,38] If a proximal tourniquet is used for the procedure, the antibiotic infusion must be completed prior to its inflation. A prospective randomized study in patients undergoing diagnostic and operative **arthroscopic surgery** concluded that antibiotic prophylaxis is not indicated.[39]

Thoracic (Non-Cardiac) Surgery – Antibiotic prophylaxis is given routinely in thoracic surgery, but supporting data are sparse. In one study, a single preoperative dose of cefazolin before **pulmonary resection** led to a decrease in the incidence of surgical site infection, but not of pneumonia or empyema.[40] Other trials have found that multiple doses of a cephalosporin can prevent infection after **closed-tube thoracostomy** for chest trauma with hemo- or pneumothorax.[41] Insertion of chest tubes for other indications, such as spontaneous pneumothorax, does not require antimicrobial prophylaxis.

Vascular Surgery – Preoperative administration of a cephalosporin decreases the incidence of postoperative surgical site infection after arterial reconstructive surgery on the abdominal aorta, vascular operations on the leg that include a groin incision, and amputation of the lower extremity for ischemia. Many experts also recommend prophylaxis for implantation of any vascular prosthetic material, such as grafts for vascular access in hemodialysis. Prophylaxis is not indicated for carotid endarterectomy or brachial artery repair without prosthetic material.

Other Procedures – Antimicrobial prophylaxis is generally **not indicated** for **cardiac catheterization**, **varicose vein** surgery, most **dermatologic and plastic** surgery, **arterial puncture**, **thoracentesis**, **paracentesis**, repair of **simple lacerations**, **outpatient treatment of burns**, **dental extractions** or **root canal therapy** because the incidence of surgical site infections is low. A study in patients undergoing cosmetic procedures who did not receive prophylactic antibiotics found that infection was more common after longer operations; the authors concluded that a single dose of cefazolin might be helpful before operations that will last more than 3 hours.[42]

The need for prophylaxis in **breast surgery**, **herniorraphy** and other "clean" surgical procedures has been **controversial**. Medical Letter consultants generally do not recommend surgical prophylaxis for these procedures because of the low rate of infection, the low morbidity of these infections and the potential adverse effects with use of prophylaxis in such a large number of patients; some recommend prophylaxis for procedures involving placement of prosthetic material (synthetic mesh, saline implants, tissue expanders).

1. www.ashp.org/shortage
2. DW Bratzler and DR Hunt. The surgical infection prevention and surgical care improvement projects: national initiatives to improve outcomes for patients having surgery. Clin Infect Dis 2006; 43:322.
3. ME Pichichero. A review of evidence supporting the American Academy of Pediatrics recommendation for prescribing cephalosporin antibiotics for penicillin-allergic patients. Pediatrics 2005; 115:1048
4. G Zanetti and R Platt. Antibiotic prophylaxis for cardiac surgery: does the past predict the future? Clin Infect Dis 2004; 38:1364.
5. R Finkelstein et al. Vancomycin versus cefazolin prophylaxis for cardiac surgery in the setting of a high prevalence of methicillin-resistant staphylococcal infections. J Thorac Cardiovasc Surg 2002; 123:326.
6. NK Shrestha et al. Safety of targeted perioperative mupirocin treatment for preventing infections after cardiac surgery. Ann Thorac Surg 2006; 81:2183.
7. DW Bratzler et al. Antimicrobial prophylaxis for surgery: an advisory statement from the National Surgical Infection Prevention Project. Clin Infect Dis 2004; 38:1706.
8. G Zanetti et al. Intraoperative redosing of cefazolin and risk for surgical site infection in cardiac surgery. Emerg Infect Dis 2001; 7:828.
9. LM Baddour et al. Nonvalvular cardiovascular device-related infections. Circulation 2003; 108:2015.
10. E Bertaglia et al. Antibiotic prophylaxis with a single dose of cefazolin during pacemaker implantation: incidence of long-term infective complications. Pacing Clin Electrophysiol 2006; 29:29.
11. AJ Chong and EP Dellinger. Infectious complications of surgery in morbidly obese patients. Curr Treat Options Infect Dis 2003; 5:387.
12. WK Hirota et al. Guidelines for antibiotic prophylaxis for GI endoscopy. Gastrointest Endosc 2003; 58:475.

Antimicrobial Prophylaxis for Surgery

13. I Ahmad et al. Antibiotic prophylaxis for percutaneous endoscopic gastrostomy - a prospective, randomised, double-blind trial. Aliment Pharmacol Ther 2003; 18:209.

14. JS Mallery et al. Complications of ERCP. Gastrointest Endosc 2003; 57:633.

15. M Koc et al. A prospective randomized study of prophylactic antibiotics in elective laparoscopic cholecystectomy. Surg Endosc 2003; 17:1716.

16. WT Chang et al. The impact of prophylactic antibiotics on postoperative infection complication in elective laparoscopic cholecystectomy: a prospective randomized study. Am J Surg 2006; 191:721.

17. RT Lewis. Oral versus systemic antibiotic prophylaxis in elective colon surgery: a randomized study and meta-analysis send a message from the 1990s. Can J Surg 2002; 45:173.

18. BR Andersen et al. Antibiotics versus placebo for prevention of postoperative infection after appendicectomy. Cochrane Database Syst Rev 2003; 2:CD001439.

19. EP Dellinger et al. Efficacy of short-course antibiotic prophylaxis after penetrating intestinal injury. A prospective randomized trial. Arch Surg 1986; 121:23.

20. A Bozorgzadeh et al. The duration of antibiotic administration in penetrating abdominal trauma. Am J Surg 1999; 177:125.

21. EE Cornwell 3rd et al. Duration of antibiotic prophylaxis in high-risk patients with penetrating abdominal trauma: a prospective randomized trial. J Gastrointest Surg 1999; 3:648.

22. A Berry and A Barratt. Prophylatic antibiotic use in transurethral prostatic resection: a meta-analysis. J Urol 2002; 167:571.

23. M Aron et al. Antibiotic prophylaxis for transrectal needle biopsy of the prostate: a randomized controlled study. BJU Int 2000; 85:682.

24. A Gomelsky and RR Dmochowski. Antibiotic prophylaxis in urologic prosthetic surgery. Curr Pharm Des 2003; 9:989.

25. EL Eason et al. Prophylactic antibiotics for abdominal hysterectomy: indication for low-risk Canadian women. J Obstet Gynaecol Can 2004; 26:1067.

26. F Smaill and GJ Hofmeyr. Cochrane Database Syst Rev 2002; 3:CD000933.

27. D Chelmow et al. Prophylactic use of antibiotics for nonlaboring patients undergoing cesarean delivery with intact membranes: a meta-analysis. Am J Obstet Gynecol 2001; 184:656.

28. L French. Prevention and treatment of postpartum endometritis. Curr Womens Health Rep 2003; 3:274.

29. GF Sawaya et al. Antibiotics at the time of induced abortion: the case for universal prophylaxis based on a meta-analysis. Obstet Gynecol 1996; 87:884.

30. FG Barker II. Efficacy of prophylactic antibiotic therapy in spinal surgery: a meta-analysis. Neurosurgery 2002; 51:391.

31. JB Dimick et al. Spine update: antimicrobial prophylaxis in spine surgery: basic principles and recent advances. Spine 2000; 25:2544.

32. DV Leaming. Practice styles and preferences of ASCRS members - 2003 survey. J Cataract Refract Surg 2004; 30:892.

33. TJ Liesegang. Perioperative antibiotic prophylaxis in cataract surgery. Cornea 1999; 18:383.

34. TA Ciulla et al. Bacterial endophthalmitis prophylaxis for cataract surgery: an evidence-based update. Ophthalmology 2002; 109:13.
35. H Boxma et al. Randomised controlled trial of single-dose antibiotic prophylaxis in surgical treatment of closed fractures: the Dutch Trauma Trial. Lancet 1996; 347:1133.
36. JP Southwell-Keely et al. Antibiotic prophylaxis in hip fracture surgery: a metaanalysis. Clin Orthop Relat Res 2004; 419:179.
37. A Trampuz and W Zimmerli. Antimicrobial agents in orthopaedic surgery: Prophylaxis and treatment. Drugs 2006; 66:1089.
38. CJ Hauser et al. Surgical Infection Society guideline: prophylactic antibiotic use in open fractures: an evidence-based guideline. Surg Infect 2006; 7:379.
39. JA Wieck et al. Efficacy of prophylactic antibiotics in arthroscopic surgery. Orthopedics 1997; 20:133.
40. R Aznar et al. Antibiotic prophylaxis in non-cardiac thoracic surgery: cefazolin versus placebo. Eur J Cardiothorac Surg 1991; 5:515.
41. RP Gonzalez and MR Holevar. Role of prophylactic antibiotics for tube thoracostomy in chest trauma. Am Surg 1998; 64:617.
42. CA Fatica et al. The role of preoperative antibiotic prophylaxis in cosmetic surgery. Plast Reconstr Surg 2002; 109:2570.

Major Changes in Endocarditis Prophylaxis for Dental, GI and GU Procedures
Originally published in The Medical Letter – December 2007; 49:99

The American Heart Association has issued its revised guidelines for prevention of infective endocarditis.[1] Antimicrobial prophylaxis for dental procedures is now recommended only for patients at the highest risk of severe consequences from endocarditis who are undergoing the highest-risk procedures. Endocarditis prophylaxis is no longer recommended for gastrointestinal (GI) and genitourinary (GU) procedures. When these changes are implemented, the number of patients receiving antimicrobial prophylaxis to prevent endocarditis should decline sharply.

HIGHEST-RISK PATIENTS — The risk of severe consequences from endocarditis after dental procedures is highest in patients with previous bacterial endocarditis, prosthetic heart valves, or unrepaired cyanotic congenital heart disease such as tetralogy of Fallot, including those with surgically constructed palliative shunts or conduits. Patients are also at highest risk during the first 6 months after repair of congenital heart defects with prosthetic material or a prosthetic device, at any time after a congenital heart repair that left a residual defect at the site of or adjacent to a prosthetic patch or device, or when they develop cardiac valvulopathy after cardiac transplant.

HIGHEST-RISK PROCEDURES — The dental procedures now thought to justify prophylaxis (and then only in the highest-risk patients) are those that involve manipulation of gingival tissues or periapical regions of teeth (cleaning, extractions, suture removal, biopsies, placement of orthodontic bands) or perforation of the oral mucosa, but not routine anesthetic injections, dental radiographs, adjustment of orthodontic appliances or placement of orthodontic brackets.

ENDOCARDITIS PROPHYLAXIS FOR DENTAL PROCEDURES[1]

	Adult Dosage (30-60 minutes before procedure)	Pediatric Dosage (30-60 minutes before procedure)
ORAL		
Amoxicillin[2,3] (*Amoxil*, and others)	2 g	50 mg/kg
Penicillin allergy:		
Cephalexin[4,5] (*Keflex*, and others) OR	2 g	50 mg/kg
Clindamycin (*Cleocin*, and others) OR	600 mg	20 mg/kg
Azithromycin[3] (*Zithromax*, and others) or clarithromycin[3] (*Biaxin*, and others)	500 mg	15 mg/kg
PARENTERAL (FOR PATIENTS UNABLE TO TAKE ORAL DRUGS)		
Ampicillin[3] OR	2 g IM or IV	50 mg/kg IM or IV
Cefazolin or ceftriaxone (*Rocephin*, and others)	1 g IM or IV	50 mg/kg IM or IV
Penicillin allergy:		
Cefazolin[4] or ceftriaxone[4] (*Rocephin*, and others) OR	1 g IM or IV	50 mg/kg IM or IV
Clindamycin (*Cleocin Phosphate*, and others)	600 mg IM or IV	20 mg/kg IV

1. Viridans streptococci are the most common cause of endocarditis after dental procedures.
2. Amoxicillin remains the drug of choice for patients without penicillin allergy because of its excellent bioavailability and generally good activity against streptococci.
3. Resistance and tolerance to penicillins and macrolides are increasing among viridans streptococci, but failure of prophylaxis has been rare (RM Prabhu et al. Antimicrob Agents Chemother 2004; 48:4463; MJ Kennedy et al. Clin Pediatr 2004; 43:773).
4. Not recommended for patients with history of severe or immediate-type (urticaria, angioedema, anaphylaxis) allergy to penicillin.
5. Or another first- or second-generation oral cephalosporin in equivalent dosage.

Major Changes in Endocarditis Prophylaxis

1. W Wilson et al. Prevention of infective endocarditis: guidelines from the American Heart Association: a guideline from the American Heart Association Rheumatic Fever, Endocarditis, and Kawasaki Disease Committee, Council on Cardiovascular Disease in the Young, and the Council on Clinical Cardiology, Council on Cardiovascular Surgery and Anesthesia, and the Quality of Care and Outcomes Research Interdisciplinary Working Group. Circulation 2007; 116:1736.

Antifungal Drugs

Original publication date – January 2008

The drugs of choice for treatment of some fungal infections are listed in the tables that begin on the next page. Some of the indications and dosages recommended here have not been approved by the FDA. Other guidelines are available from the Infectious Diseases Society of America (www.idsociety.org).

AZOLES

Azole antifungals inhibit synthesis of ergosterol, an essential component of the fungal cell membrane.

FLUCONAZOLE — Fluconazole is active against most *Candida* species other than *C. krusei*, which is intrinsically resistant, and many strains of *C. glabrata*, which are increasingly resistant. Fluconazole has good activity against *Coccidioides*, *Histoplasma* and *Cryptococcus* spp., but high doses are needed. The drug has no clinically significant activity against most molds, including *Aspergillus* spp., *Fusarium* spp. and Zygomycetes.

Adverse Effects – Fluconazole is generally well tolerated. Headache, gastrointestinal distress and rash can occur. Stevens-Johnson syndrome, anaphylaxis and hepatic toxicity have been reported. Fluconazole is teratogenic in animals (pregnancy category C).

AZOLES

Drug	Usual Dosage	Cost[1]
PARENTERAL		
Fluconazole – *Diflucan* (Pfizer)	100-800 mg 1x/d	$357.62
Voriconazole – *Vfend* (Pfizer)	4 mg/kg bid	364.89
ORAL		
Fluconazole –	100-800 mg 1x/d	
generic		57.20
Diflucan (Pfizer)		71.15
Itraconazole – *Sporanox* (Janssen)	200 mg 1x/d-bid	43.76
Posaconazole – *Noxafil* (Schering)	100 mg 1x/d-200 mg qid	145.80
Voriconazole – *Vfend* (Pfizer)	200-300 mg bid	116.97[2]

1. For one day's treatment of a 70-kg patient at the highest usual dosage, according to AWP listings in *Red Book* 2007 and *Update* December 2007. Cost may vary among institutions based on formulary contracts.
2. Cost of three 200 mg tablets.

Drug Interactions – Fluconazole is a moderate inhibitor of CYP3A4 and may increase serum concentrations of drugs metabolized by 3A4, such as cyclosporine (*Sandimmune*, and others), tacrolimus (*Prograf*), carbamazepine (*Tegretol*, and others), and lovastatin (*Mevacor*, and others).[1] Fluconazole is a strong inhibitor of CYP2C9 and can increase serum concentrations of phenytoin (*Dilantin*, and others), zidovudine (*Retrovir*), warfarin (*Coumadin*, and others) and other drugs metabolized by 2C9. Concomitant administration of rifampin (*Rifadin*, and others) can lower serum concentrations of fluconazole.

ITRACONAZOLE — Itraconazole has a broader spectrum of activity than fluconazole. It is active against a wide variety of fungi including *Cryptococcus neoformans*, *Aspergillus* spp., *Blastomyces dermatitidis*,

Coccidioides immitis, Histoplasma capsulatum, Paracoccidioides brasiliensis, Scedosporium apiospermum (the asexual form of *Pseudallescheria boydii*), *Sporothrix* spp., and dermatophytes. It also has good activity against most *Candida* spp. Itraconazole has no clinically meaningful activity against *Fusarium* spp. or Zygomycetes.

Itraconazole is available orally in both capsules and solution. The IV formulation will no longer be available after February 2008. Absorption after oral dosing is variable; the solution is more bioavailable than the capsules and is generally preferred. The capsules should be taken with food, while the solution is absorbed best without food.

The absorption of itraconazole capsules is reduced by drugs that decrease gastric acidity, such as antacids, H_2-receptor blockers or proton pump inhibitors.

Adverse Effects – The most common adverse effects of itraconazole are dose-related nausea and abdominal discomfort. Rash, including Stevens-Johnson syndrome, and serious hepatic toxicity can occur. The drug can cause hypokalemia, edema and hypertension. Congestive heart failure has been reported, and the drug should not be used in patients with ventricular dysfunction. Itraconazole is teratogenic in rats (pregnancy category C).

Drug Interactions – Itraconazole is a strong inhibitor of CYP3A4 and may increase serum concentrations of cyclosporine, tacrolimus and other drugs metabolized by this enzyme.[1] It is contraindicated for use with cisapride *(Propulsid)*, dofetilide *(Tikosyn)*, ergot alkaloids, levomethadyl *(Orlaam),* lovastatin *(Mevacor*, and others), oral midazolam (*Versed*, and others), pimozide *(Orap)*, quinidine, simvastatin (*Zocor*, and others), and triazolam (*Halcion*, and others).

Itraconazole is also a substrate of CYP3A4; its metabolism may be affected by both inducers of the enzyme, such as rifampin, phenytoin or carbamazepine, and by other inhibitors. When some protease inhibitors,

TREATMENT OF CANDIDA INFECTIONS

Infection		Drug
CANDIDIASIS		
Vaginal [3]		
Topical therapy (intravaginal creams, ointments, tablets, ovules or suppositories)		Butoconazole, clotrimazole, miconazole, tioconazole, or terconazole
Systemic therapy		Fluconazole
Recurrent [6]		Fluconazole
Urinary [7]		Fluconazole
Oropharyngeal or Esophageal [11,12,13]		Fluconazole
	or	An echinocandin Caspofungin Micafungin Anidulafungin
Candidemia[12]		Fluconazole[19]
	or	An echinocandin Caspofungin[22]
		Anidulafungin
		Micafungin[5]
	or	Amphotericin B

Dosage/Duration[1,2]	Alternatives
1x/d x 1-7d	
150 mg PO once[4] x 1d	Itraconazole[5] 200 mg PO bid x 1d Ketoconazole[5] 200 mg PO bid x 5d
150 mg PO 1x/wk	
200 mg IV or PO 1x/d x 7-14d	Amphotericin B[8] 0.3-0.5 mg/kg/d IV[9] x 1-7d Flucytosine 25 mg/kg PO qid x 5-7d[10]
200-400 mg IV or PO once, then 100-200 mg 1x/d x 1-3 wks[14,15]	Other Azoles: Voriconazole[16] 200 mg PO bid x 1-3 wks[14] Itraconazole[17] 200 mg PO 1x/d x 1-3 wks[14] Posaconazole 100 mg bid x 1d then 100 mg 1x/d x 1-3 wks[14,18]
	Amphotericin B 0.3-0.5 mg/kg/d IV x 1-3 wks[9,14]
50 mg IV 1x/d x 1-3 wks[14] 150 mg IV 1x/d x 1-3 wks[14] 100 mg IV once, then 50 mg 1x/d x 1-3 wks[14]	
400-800 mg 1x/d IV, then PO[20,21]	Voriconazole 6 mg/kg IV q12h x 1d then 4 mg/kg IV bid then 200-300 mg PO bid[21]
70 mg IV x 1d, then 50 mg IV 1x/d[21] 200 mg IV once, then 100 mg 1x/d[21] 100 mg IV 1x/d[21]	
0.5-1 mg/kg/d IV[9,21]	

Continued on next page.

TREATMENT OF CANDIDA INFECTIONS (continued)

1. Usual adult dosage. Some patients may need dosage adjustment for renal or hepatic dysfunction or when used with interacting drugs.
2. The optimal duration of treatment with antifungal drugs is often unclear. Depending on the disease and its severity, they may be continued for weeks or months or, particularly in immunocompromised patients, indefinitely.
3. Non-albicans species, such as *C. glabrata* and *C. krusei*, respond to boric acid 600 mg intravaginally daily x 14d or to topical flucytosine cream (JD Sobel et al, Am J Obstet Gynecol 2003; 189:1297).
4. May be repeated in 72 hours if patient remains symptomatic.
5. Not FDA-approved for this indication.
6. JD Sobel et al, N Engl J Med 2004; 351:876.
7. Asymptomatic candiduria usually does not require treatment. Patients who are symptomatic, neutropenic, have renal allografts or are undergoing urologic manipulation, and infants with low birth weight, should be treated (PG Pappas et al, Clin Infect Dis 2004; 38:161).
8. Bladder irrigation with amphotericin B has been used to treat candidal cystitis, but does not treat disease beyond the bladder, and is generally not recommended.
9. Dosage of amphotericin B deoxycholate given once daily. For safety reasons, lipid-based formulations may be preferred. Usual doses of lipid-based formulations for treatment of invasive fungal infection are: amphotericin B lipid complex *(Abelcet)* 5 mg/kg/d; liposomal amphotericin B *(AmBisome)* 3-5 mg/kg/d; amphotericin B cholesteryl sulfate *(Amphotec)* 3-6 mg/kg/d.
10. Dosage must be decreased in patients with diminished renal function.

such as ritonavir *(Norvir)* or indinavir *(Crixivan),* are taken with itraconazole, serum concentrations of both drugs may increase. Itraconazole can increase serum concentrations of digoxin *(Lanoxin,* and others). A decreased contraceptive effect has been reported in patients taking oral contraceptives with itraconazole.

VORICONAZOLE — Voriconazole has a spectrum of activity similar to that of itraconazole but appears to be more active against *Aspergillus* spp. and some species of *Candida,* including *C. glabrata* and *C. krusei.* Unlike itraconazole, voriconazole is active against *Fusarium.* It is not active against zygomycetes, such as *Mucor* and *Rhizomucor* spp.; infection with these organisms has developed during treatment with the drug. In a randomized trial of initial treatment of invasive aspergillosis, voriconazole was shown to improve survival more than amphotericin B and was associated with fewer severe adverse effects.[2] Serum concentrations of voriconazole vary from patient to patient and may need monitoring.[3,4]

11. For uncomplicated oropharyngeal thrush, clotrimazole troches (10 mg) 5x/d or nystatin suspension 500,000 units (5 mL) qid can also be used. Azole-resistant oropharyngeal or esophageal candidiasis usually responds to amphotericin B or an echinocandin.

12. *Candida albicans* is generally highly susceptible to fluconazole. *C. krusei* infections are resistant to fluconazole. *C. glabrata* infections are often resistant to low doses, but may be susceptible to high doses of fluconazole. *C. lusitaniae* may be resistant to amphotericin B.

13. HIV-infected patients with frequent or severe recurrences of oral or esophageal candidiasis may require prophylaxis. For patients with organisms that are still susceptible, the regimen of choice is fluconazole 100-200 mg PO once daily.

14. Duration of treatment for esophageal candidiasis is 14 to 21 days after clinical improvement.

15. Use higher end of range for esophageal candidiasis.

16. R Ally et al, Clin Infect Dis 2001; 33:1447.

17. For patients with oropharyngeal disease, itraconazole oral solution 200 mg (20 mL) given once daily without food is more effective than itraconazole capsules.

18. For refractory oropharyngeal candidiasis, use 400 mg once/d or bid.

19. Non-neutropenic patients only.

20. In general, a loading dose of twice the daily dose is recommended on the first day of therapy.

21. For 2 weeks after afebrile and blood cultures negative.

22. In a large controlled trial, caspofungin was at least as effective as amphotericin B for treatment of invasive candidiasis or candidemia (J Mora-Duarte et al, N Engl J Med 2002; 347:2020).

Adverse Effects – Transient visual disturbances, including blurred vision, photophobia and altered perception of color or image, can occur with voriconazole. Rash (including Stevens-Johnson syndrome) photosensitivity, increased transaminase levels, confusion and hallucinations have also occurred. In patients with creatinine clearance <50 mL/min, the oral drug is preferred because the solubilizing agent in the IV formulation (sulfobutyl ether ß-cyclodextrin) can accumulate. Patients with mild to moderate hepatic cirrhosis should receive a normal loading dose of voriconazole, but half the maintenance dose. Voriconazole is teratogenic in animals (pregnancy category D).

Drug Interactions – Voriconazole is metabolized in the liver by, and is an inhibitor of, CYP2C19, 2C9 and 3A4. CYP2C19 is genetically variable (about 3% to 5% of Caucasians and African-Americans and about 15% of Asians do not express it) and patients deficient in this enzyme may be exposed to higher concentrations of the drug. Voriconazole is contraindicated in patients taking rifampin, rifabutin *(Mycobutin)*, ergot alkaloids, long-acting barbiturates, carbamazepine, pimozide, quinidine, cisapride or sirolimus *(Rapamune)*. Clinical monitoring or dose adjustment may be required in patients taking warfarin, sulfonylureas, statins, benzodiazepines, vinca alkaloids, nevirapine *(Viramune)* and HIV protease inhibitors other than indinavir. Omeprazole *(Prilosec*, and others), efavirenz *(Sustiva)*, cyclosporine and tacrolimus require dose reductions when given with voriconazole. Patients taking phenytoin require increased doses of voriconazole and more frequent monitoring for phenytoin toxicity.

POSACONAZOLE — Posaconazole, one of the newer triazole antifungals,[5] has an antifungal spectrum similar to that of itraconazole, but unlike other azoles it has *in vitro* activity against Zygomycetes such as *Mucor*. Before approval of posaconazole, amphotericin B formulations were the only products available for treatment of Zygomycete infections. Posaconazole is only available as an oral suspension and must be taken with high-fat meals for adequate absorption. Monitoring of serum concentrations may be helpful.

Clinical Use – A randomized, open-label clinical trial found that adults who were neutropenic due to acute myelogenous leukemia or myelodysplastic syndrome had fewer invasive mycoses and lower mortality when receiving posaconazole prophylaxis compared to those receiving fluconazole or itraconazole.[6] A double-blind randomized trial in adults with graft-versus-host disease following allogeneic hematopoietic stem cell transplantation (HSCT) found posaconazole similar to fluconazole in preventing invasive mycoses and superior in preventing invasive aspergillosis.[7] Oropharyngeal and esophageal candidiasis refractory to treatment with fluconazole or itraconazole have responded to posaconazole.[8] Posaconazole has also been used in therapy of other refractory mycoses, including aspergillosis, coccidioidomycosis and zygomycosis.[9-11]

Adverse Effects – Posaconazole has a safety profile comparable to that of fluconazole; dry mouth, rash, headache, diarrhea, fatigue, nausea, vomiting, QT prolongation, and abnormal liver function have been reported, but infrequently led to drug discontinuation. Arrhythmias, toxic epidermal necrolysis, angioedema and anaphylaxis have been rare. Posaconazole causes skeletal malformations in rats (pregnancy category C).

Drug Interactions – Posaconazole inhibits CYP3A4; doses of coadministered drugs that are metabolized by this isozyme, such as cyclosporine or tacrolimus, should be reduced.[1]

KETOCONAZOLE — Ketoconazole is now seldom used. The other azoles have fewer adverse effects and are generally preferred.

Adverse Effects – Anorexia, nausea and vomiting are common with higher doses (>400 mg/day) of ketoconazole; taking the drug with food or at bedtime may improve tolerance. Pruritus, rash and dizziness may occur. Ketoconazole can decrease plasma testosterone concentrations and cause gynecomastia, decreased libido and loss of potency in men and menstrual irregularities in women. High doses may inhibit adrenal steroidogenesis and decrease plasma cortisol concentrations. Hepatic toxicity, including fatal hepatic necrosis, can occur. Ketoconazole is teratogenic in animals (pregnancy category C).

Drug Interactions – Ketoconazole is a strong inhibitor of CYP3A4. Drug interactions with ketoconazole are similar to those with itraconazole.

ECHINOCANDINS

Echinocandins inhibit synthesis of ß (1, 3)-D-glucan, an essential component of the fungal cell wall. Their potential for adverse effects in humans is low due to the absence in mammalian cells of enzymes involved in glucan synthesis. Caspofungin, anidulafungin and micafungin all have activity against most *Candida* species, including those

ECHINOCANDINS

Drug	Dosage	Cost[1]
Caspofungin – *Cancidas* (Merck)	50 mg IV once/d	$395.36
Anidulafungin – *Eraxis* (Pfizer)	100 mg IV once/d	216.00
Micafungin – Mycamine (Astellas)	100 mg IV once/d	224.40

1. For one day's treatment according to AWP listings in *Red Book* 2007 and *Update* December 2007. Cost may vary among institutions based on formulary contracts.

resistant to azoles. Their activity against molds appears confined to *Aspergillus*. All three echinocandins are given intravenously once daily, do not require dose adjustment for renal failure and appear to be similar in efficacy and safety.[12]

CASPOFUNGIN — Caspofungin is FDA-approved for treatment of esophageal candidiasis, candidemia, intra-abdominal abscesses, peritonitis, and pleural space infections due to *Candida*. It is also approved for empiric treatment of presumed fungal infections in febrile, neutropenic patients and for treatment of invasive aspergillosis in patients who are refractory to or intolerant of other therapies. Data on its use for primary treatment of aspergillosis are lacking.

Adverse Effects – Although generally well tolerated, caspofungin occasionally causes rash, fever and mild hepatic toxicity. Anaphylaxis has occurred. Dosage should be reduced in patients with moderate hepatic dysfunction. Caspofungin is embryotoxic in animals (pregnancy category C).

Drug Interactions – Rifampin, carbamazepine, dexamethasone, efavirenz, nevirapine and phenytoin may increase clearance of caspofungin. An increase in caspofungin dosage to 70 mg should be considered when it is co-administered with these drugs. Caspofungin can decrease serum concentrations of tacrolimus. Liver function tests should be monitored in patients taking cyclosporine with caspofungin.

MICAFUNGIN — Micafungin is FDA-approved for treatment of esophageal candidiasis and prevention of invasive candidiasis in autologous or allogeneic stem cell transplant recipients. In one trial in patients with candidemia and deeply invasive candidiasis, micafungin was noninferior to liposomal amphotericin B (success rate of 89.6% vs. 89.5%).[13]

Adverse Effects – Micafungin is well tolerated. Possible histamine-like effects, as with other echinocandins, have included rash, pruritus and facial swelling. Anaphylaxis has been rare. Fever, hepatic function abnormalities, headache, nausea, vomiting and diarrhea have been reported, but rarely limit therapy. Micafungin is teratogenic in animals (pregnancy category C).

ANIDULAFUNGIN — Anidulafungin[14] is approved by the FDA for treatment of esophageal candidiasis and candidemia. It was as effective as fluconazole for invasive candidiasis in a randomized, double-blind trial.[15]

Adverse Effects – Anidulafungin has a low incidence of adverse effects similar to those of caspofungin and micafungin. Its safety in pregnancy has not been established (pregnancy category C).

AMPHOTERICIN B

Amphotericin B binds to ergosterol in the fungal cell membrane, leading to loss of membrane integrity and leakage of cell contents. Conventional amphotericin B and the newer lipid-based formulations have the same spectrum of activity and are active against most pathogenic fungi and some protozoa. They are not active against most strains of *Aspergillus terreus*, *Scedosporium apiospermum* (the asexual form of *Pseudallescheria*

TREATMENT OF ONYCHOMYCOSIS AND TINEA PEDIS

Infection		Drug
ONYCHOMYCOSIS[3, 4]		
		Terbinafine
	or	Itraconazole
TINEA PEDIS[7]		
		Terbinafine cream[8]
	or	Topical azoles (i.e. clotrimazole, miconazole, econazole)

1. Usual adult dosage. Some patients may need dosage adjustment for renal or hepatic dysfunction or when used with interacting drugs.
2. The optimal duration of treatment with antifungal drugs is often unclear. Depending on the disease and its severity, they may be continued for weeks or months or, particularly in immunocompromised patients, indefinitely.
3. Nail specimens should be obtained prior to any drug therapy to confirm the diagnosis of onychomycosis.
4. Topical treatment with ciclopirox 8% nail laquer *(Penlac)* is indicated for treatment of mild-to-moderate onychomycosis caused by *T. rubrium* that does not involve the lunula. Ciclopirox is less effective than systemic therapy, but has no systemic side effects or drug interactions.

boydii), Trichosporon and *Candida lusitaniae.* Amphotericin B is the preferred treatment for deep fungal infections during pregnancy.

Conventional Amphotericin B – Amphotericin B deoxycholate, the non-lipid formulation of amphotericin, is the least expensive but also the most toxic, particularly to the kidney. The development of better tolerated lipid-based formulations has led to a decrease in its use. Intravenous infusion of amphotericin B deoxycholate frequently causes fever and chills, and sometimes headache, nausea, vomiting, hypotension and tachypnea, usually beginning 1 to 3 hours after starting the infusion and lasting about 1 hour. The intensity of these infusion-related acute reactions tends to decrease after the first few doses. Pretreatment with acet-

Dosage/Duration[1,2]	Alternatives
250 mg PO once/d x 12 wks[5]	
200 mg PO once/d x 3 mos[5] or 200 mg PO bid 1 wk/mo x 3 mos[5]	Fluconazole[6] 150-300 mg PO once wkly x 6-12 mos[5]
twice daily application x 1-2 wks	Fluconazole[6] 150 mg PO once/wk x 1-4 wks
once or twice daily application x 4 wks	

5. Duration for toenail infection. Duration of treatment for fingernail infection: 6 weeks with terbinafine, 2 months with itraconazole and 3-6 months with fluconazole.
6. Not FDA-approved for this indication.
7. Topical treatment of "athlete's foot" is adequate for mild cases. Relapse is common and requires prolonged treatment (>4 wks).
8. Other topical non-azoles, including butenafine and naftifine may also be used, but the duration of treatment should then be increased to 2-4 weeks.

aminophen (*Tylenol*, and others) or a nonsteroidal anti-inflammatory drug (NSAID) such as ibuprofen, diphenhydramine (*Benadryl*, and others) 25 mg IV and/or hydrocortisone 25 mg IV can decrease the severity of the reaction. Treatment with meperidine (*Demerol*, and others) 25-50 mg IV can shorten the duration of rigors.

Nephrotoxicity is the major dose-limiting toxicity of amphotericin B deoxycholate; sodium loading with normal saline may prevent or ameliorate it and is generally recommended for patients who can tolerate a fluid load. The nephrotoxicity of amphotericin B may add to the nephrotoxicity of other drugs including cyclosporine, tacrolimus and aminoglycoside antibiotics such as gentamicin (*Garamycin*, and others). Hypokalemia and

AMPHOTERICIN B FORMULATIONS

Drug	Daily Dosage	Cost[1]
Amphotericin B deoxycholate generic (Abbott)	1-1.5 mg/kg IV	$ 34.92
Amphotericin B lipid complex (ABLC) *Abelcet* (Enzon)	5 mg/kg IV	960.00
Liposomal amphotericin B (L-AmB) *AmBisome* (Astellas)	3-6 mg/kg IV	1318.80
Amphotericin B colloidal dispersion (ABCD) *Amphotec* (Three Rivers)	3-4 mg/kg IV	480.00

1. For one day's treatment of a 70-kg patient at the highest usual dosage, according to AWP listings in *Red Book* 2007. Cost may vary among institutions based on formulary contracts.

hypomagnesemia are common and are usually due to a mild renal tubular acidosis. Weight loss, malaise, anemia, thrombocytopenia and mild leukopenia can occur. Cardiac toxicity and myopathy have been reported.

Lipid Formulations – The 3 lipid formulations of amphotericin B marketed in the US appear to be as effective as amphotericin B deoxycholate. Compared to conventional amphotericin B, acute infusion-related reactions are more severe with *Amphotec*, less severe with *Abelcet*, and least severe with *AmBisome*. Nephrotoxicity is less common with lipid-based products than with amphotericin B deoxycholate and, when it occurs, less severe. Liver toxicity, which is generally not associated with amphotericin B deoxycholate, has been reported with the lipid formulations.

Cost comparisons of amphotericin B formulations should take into account the fact that conventional amphotericin B deoxycholate may cause renal failure, which can increase the length of hospital stays, healthcare costs and mortality rates.[16]

OTHER DRUGS

FLUCYTOSINE *(Ancobon)* – Potentially lethal, dose-related bone marrow toxicity and rapid development of resistance with monotherapy have limited use of flucytosine mainly to combination use with amphotericin B for treatment of cryptococcal meningitis. Keeping serum concentrations below 100 mcg/mL (some clinicians recommend staying below 50 mcg/mL) decreases toxicity, but delays in obtaining assay results often limit their utility. Flucytosine is only available for oral use.

TERBINAFINE *(Lamisil)* – Terbinafine is a synthetic allylamine approved by the FDA for treatment of onychomycosis of the toenail or fingernail due to dermatophytes. It probably acts by inhibiting squalene epoxidase and blocking ergosterol synthesis.

The most common adverse effects of oral terbinafine have been headache, gastrointestinal symptoms including diarrhea, dyspepsia and abdominal pain, and occasionally a taste disturbance that may persist for weeks after the drug is stopped. Rash, pruritus and urticaria, usually mild and transient, have occurred. Toxic epidermal necrolysis and erythema multiforme have been reported. Increased aminotransferase levels and serious hepatic injury have occurred. Liver function should be assessed before initiation and periodically during treatment with terbinafine. Anaphylaxis, pancytopenia and severe neutropenia have also been reported.

Drug Interactions – Terbinafine is an inhibitor of CYP2D6 and may increase the effect or toxicity of drugs metabolized by this enzyme, including tricyclic antidepressants. Cimetidine *(Tagamet*, and others) may reduce the clearance of terbinafine. Enzyme inducers such as rifampin may increase terbinafine clearance.

TREATMENT OF OTHER FUNGAL INFECTIONS

Infection		Drug
ASPERGILLOSIS		Voriconazole[3]
	or	Amphotericin B
BLASTOMYCOSIS[6]		Itraconazole
	or	Amphotericin B
COCCIDIOIDOMYCOSIS[9]		Itraconazole[8]
	or	Fluconazole[8]
	or	Amphotericin B
CRYPTOCOCCOSIS		Amphotericin B
		±Flucytosine
	followed by	Fluconazole
	Chronic suppression[11]	Fluconazole
FUSARIOSIS		Amphotericin B
	or	Voriconazole

Dosage/Duration[1,2]	Alternatives
6 mg/kg IV q12h x 1d, then 4 mg/kg IV bid or 200-300 mg PO bid ≥10 wks	
1-1.5 mg/kg/d IV[4]	Posaconazole 200 mg PO tid-qid Itraconazole 200 mg PO tid x 3d followed by 200 mg PO bid Caspofungin[5] 70 mg IV x 1d, then 50 mg IV 1x/d
200 mg PO bid x 6-12 mos	Fluconazole 400-800 mg PO 1x/d[7,8]
0.5-1.0 mg/kg/d IV[4]	
200 mg PO bid x >1 yr	
400-800 mg PO 1x/d x >1 yr[7]	
0.5-1.5 mg/kg/d IV[4] x >1 yr	
0.5-1 mg/kg/d IV[4] x 2 wks	
25 mg/kg PO qid[10]	
400 mg PO 1x/d x 10 wks[7]	Itraconazole[8] 200 mg PO bid
200 mg PO 1x/d	Itraconazole[8] 200 mg PO bid Amphotericin B 0.5-1 mg/kg IV wkly[4]
1-1.5 mg/kg/d IV[4]	
6 mg/kg IV q12h x 1d, then 4 mg/kg q12h or 200 mg PO bid	

Continued on next page.

Antifungal Drugs

Infection		Drug
HISTOPLASMOSIS		
		Amphotericin B[12]
	or	Itraconazole
Chronic suppression[11]		Itraconazole[8]
PARACOCCIDIOIDOMYCOSIS[6]		
		Itraconazole[8]
	or	Amphotericin B[14]
SCEDOSPORIOSIS (asexual form of Pseudallescheriasis)		
		Voriconazole
SPOROTRICHOSIS		
Cutaneous		Itraconazole[8]
Extracutaneous[6]		Amphotericin B
	or	Itraconazole[8]
ZYGOMYCOSIS		
		Amphotericin B

1. Usual adult dosage. Some patients may need dosage adjustment for renal or hepatic dysfunction or when used with interacting drugs.
2. The optimal duration of treatment with antifungal drugs is often unclear. Depending on the disease and its severity, they may be continued for weeks or months or, particularly in immunocompromised patients, indefinitely.
3. In one large controlled trial, voriconazole was more effective than amphotericin B for treatment of invasive aspergillosis (R Herbrecht et al, N Engl J Med 2002; 347:408).
4. Dosage of amphotericin B deoxycholate given once daily. For safety reasons, lipid-based formulations may be preferred. Usual doses of lipid-based formulations for treatment of invasive fungal infection are: amphotericin B lipid complex *(Abelcet)* 5 mg/kg/d; liposomal amphotericin B *(AmBisome)* 3-5 mg/kg/d; amphotericin B cholesteryl sulfate *(Amphotec)* 3-6 mg/kg/d. For treatment of zygomycosis, the dosage of *AmBisome* is 5 mg/kg/d. For treatment of cryptococcal meningitis in HIV patients, the dosage of *AmBisome* is 4-6 mg/kg/d.
5. Micafungin and anidulafungin are also active against *Aspergillus.*
6. Patients with severe illness or CNS involvement should receive amphotericin B.
7. In general, a loading dose of twice the daily dose is recommended on the first day of therapy.
8. Not FDA-approved for this indication.

Dosage/Duration[1,2]	Alternatives
0.5-1.0 mg/kg/d IV[4] x 2 wks	
200 mg tid x 3d then 200 mg PO bid x 6 wks-$\geq$12 mos	Fluconazole[8] 400-800 mg PO 1x/d[7,13]
200 mg PO 1x/d or bid	Amphotericin[8] B 0.5-1 mg/kg IV wkly[4]
100-200 mg PO 1x/d x 6-12 mos	Ketoconazole 200-400 mg PO 1x/d
0.4-0.5 mg/kg/d IV[4]	
6 mg/kg IV q12h x 1d, then 4 mg/kg IV bid, or 200 mg PO bid x 12 wks	Itraconazole[8] 200 mg PO tid x 3d, then 200 mg PO bid Posaconazole[8] 200 mg PO qid
200 mg PO 1x/d x 3-6 mos	Terbinafine[8] 500 mg PO bid Saturated solution of potassium iodide 1-5 mL PO tid Fluconazole[7,8] 400-800 mg 1x/d
0.7-1 mg/kg/d IV[4] x 6-12 wks 200 mg PO bid x 12 mos	
1-1.5 mg/kg/d IV[4] x 6-10 wks	Posaconazole[8,15] 200 mg PO qid

9. Itraconazole is the drug of choice for non-meningeal coccidioidomycosis. Fluconazole is preferred for coccidioidal meningitis. Patients with meningitis who do not respond may require intrathecal amphotericin B. One patient with meningitis was successfully treated with voriconazole (KJ Cortez et al, Clin Infect Dis 2003; 36:1619).
10. Dosage must be decreased in patients with diminished renal function. When given with amphotericin B, some Medical Letter consultants recommend beginning flucytosine at 75 mg/kg/day divided q6h, until the degree of amphotericin nephrotoxicity becomes clear or flucytosine blood levels can be determined.
11. Suppressive for patients with HIV infection.
12. For severe disease, before switching to itraconazole. Amphotericin B should be continued for 4-6 weeks in patients with CNS involvement. In one study, liposomal amphotericin B (AmBisome) was associated with greater improvement in survival compared to amphotericin B deoxycholate (PC Johnson et al, Ann Intern Med 2002; 137:105).
13. For use only in patients who cannot tolerate itraconazole or amphotericin B.
14. Initial treatment of severely ill patients. To be followed by itraconazole.
15. Posaconazole has been used after mucormycosis was clinically improved and oral alimentation was sufficient to enhance absorption (AM Tobon et al, Clin Infect Dis 2003; 36:1488).

COMBINATION THERAPY

Use of combination therapy for treatment of immunosuppressed patients with invasive aspergillosis (IA), which has a high morbidity and mortality despite current treatments, is controversial. *In vitro* studies and animal data suggest a potential benefit of combining an echinocandin with either an azole or amphotericin B, but clinical studies are lacking.

NEUTROPENIA

PROPHYLAXIS — High-risk neutropenic patients, such as those undergoing allogeneic and certain autologous stem cell transplants, and those with hematologic malignancy who are expected to have prolonged profound neutropenia, may require prophylactic treatment with antifungal drugs. Fluconazole 400 mg PO or IV once daily has been used, but because of the high risk of invasive aspergillosis in these patients, many clinicians now use voriconazole or posaconazole instead. Itraconazole solution, 200 mg once daily, is an alternative but may not be well tolerated. Micafungin has also been effective in this population. In a prospective randomized trial for prevention of invasive fungal infections in neutropenic patients with acute myelogenous leukemia or myelodysplastic syndrome undergoing chemotherapy, posaconazole was superior to fluconazole or itraconazole and improved survival.[6]

FEVER AND NEUTROPENIA — For neutropenic patients with fever that persists despite treatment with antibacterial drugs, empiric addition of an antifungal drug is common practice. Caspofungin and voriconazole appear to be as effective as liposomal amphotericin B. Fluconazole and itraconazole have also been used for this indication.

1. CYP3A and drug interactions. Med Lett Drugs Ther 2005; 47:54.
2. R Herbrecht et al. Voriconazole versus amphotericin B for primary therapy of invasive aspergillosis. N Engl J Med 2002; 347:408.
3. J Smith et al. Voriconazole therapeutic drug monitoring. Antimicrob Agents Chemother 2006; 50:1570.

4. S Trifilio et al. Monitoring plasma voriconazole levels may be necessary to avoid subtherapeutic levels in hematopoietic stem cell transplant recipients. Cancer 2007; 109:1532.

5. Posaconazole *(Noxafil)* for invasive fungal infections. Med Lett Drugs Ther 2006; 48:93.

6. OA Cornely et al. Posaconazole vs. fluconazole or itraconazole prophylaxis in patients with neutropenia. N Engl J Med 2007; 356:348.

7. AJ Ullmann et al. Posaconazole or fluconazole for prophylaxis in severe graft-versus-host disease. N Engl J Med 2007; 356:335.

8. DJ Skiest et al. Posaconazole for the treatment of azole-refractory oropharyngeal and esophageal candidiasis in subjects with HIV infection. Clin Infect Dis 2007; 44:607.

9. TJ Walsh et al. Treatment of invasive aspergillosis with posaconazole in patients who are refractory to or intolerant of conventional therapy: an externally controlled trial. Clin Infect Dis 2007; 44:2.

10. DA Stevens et al. Posaconazole therapy for chronic refractory coccidioidomycosis. Chest 2007; 132:952.

11. JA Van Burik et al. Posaconazole is effective as salvage therapy in zygomycosis: a retrospective summary of 91 cases. Clin Infect Dis 2006; 42:e61.

12. C Wagner et al. The echinocandins: comparison of their pharmacokinetics, pharmacodynamics and clinical applications. Pharmacology 2006; 78:161.

13. ER Kuse et al. Micafungin versus liposomal amphotericin B for candidaemia and invasive candidosis: a phase III randomised double-blind trial. Lancet 2007; 369:1519.

14. Anidulafungin (Eraxis) for Candida infections. Med Lett Drugs Ther 2006; 48:43.

15. AC Reboli et al. Anidulafungin versus fluconazole for invasive candidiasis. N Engl J Med 2007; 356:2472.

16. AJ Ullmann et al. Prospective study of amphotericin B formulations in immunocompromised patients in 4 European countries. Clin Infect Dis 2006; 43:e29.

DRUGS FOR
HIV Infection

Original publication date – October 2006

The approval of new drugs and continuing concerns about drug toxicity and resistance have prompted new antiretroviral treatment guidelines.[1,2] Resistance testing is now recommended before starting antiretroviral therapy. HIV infection is treated with combinations of antiretroviral drugs while monitoring the patient's HIV RNA levels ("viral load") and CD4 cell count. Increases in viral load while on therapy may indicate development of drug resistance requiring further testing and a change in treatment regimen.

The dosage and cost of drugs for HIV infection are listed in the tables on pages 168 and 174. The regimens of choice are listed on page 182 and drugs that should not be used together on page 187. Antiretroviral drugs interact with each other and with many other drugs. Most of these interactions are not included here. For more information, see *The Medical Letter Adverse Drug Interactions Program.*

NUCLEOSIDE REVERSE TRANSCRIPTASE INHIBITORS (NRTIs)

Nucleoside analogs inhibit HIV reverse transcriptase and decrease or prevent HIV replication in infected cells. All NRTIs except didanosine generally do not interact with other drugs and can be taken without regard to meals.

Class Adverse Effects – According to the labeling for these drugs, all NRTIs can cause a potentially fatal syndrome of lactic acidosis with hepatic steatosis, probably due to mitochondrial toxicity, and have also been associated with peripheral lipoatrophy, central fat accumulation and hyperlipidemia, but, according to Medical Letter consultants, these adverse effects occur rarely, if at all, with NRTIs other than stavudine and zidovudine.

Abacavir (ABC, *Ziagen*) – Abacavir is available alone and in fixed-dose combinations with lamivudine *(Epzicom)* and with lamivudine and zidovudine *(Trizivir)*. It can be administered once or twice daily. Abacavir should not be used in a three-drug combination with lamivudine (or emtricitabine) and tenofovir because of high rates of virologic failure.[3] Treatment with *Trizivir* alone has been associated with higher rates of virologic failure than with *Trizivir*/efavirenz or lamivudine/zidovudine/efavirenz.[4] Patients with extensive prior NRTI therapy are less likely to respond to abacavir.

Adverse Effects – In 3-9% of patients treated with abacavir, a severe hypersensitivity reaction, usually with rash, fever and malaise, and sometimes with respiratory or gastrointestinal symptoms develops early in treatment (median of 11 days), but can occur at any time. Patients who have a hypersensitivity reaction should not be rechallenged. When rash occurs without systemic symptoms, the drug can sometimes be continued with close monitoring. Whether hypersensitivity reactions can occur when restarting abacavir after a hiatus in patients who previously tolerated the drug is controversial.

Didanosine (ddl, *Videx*) – Didanosine is available in enteric-coated capsules *(Videx EC*, and others) and as a pediatric powder for oral solution. The chewable buffered tablet formulation has been discontinued.

Patients with extensive prior NRTI therapy are less likely to respond to didanosine.

Adverse Effects – Dose-related peripheral neuropathy, pancreatitis and gastrointestinal disturbances are treatment-limiting toxicities of didanosine. Gastrointestinal tolerance is better with the enteric-coated capsules than with earlier formulations. Retinal changes and optic neuritis have been reported.

The combination of didanosine, tenofovir and a non-nucleoside reverse transcriptase inhibitor (NNRTI) is no longer recommended for initial antiretroviral therapy because of a high rate of virologic failure and rapid emergence of resistance.[5] Paradoxical CD4 cell count decline has been described in patients taking concurrent didanosine and tenofovir, despite virologic suppression.[6]

Drug Interactions – Didanosine buffered tablets (discontinued) and the pediatric powder formulation interfere with absorption of drugs that require gastric acidity, including delavirdine, indinavir, and atazanavir. Use of the enteric-coated preparation appears to eliminate this problem. Tenofovir inhibits metabolism of didanosine; if they are used together, the dose of didanosine should be decreased.

The risk of pancreatitis, neuropathy and lactic acidosis is increased when didanosine is combined with stavudine; the combination of didanosine and stavudine is no longer recommended for initial treatment or for treatment during pregnancy.

Emtricitabine (FTC, *Emtriva*) – Emtricitabine is the 5-fluorinated derivative of lamivudine.[7] It is similar to lamivudine in safety and efficacy, and can be given once daily. Emtricitabine is also available in fixed-dose combinations with tenofovir *(Truvada)* and with tenofovir and efavirenz *(Atripla)*. Resistance to emtricitabine is conferred by the

NRTIs/NNRTIs FOR HIV INFECTION

Drug	Usual adult dosage
NUCLEOSIDE REVERSE TRANSCRIPTASE INHIBITORS (NRTIs)	
Abacavir (ABC)	
Ziagen – GlaxoSmithKline*	300 mg bid[2] or 600 mg once/d[2]
Didanosine (ddI) enteric-coated capsules	
generic	400 mg once/d[3,18]
Videx EC – Bristol-Myers Squibb*	
Emtricitabine (FTC)	
Emtriva – Gilead	200 mg once/d[4,18]
Lamivudine (3TC)	
Epivir – GlaxoSmithKline*	150 mg bid[5,18] or 300 mg once/d[5,18]
Stavudine (d4T)	
Zerit – Bristol-Myers Squibb*	40 mg bid[6,18]
Zalcitabine (ddC)	
Hivid – Roche	0.75 mg tid[7,18]
Zidovudine (AZT, ZDV)	
generic	300 mg bid[8,18]
Retrovir – GlaxoSmithKline*	

* Also available in a liquid or oral powder formulation.
1. Daily cost according to most recent data (July 31, 2006) available from Wolters Kluwer Health.
2. With or without food. Available in 300-mg tablets. Dosage for mild hepatic impairment is 200 mg bid.
3. Doses should be taken on an empty stomach. Available in 125- (only *Videx EC*), 200-, 250- and 400-mg capsules; for patients <60 kg, 250 mg once daily, ≥60 kg, 400 mg once daily. The dose of didanosine should be decreased to 250 mg/d for adults weighing ≥60 kg and to 200 mg/d for those weighing <60 kg when combined with tenofovir, which increases didanosine serum concentrations.

Total tablets or capsules/day	Cost[1]
2	$15.50
1	9.95
	11.15
1	11.49
2	11.52
1	11.53
2	12.66
3	7.98
2	10.70
	13.24

4. With or without food. Available in 200-mg capsules.
5. With or without food. For patients <50 kg, 2 mg/kg bid. Available in 150- and 300-mg tablets.
6. With or without food. For patients <60 kg, 30 mg bid. Available in 15-, 20-, 30- and 40-mg capsules.
7. With or without food. Available in 0.375- and 0.75-mg tablets.
8. With or without food. Available in 100-mg capsules and 300-mg tablets. Can also be given as 200 mg tid. Also available in a parenteral preparation for intrapartum use, the dose during labor is a 2 mg/kg load the first hour, and then 1 mg/kg/hour throughout the duration of labor.

Continued on next page.

NRTIs/NNRTIs FOR HIV INFECTION (continued)

Drug	Usual adult dosage
NUCLEOTIDE REVERSE TRANSCRIPTASE INHIBITOR (NRTI)	
Tenofovir DF (TDF)	
Viread – Gilead	300 mg once/d[9,18]
NON-NUCLEOSIDE REVERSE TRANSCRIPTASE INHIBITORS (NNRTIs)	
Delavirdine (DLV)	
Rescriptor – Pfizer	400 mg tid[10]
Efavirenz (EFV)	
Sustiva – Bristol-Myers Squibb	600 mg once/d[11]
Nevirapine (NVP)	
Viramune – Boehringer Ingelheim*	200 mg bid[12]
FIXED-DOSE NRTI COMBINATIONS	
Zidovudine/lamivudine	300 mg/150 mg bid[13]
Combivir – GlaxoSmithKline	
Zidovudine/lamivudine/abacavir	200 mg/150 mg/300 mg bid[14]
Trizivir – GlaxoSmithKline	
Abacavir/lamivudine	600 mg/300 mg once/d[15]
Epzicom – GlaxoSmithKline	
Emtricitabine/tenofovir DF	200 mg/300 mg once/d[16]
Truvada – Gilead	
FIXED-DOSE NNRTI/NRTI COMBINATION	
Efavirenz/emtricitabine/tenofovir DF	
Atripla – Gilead/Bristol-Myers Squibb	600 mg/200 mg/300 mg once/d[17]

* Also available in a liquid or oral powder formulation.
9. May be taken with or without food. Available in 300-mg tablets.
10. With or without food. Available in 100- and 200-mg tablets.
11. At bedtime for at least the first 2 to 4 weeks; taken on an empty stomach. Available in 50-, 100-, and 200-mg capsules and 600-mg tablets.
12. With or without food. 200 mg once/day for the first 2 weeks of treatment to decrease the risk of rash. Available in 200-mg tablets.

Total tablets or capsules/day	Cost[1]
1	17.43
6	9.96
1	16.41
2	14.56
2	25.08
2	40.58
1	26.99
1	28.98
1	46.07

13. Each tablet contains 300 mg of zidovudine and 150 mg of lamivudine.
14. Each tablet contains 300 mg of zidovudine, 150 mg of lamivudine and 300 mg of abacavir.
15. Each tablet contains 600 mg of abacavir and 300 mg of lamivudine.
16. Each tablet contains 200 mg of emtricitabine and 300 mg of tenofovir.
17. Each tablet contains 600 mg of efavirenz, 200 mg of emtricitabine, and 300 mg tenofovir. Should be taken without food. Dosing at bedtime may diminish CNS side effects.
18. Dosage adjustment required for renal impairment.

M184V mutation, which is the main cause of resistance to lamivudine, so cross-resistance is complete.

Adverse Effects – Emtricitabine is among the best tolerated NRTIs. It can cause hyperpigmentation of the palms and soles, particularly in dark-skinned patients. Because emtricitabine is also active against hepatitis B virus (HBV), HIV-positive patients with chronic HBV infection may experience a flare of hepatitis if emtricitabine is withdrawn or if their HBV strain becomes resistant to the drug.

Lamivudine (3TC, *Epivir*) – Lamivudine, like emtricitabine, is among the best tolerated of the NRTIs. It can be taken once or twice daily. Lamivudine is also available in fixed-dose combinations with abacavir *(Epzicom)*, zidovudine *(Combivir)*, and zidovudine and abacavir *(Trizivir)*. An increase in viral load during treatment with a lamivudine-containing regimen is often an indication of resistance to lamivudine. Lamivudine-resistant strains are cross-resistant to emtricitabine, and may have a modest decrease in susceptibility to abacavir and didanosine.

A lower-dose lamivudine tablet is approved for treatment of chronic hepatitis B *(Epivir-HBV)*.

Adverse Effects – Because lamivudine is also active against hepatitis B virus (HBV), HIV-positive patients with chronic HBV infection may experience a flare of hepatitis if lamivudine is withdrawn or if their HBV strain becomes resistant to the drug. Other adverse effects are uncommon; pancreatitis has been reported rarely in children.

Stavudine (d4T, *Zerit*) – Stavudine can be given either in initial combination therapy or after failure of regimens containing other NRTIs, but cross-resistance with zidovudine is virtually complete. Concurrent administration of zidovudine causes antagonism.

Adverse Effects – Fatal lactic acidosis may occur more frequently with stavudine than with other NRTIs. Serum aminotransferase activity may increase with stavudine treatment, and pancreatitis has occurred rarely. Lactic acidosis and pancreatitis are more common when stavudine is combined with didanosine; this regimen is no longer recommended for initial treatment or treatment of pregnant women. Stavudine commonly causes peripheral sensory neuropathy, which often disappears when the drug is stopped and may not recur when it is restarted at a lower dose. Stavudine causes lipoatrophy, raises serum lipid concentrations, and has been associated with development of diabetes.

Zalcitabine (ddC, *Hivid*) – Zalcitabine is less effective, less convenient and more toxic than the other NRTIs; it is used rarely. The manufacturer will discontinue distribution of the drug by December 31, 2006.

Zidovudine (AZT, ZDV, *Retrovir*, and others) – Zidovudine is available alone and in fixed-dose combinations with lamivudine *(Combivir)* and with lamivudine and abacavir *(Trizivir)*. It can be given in combination with any other NRTI except stavudine, which causes antagonism. Non-suppressive therapy with a zidovudine-containing regimen results in resistance to zidovudine and cross-resistance to other NRTIs.

Adverse Effects – Adverse effects of zidovudine include anemia, neutropenia, nausea, vomiting, headache, fatigue, confusion, malaise, myopathy, hepatitis, and hyperpigmentation of the oral mucosa and nail beds. It may be better tolerated when taken without food. Zidovudine is less likely than stavudine to cause lipoatrophy, lactic acidosis and hepatic steatosis.

NUCLEOTIDE REVERSE TRANSCRIPTASE INHIBITOR (NRTI)

Nucleotides are phosphorylated nucleosides; nucleoside and nucleotide RTIs have similar mechanisms of action.

PIs/FUSION INHIBITOR FOR HIV INFECTION

Drug	Usual adult dosage
PROTEASE INHIBITORS	
Amprenavir (APV)	
Agenerase – GlaxoSmithKline*	1200 mg bid[2,9]
Atazanavir (ATV)	
Reyataz – Bristol-Myers Squibb	300 mg/100 mg RTV once/d[3,4,9]
Darunavir (DRV)	
Prezista – Tibotec	600 mg/100 mg RTV bid[4,5]
Fosamprenavir (FPV)	
Lexiva – GlaxoSmithKline	1400 mg/200 mg RTV once/d[4,6,9]
Indinavir (IDV)	
Crixivan – Merck	800 mg tid or 800 mg/100 mg RTV bid[4,7,9]
Lopinavir/ritonavir (LPV/RTV)	
Kaletra – Abbott*	400/100 mg bid[8] or 800/200 mg once/d[8]

* Also available in a liquid or oral powder formulation.
1. Daily cost according to most recent data (July 31, 2006) available from Wolters Kluwer Health.
2. With or without food, but not with a fatty meal. Now available only in 50-mg capsules or as an oral solution. Capsules are also FDA-approved for administration with ritonavir: 1200 mg APV/200 mg RTV once/day or 600 mg APV/100 mg RTV bid. Dose for oral solution is 1400 mg bid.
3. *Reyataz* is taken with food. Available in 100-, 150- and 200-mg capsules. For therapy-experienced patients and when taken with EFV or TDF, the FDA-approved dose is 300 mg ATV/100 mg RTV. For therapy-naïve patients, the FDA-approved dose is 400 mg once/d (300 mg/100 mg RTV once/d is also used).
4. RTV = Ritonavir (*Norvir* – Abbott). Available as a 100-mg soft-gelatin capsule. The liquid formulation has an unpleasant taste; the manufacturer suggests taking it with chocolate milk or a liquid nutritional supplement.
5. *Prezista* is taken with food. Available in 300-mg tablets.

Total tablets or capsules/day	Cost[1]
48	26.88
3	39.31
6	49.78
4	42.24
6	18.06
6	32.34
4	25.16
4	

6. *Lexiva* is taken with or without food. Can also be given as 1400 mg bid or 700 mg/100 mg RTV bid in treatment-naïve patients and 700 mg/100 mg RTV bid in PI-experienced patients. When taken once daily with efavirenz, the recommended dosage is 1400 mg/300 mg RTV.

7. RTV-boosted dosage is not FDA-approved. *Crixivan* is taken with water or other liquids, 1 hour before or 2 hours after a meal, or with a light meal. Available in 100-, 200-, 333- and 400-mg capsules. Dosage is 600 mg q8h when taken with DLV. Patients should drink at least 48 ounces (1.5 L) of water daily.

8. Each tablet contains 200 mg of lopinavir and 50 mg of ritonavir. The recommended dose is 600/150 mg bid when taken with EFV, NVP, FPV or NFV in treatment-experienced pateints. The higher dose can also be tried if lopinavir resistance is suspected. Once-daily dosing in treatment-naive patients only. With or without food. No refrigeration.

9. Dosage adjustment required for hepatic impairment.

Continued on next page.

PIs/FUSION INHIBITOR FOR HIV INFECTION (continued)

Drug	Usual adult dosage
PROTEASE INHIBITORS (continued)	
Nelfinavir (NFV)	
Viracept – Pfizer*	1250 mg bid[10] or 750 mg tid[10]
Saquinavir (SQV)	
Invirase – Roche	1000 mg/100 mg RTV bid[4,11]
Tipranavir (TPV)	
Aptivus – Boehringer Ingelheim	500 mg/200 mg RTV bid[4,12]
FUSION INHIBITOR	
Enfuvirtide (T20)	
Fuzeon – Roche	90 mg SC bid[13]

* Also available in a liquid or oral powder formulation.
10. *Viracept* is available in 250- and 625-mg tablets and should be taken with food.
11. *Invirase* should be taken within 2 hours after a full meal. Available in 200-mg capsules and 500-mg tablets. Dosage is 1000 mg bid (without RTV) when taken with LPV/RTV.

Tenofovir disoproxil fumarate (TDF, *Viread*) – Tenofovir DF is the only nucleotide RTI available for treatment of HIV. It is a prodrug of tenofovir, a potent inhibitor of HIV replication. Tenofovir DF is given once daily. It is effective as part of initial HIV therapy and has activity against some HIV strains that are resistant to other NRTIs.

Tenofovir DF is available alone and in fixed-dose combinations with emtricitabine *(Truvada)* and with emtricitabine and efavirenz *(Atripla)*.

Tenofovir should not be used in three-drug combinations with abacavir/lamivudine or didanosine/lamivudine because of high rates of virologic failure. The combination of tenofovir with didanosine and an NNRTI has

Total tablets or capsules/day	Cost[1]
4 (625-mg tablets)	23.96
9 (250-mg tablets)	21.60
6	46.70
8	75.68
—	66.51

12. With food. Available in 250-mg capsules.
13. Available in kits containing a one-month supply of syringes and single-use vials with powder for a 90-mg dose and sterile water for reconstitution.

been associated with early virologic failure and is not recommended for initial antiretroviral therapy.[5]

Adverse Effects – Tenofovir is generally well tolerated. Renal toxicity, including a Fanconi-like syndrome and progression to renal failure, has been reported. Tenofovir dosage must be decreased in patients with diminished renal function. Tenofovir is also active against HBV[8,9]; in patients with chronic HBV infection, a hepatitis flare can occur if it is discontinued.

Drug Interactions – If tenofovir is used in combination with didanosine, the dose of didanosine should be decreased. Tenofovir lowers serum concentrations of atazanavir; ritonavir should be added (100 mg with

300 mg daily of atazanavir) to boost atazanavir levels when given in combination with tenofovir.

FIXED-DOSE NRTI COMBINATIONS

Four different fixed-dose NRTI combinations are available (see table on page 170). They offer the advantage of simplifying dosing schedules and reducing pill burden, but they are less flexible in terms of dosage adjustment. Some patients with hepatic or renal impairment will not be able to take them.

NON-NUCLEOSIDE REVERSE TRANSCRIPTASE INHIBITORS (NNRTIs)

These drugs are direct, non-nucleoside inhibitors of HIV-1 reverse transcriptase. Combinations of an NNRTI with NRTIs tend to be at least additive in reducing HIV replication *in vitro*.

HIV isolates that are resistant to NRTIs and to protease inhibitors (PI) may remain sensitive to NNRTIs, but cross-resistance is common within the NNRTI class. Resistance to NNRTIs develops rapidly if they are used alone or in combinations that do not completely suppress viral replication. Because of their relatively long plasma half-life, further increased in patients with genetic polymorphisms of CYP450 isoenzymes, discontinuation of NNRTI-based regimens (particularly when efavirenz is the NNRTI) should be approached in a step-wise fashion or by substituting a PI for up to one month to let the NNRTI "wash out".[10]

Class Adverse Effects – All NNRTIs, especially nevirapine, can cause a rash that is sometimes severe. NNRTIs are metabolized by and can affect hepatic CYP450 isozymes; they can interact with PIs and many other drugs.[11]

Delavirdine (DLV, *Rescriptor*) – Delavirdine is the least potent NNRTI and is given 3 times daily. It is rarely used. Unlike efavirenz and nevirapine, delavirdine inhibits the metabolism and increases serum concentrations of PIs.

Efavirenz (EFV, *Sustiva*) – Efavirenz is the only NNRTI approved for once-daily dosing. In previously untreated patients, the combination of efavirenz with zidovudine/lamivudine has been more effective than indinavir/zidovudine/lamivudine, nelfinavir/zidovudine/lamivudine or abacavir/zidovudine/lamivudine in lowering HIV RNA concentrations, even among patients with high baseline levels (>100,000 copies/mL), and has been better tolerated. Brief studies in treatment-experienced patients or those failing other regimens have shown that efavirenz in combination with at least two other new agents can be effective in suppressing plasma HIV RNA levels and raising CD4 cell counts. Efavirenz is available alone and in a fixed-dose combination with emtricitabine and tenofovir *(Atripla)*.

Adverse Effects – The most common adverse effects of efavirenz have been rash, dizziness, headache, insomnia and inability to concentrate. Vivid dreams and nightmares can occur. Hallucinations, psychosis, depression and suicidal ideation have been reported. CNS effects tend to occur between 1 and 3 hours after each dose. They may stop within a few days or weeks, but can persist for months or years, particularly in patients with high efavirenz serum concentrations.[12,13] When the dose is taken at bedtime, CNS effects may still be present in the morning on awakening and may impair driving; this effect generally wanes with time and can be ameliorated by taking the drug earlier in the evening. Hypertriglyceridemia has occurred. Fetal abnormalities have occurred in pregnant monkeys exposed to efavirenz, and neural tube defects have been reported in women who took the drug during the first trimester of pregnancy; the drug should not be given to women who are, or are considering becoming, pregnant.

Drug Interactions – Efavirenz is an inducer of CYP3A4. Methadone dosage often needs to be increased if efavirenz is used concurrently. Efavirenz decreases serum concentrations of some protease inhibitors. It also decreases serum concentrations of voriconazole *(Vfend)*; they should not be taken together.

Nevirapine (NVP, *Viramune*) – Nevirapine appears to be comparable to efavirenz in effectiveness, but must be dosed twice daily and has greater potential for serious adverse effects.

Adverse Effects – Nevirapine can cause severe hepatotoxicity, hepatic failure and death, particularly in patients with previously elevated transaminases or underlying hepatitis B or C. Hepatotoxicity has also occurred when the drug was used for post-exposure prophylaxis in HIV-negative patients. Fever, nausea and headache can occur. Rash is common early in treatment with nevirapine and can be more severe than with other NNRTIs; it may progress to Stevens-Johnson syndrome. To decrease the incidence of rash and hepatic toxicity, the dose of nevirapine should be 200 mg once daily for the first 2 weeks, and then 200 mg twice daily. Women with CD4 counts >250 cells/mm^3 and men with baseline CD4 counts >400 cells/mm^3 are at increased risk of nevirapine-associated hepatotoxicity.[14]

Drug Interactions – As with efavirenz, the dose of methadone often needs to be increased if nevirapine is used concurrently. Nevirapine decreases serum concentrations of some protease inhibitors.

FIXED-DOSE NNRTI/NRTI COMBINATION

Atripla is the first fixed-dose antiretroviral combination to contain antiretrovirals from two different classes (1 NNTRI/2 NRTIs). Each tablet contains 600 mg of **efavirenz**, 200 mg of **emtricitabine** and 300 mg of **tenofovir DF**. The dose is one tablet once daily.

An open-label, randomized noninferiority study in 517 treatment-naïve patients compared the combination of efavirenz, emtricitabine and tenofovir once daily (separately, not in the combination tablet) with fixed-dose zidovudine and lamivudine *(Combivir)* twice daily plus efavirenz once daily. At week 48, significantly more patients taking emtricitabine/tenofovir/efavirenz achieved and maintained HIV viral loads <400 copies/mL (84% vs. 73%) and <50 copies/mL (80% vs. 70%).[15] At week 96, the percentages of patients with HIV RNA <400 copies/mL were 76% vs. 64%, and with <50 copies/mL were 69% vs. 63%.[16]

Adverse Effects – Adverse effects for *Atripla* are generally similar to those with the drugs taken separately. Patients with renal impairment who require dose adjustments and women who are or might become pregnant will not be able to take *Atripla*.

PROTEASE INHIBITORS (PIs)

Protease inhibitors prevent cleavage of protein precursors essential for HIV maturation, infection of new cells and viral replication. Use of a PI in combination with other drugs has led to marked clinical improvement and prolonged survival even in patients with advanced HIV infection. Most PIs potently suppress HIV replication *in vivo*. Low-dose ritonavir taken with some other PIs inhibits the metabolism and increases serum concentrations of the other PI ("ritonavir boosting"); this technique is increasingly used.

Class Adverse Effects – Many PIs can cause gastrointestinal distress, increased bleeding in hemophiliacs, hyperglycemia, insulin resistance and hyperlipidemia and have been associated with an increased risk of coronary artery disease. They have also been associated with peripheral lipoatrophy and central fat accumulation. All, especially tipranavir, can cause hepatotoxicity, which may occasionally be severe and is more common in patients who are co-infected with HBV or hepatitis C virus (HCV). All PIs are metabolized by and are inhibitors of hepatic CYP3A4; drug interactions are common and can be severe.[11]

ANTIRETROVIRAL REGIMENS FOR TREATMENT-NAÏVE PATIENTS

NNRTI-BASED (1 NNRTI + 2 NRTIs)
  Regimen of Choice
    Efavirenz[1] + (lamivudine or emtricitabine) + (zidovudine or tenofovir)

  Substitutes
    For the NNRTI: nevirapine
    For the NRTIs: (lamivudine or emtricitabine) + (abacavir or didanosine or
      stavudine)

PI-BASED (1 OR 2 PIs + 2 NRTIs)
  Regimen of Choice
    (Lopinavir/ritonavir or atazanavir/ritonavir) + (lamivudine or emtricitabine)
      + zidovudine

  Substitutes
    For the PI(s): fosamprenavir/ritonavir or saquinavir/ritonavir or
      indinavir/ritonavir or nelfinavir
    For the NRTIs: (lamivudine or emtricitabine) + (abacavir or didanosine or
      stavudine or tenofovir)

TRIPLE NRTI[2]
  Regimen of Choice
    Abacavir + lamivudine + zidovudine

1. Except in pregnant women or women who might become pregnant because efavirenz is contraindicated in pregnancy.
2. Should only be considered after NNRTI- and PI-based regimens have been excluded.

Amprenavir (APV, *Agenerase*) – Amprenavir is available in capsules and in an oral solution; full doses taken without ritonavir would require 48 capsules or 187 mL daily. It has largely been replaced by fosamprenavir.

Adverse Effects – The most common adverse effects of amprenavir have been nausea, vomiting (especially in combination with zidovudine), perioral paresthesias and rash. Many patients with rash can continue or restart amprenavir if the rash is mild or moderate, but about 1% of patients have developed severe rash, including Stevens-Johnson syndrome.

Atazanavir (ATV, *Reyataz*) – Atazanavir is a PI with once-daily dosing.[7] Most clinicians prefer to use boosted atazanavir whenever possible; atazanavir/ritonavir has been comparable to lopinavir/ritonavir in treatment-experienced patients.

Adverse Effects – Atazanavir causes an asymptomatic indirect hyperbilirubinemia. Unboosted, it has had fewer adverse effects than other PIs on lipid profiles, fat accumulation or glucose metabolism. It can cause PR prolongation and should be used with caution in patients with cardiac conduction abnormalities.

Darunavir *(Prezista)* – Darunavir, like tipranavir, has been effective in treatment-experienced patients infected with HIV strains resistant to other protease inhibitors. It must be taken with ritonavir to achieve adequate bioavailability.[17] Patients on darunavir who also received the fusion inhibitor enfuvirtide as part of their regimen have had better response rates.

Adverse Effects – The incidence of adverse effects with darunavir, including diarrhea, nausea, headache, nasopharyngitis and increased aminotransferase activity, has been similar to that with other boosted protease inhibitors. It appears to be better tolerated than tipranavir, but no direct comparision is available. In clinical trials, rash occurred in 7% of patients treated with darunavir and severe rash, including erythema multiforme and Stevens-Johnson syndrome, has been reported. Like tipranavir and fosamprenavir, darunavir contains a sulfonamide moiety; it should be used with caution in patients with sulfonamide allergy.

Fosamprenavir calcium (FPV, *Lexiva*) – Fosamprenavir calcium, a prodrug of amprenavir, is available in 700-mg tablets equivalent to 600 mg of amprenavir. In patients who have not previously been treated with a PI, fosamprenavir can be taken once daily combined with ritonavir, or twice daily with or without ritonavir. In patients who are treatment-experienced, it should be taken twice daily with ritonavir. Fosamprenavir/ritonavir was as effective and as well tolerated as lopinavir/ritonavir, each in combination with abacavir/lamivudine, in treatment-naïve patients.[18] If fosamprenavir/ritonavir once daily is coadministered with efavirenz, the ritonavir dosage should be increased. Fosamprenavir has largely replaced amprenavir.

Adverse Effects – Adverse effects are similar to those with amprenavir, but in clinical studies the incidence of nausea, vomiting and severe rash was lower. Unlike amprenavir, which should not be taken with a fatty meal, fosamprenavir has no food restrictions. Like tipranavir and darunavir, it contains a sulfonamide moiety and should be used with caution in patients with sulfonamide allergy.

Indinavir (IDV, *Crixivan*) – Indinavir has good oral bioavailability and has been effective taken twice daily when combined with low-dose ritonavir, but it is used uncommonly because of its toxicity.

Adverse Effects – In addition to adverse effects similar to those of other protease inhibitors, indinavir causes asymptomatic elevation of indirect bilirubin, indinavir-containing kidney stones and renal insufficiency, dermatologic changes including alopecia, dry skin and mucous membranes, and paronychia and ingrown toenails. Patients should drink at least 1.5-2 liters of water daily to minimize renal adverse effects. Ritonavir boosting increases the risk of nephrolithiasis. Gallstones have also been reported.[19]

Lopinavir/ritonavir (LPV/RTV, *Kaletra*) – Lopinavir is available in the US only in a fixed-dose combination with ritonavir.[20] A new tablet formulation has replaced the previous capsule formulation; this new formulation has a lower daily pill burden, does not require refrigeration, and can be taken with or without food. Though usually given twice daily, it can be offered once daily to treatment-naïve patients. Lopinavir/ritonavir has been the PI regimen of choice in both treatment-naïve patients and in those with previous HIV treatment and moderate or no PI resistance (<5 resistance mutations); atazanavir/ritonavir appears to be similarly effective in treatment-experienced patients, and in one study in treatment-naïve patients, fosamprenavir/ritonavir was not inferior.[18]

Adverse Effects – Lopinavir/ritonavir is generally well tolerated. The most common adverse effects have been diarrhea, nausea, headache and asthenia. As with other PIs, hyperlipidemia, hyperglycemia, increased aminotransferase activity and altered body fat distribution have been reported. Fatal pancreatitis has occurred.

Nelfinavir (NFV, *Viracept*) – Nelfinavir once was a commonly used PI, but it appears to be less potent than lopinavir/ritonavir, and cannot be boosted.

Adverse Effects – Nelfinavir is generally well tolerated. Diarrhea, which is nearly universal but may resolve with continued use, is its main adverse effect.

Ritonavir (RTV, *Norvir*) – Ritonavir is well absorbed from the gastrointestinal tract and at full doses potently inhibits HIV, but due to poor tolerability it is now used mainly in doses of 100-200 mg once or twice daily to increase the serum concentrations and decrease the dosage frequency of other PIs.

Adverse Effects – Adverse reactions are common with full doses of ritonavir, but less common with the low doses used in PI combinations. Ritonavir can cause hypertriglyceridemia, altered taste, nausea, vomiting and, rarely, circumoral and peripheral paresthesias. It interacts with many other drugs.

Saquinavir (SQV, *Invirase*) – *Invirase*, which is available as a hard-gel capsule or film-coated tablet, is now the only available formulation of saquinavir. Saquinavir is usually well tolerated. Saquinavir/ritonavir appears to be as effective as and better tolerated than indinavir/ritonavir.

Adverse Effects – Saquinavir occasionally causes diarrhea, abdominal discomfort, nausea, glucose intolerance, hyperlipidemia, abnormal fat distribution and increased aminotransferase activity. It can cause increased bleeding in patients with hemophilia, and rarely causes rash and hyperprolactinemia.

Tipranavir (TPV, *Aptivus*) – Tipranavir is available as a capsule and must be taken with low-dose ritonavir.[21] It can be used in treatment-experienced patients who have ongoing viral replication or in patients with HIV strains known to be resistant to multiple protease inhibitors, but darunavir may be better tolerated for the same indication. In clinical studies of patients with extensive treatment experience and drug resistance, tipranavir-containing regimens were more effective than regimens based on other ritonavir-boosted PIs, such as lopinavir/ritonavir. Patients on tipranavir who also received the fusion inhibitor enfuvirtide as a part of their background regimen had better response rates.[22]

Adverse Effects – Severe hepatitis, including some fatalities, has been reported in patients taking tipranavir. Careful monitoring of liver function tests is recommended, especially in patients with chronic HBV or HCV infection. Tipranavir may cause diarrhea, nausea, vomiting and abdominal pain. The drug contains a sulfonamide moiety; caution should be used in patients with sulfonamide allergy. Intracranial hemorrhage has been reported among patients taking tipranavir, prompting a recent safety warning from the manufacturer.

FUSION INHIBITOR — After HIV binds to the host cell surface, a conformational change occurs in the transmembrane glycoprotein subunit (gp41) of the viral envelope, facilitating fusion of the viral and host cell membranes, and entry of the virus into the cell. Fusion inhibitors bind to gp41 and prevent the conformational change.

Enfuvirtide (T-20, ENF, *Fuzeon*) – Enfuvirtide is the first fusion inhibitor approved by the FDA for treatment of HIV infection and is indicated for treatment-experienced patients with ongoing HIV replication despite current antiretroviral use.[23] It is administered twice daily by subcutaneous injection.

Adverse Effects – Almost all patients develop local injection site reactions to enfuvirtide, with mild or moderate pain, erythema, induration, nodules and cysts.[24] Other adverse effects include eosinophilia, systemic

SOME ANTIRETROVIRAL DRUGS THAT SHOULD NOT BE USED TOGETHER

Drugs	Effect	Comments
Abacavir + lamivudine (or emtricitabine) + tenofovir	Early virologic failure	Not recommended
Didanosine + lamivudine (or emtricitabine) + tenofovir	Early virologic failure	Not recommended
Didanosine + stavudine	Increased risk of peripheral neuropathy, pancreatitis and lactic acidosis	Not recommended for initial therapy or in pregnant women
Didanosine + tenofovir + NNRTI	Early virologic failure	Not recommended for initial therapy
Stavudine + zidovudine	Antagonism	Not recommended

hypersensitivity reactions, and possibly an increased incidence of bacterial pneumonia.

PREVENTION OF PERINATAL TRANSMISSION

Most perinatal transmission of HIV occurs close to the time of, or during, labor and delivery. **Zidovudine alone**, started at 14-34 weeks of gestation and continued in the infant for the first 6 weeks of life, reduced HIV transmission from 26% to 8%.[25]

Current guidelines recommend combination therapy with **zidovudine plus another NRTI plus either a PI or nevirapine** throughout pregnancy to prevent transmission of HIV to the offspring.[26] Women not already on therapy should consider waiting until after 10-12 weeks gestation to begin. Regardless of the antepartum antiretroviral regimen and the maternal HIV viral load, zidovudine administration is recommended during the intrapartum period and for the newborn for 6 weeks.

Adverse Effects – PI therapy may contribute to development of hyperglycemia in the mother. Some studies suggest that antenatal combination antiretroviral therapy including a PI may be associated with premature birth.[27] However, most clinicians believe that the overwhelming benefit of a potent antiretroviral regimen greatly outweighs the risk.

Already in Labor – For women who are already in labor and have had no antiretroviral therapy, **zidovudine** given to the mother and continued in the infant for 6 weeks or given only to the infant for 6 weeks beginning within 8-12 hours after birth, can decrease HIV transmission. A combination of **zidovudine plus lamivudine** given at the onset of labor and to the infant for one week is also effective. **Single-dose nevirapine** given to the mother at the onset of labor and to the infant at 48-72 hours after delivery, either alone or combined with zidovudine, can decrease the risk of perinatal transmission and may be more effective than zidovudine alone, but single-dose nevirapine has been associated with emergence of nevirapine-resistant strains, which could compromise future treatment of mother and child. For the mother, adding lamivudine/zidovudine and continuing for 3 to 7 days postpartum decreases the risk of nevirapine resistance.[28]

Drugs Not to be Used – Fatal lactic acidosis from the combination of stavudine and didanosine has occurred in pregnant women; this combination should not be used. Efavirenz should be avoided in pregnancy, especially in the first trimester, because of potential teratogenicity. Initiation of nevirapine in pregnancy should be avoided in women with CD4 counts >250 cells/mm^3 because of the increased risk of hepatotoxicity. This restriction does not apply to single-dose nevirapine.

SUMMARY

Depending on the results of resistance testing, reasonable first choices for initial therapy of HIV infection would include either an NNRTI, often efavirenz because it has fewer adverse effects than nevirapine, or a boosted PI combination such as lopinavir/ritonavir *(Kaletra)*, either combined with 2 NRTIs. If an NNRTI- or PI-based regimen cannot be used, a final option for initial therapy would be abacavir plus lamivudine and zidovudine. For more advanced disease, combinations should be based on resistance testing and include two or more fully active drugs. Regimens containing darunavir or tipranavir, either combined with enfuvirtide, may be particularly helpful in heavily pretreated patients. For all patients, regular monitoring of viral load and CD4 cell count should be used to guide therapy. NNRTIs and PIs have many adverse interactions with each other and with other drugs.[11]

1. Department of Health and Human Services Panel on Antiretroviral Guidelines for Adults and Adolescents. Guidelines for the use of antiretroviral agents in HIV-1-infected adults and adolescents. Revised May 4, 2006. Available at www.aidsinfo.nih.gov; accessed on September 12, 2006.
2. SM Hammer et al. Treatment for adult HIV infection: 2006 recommendations of the International AIDS Society – USA panel. JAMA 2006; 296:827.
3. JE Gallant et al. Early virological nonresponse to tenofovir, abacavir, and lamivudine in HIV-infected antiretroviral-naïve subjects. J Infect Dis 2005;192:1921.
4. RM Gulick et al. Three- vs four-drug antiretroviral regimens for the initial treatment of HIV-1 infection: a randomized controlled trial. JAMA 2006; 296:769.
5. D Maitland et al. Early virologic failure in HIV-1 infected subjects on didanosine/tenofovir/efavirenz: 12-week results from a randomized trial. AIDS 2005; 19:1183.
6. A Barrios et al. Paradoxical CD4 + T-cell decline in HIV-infected patients with complete virus suppression taking tenofovir and didanosine. AIDS 2005; 19:569.
7. Atazanavir (Reyataz) and emtricitabine (Emtriva) for HIV infection. Med Lett Drugs Ther 2003; 45:90.
8. M Nunez et al. Activity of tenofovir on hepatitis B virus replication in HIV-co-infected patients failing or partially responding to lamivudine. AIDS 2002; 16:2352.
9. R Bruno et al. Rapid hepatitis B virus-DNA decay in co-infected HIV-hepatitis B virus 'e-minus' patients with YMDD mutations after 4 weeks of tenofovir therapy. AIDS 2003; 17:783.

10. HJ Ribaudo et al. Pharmacogenetics of plasma efavirenz exposure after treatment discontinuation: an Adult AIDS Clinical Trials Group Study. Clin Infect Dis 2006; 42:401.

11. The Medical Letter Adverse Drug Interactions Program.

12. DB Clifford et al. Impact of efavirenz on neuropsychological performance and symptoms in HIV-infected individuals. Ann Intern Med 2005; 143:714.

13. F Gutierrez et al. Prediction of neuropsychiatric adverse events associated with long-term efavirenz therapy, using plasma drug level monitoring. Clin Infect Dis 2005; 41:1648.

14. BO Taiwo. Nevirapine toxicity. Int J STD AIDS 2006;17:364.

15. JE Gallant et al. Tenofovir DF, emtricitabine, and efavirenz vs. zidovudine, lamivudine, and efavirenz for HIV. N Engl J Med 2006; 354:251.

16. J Gallant et al. Efficacy and safety of tenofovir (TDF), emtricitabine (FTC) and efavirenz (EFV) compared to fixed dose zidovudine/lamivudine (CBV) and EFV through 96 weeks in antiretroviral treatment-naïve patients. 16th International AIDS Conference, August 2006; abstract TUPE0064.

17. Darunavir (Prezista) for HIV infection. Med Lett Drugs Ther 2006; 48:74.

18. J Eron Jr et al. The KLEAN study of fosamprenavir-ritonavir versus lopinavir-ritonavir, each in combination with abacavir-lamivudine, for initial treatment of HIV infection over 48 weeks: a randomised non-inferiority trial. Lancet 2006; 368:476.

19. R Verdon et al. Indinavir-induced cholelithiasis in a patient infected with human immunodeficiency virus. Clin Infect Dis 2002; 35:e57.

20. Lopinavir/ritonavir: a protease inhibitor combination. Med Lett Drugs Ther 2001; 43:1.

21. Tipranavir (Aptivus) for HIV. Med Lett Drugs Ther 2005; 47:83.

22. CB Hicks et al. Durable efficacy of tipranavir-ritonavir in combination with an optimised background regimen of antiretroviral drugs for treatment-experienced HIV-1-infected patients at 48 weeks in the Randomized Evaluation of Strategic Intervention in multidrug reSistant patients with Tipranavir (RESIST) studies: an analysis of combined data from two randomised open-label trials. Lancet 2006; 368:466.

23. Enfuviritide (Fuzeon) for HIV infection. Med Lett Drugs Ther 2003; 45:49.

24. RA Ball et al. Injection site reactions with the HIV-1 fusion inhibitor enfuvirtide. J Am Acad Dermatol 2003; 49:826.

25. EM Connor et al. Reduction of maternal-infant transmission of human immunodeficiency virus type 1 with zidovudine treatment. Pediatric AIDS Clinical Trials Group Protocol 076 Study Group. N Engl J Med 1994; 331:1173.

26. Public Health Service Task Force. Recommendations for use of antiretroviral drugs in pregnant HIV-1-infected women and for maternal health and interventions to reduce perinatal HIV-1 transmission in the United States. Revised July 6, 2006. Available at www.aidsinfo.nih.gov; accessed on September 12, 2006.

27. AM Cotter et al. Is antiretroviral therapy during pregnancy associated with an increased risk of preterm delivery, low birth weight, or stillbirth? J Infect Dis 2006; 193:1195.

28. ML Chaix et al. Low risk of nevirapine resistance mutations in the prevention of mother-to-child transmission of HIV-1: Agence Nationale de Recherches sur le SIDA Ditrame Plus, Abidjan, Cote d'Ivoire. J Infect Dis 2006; 193:482.

Two New Drugs for HIV Infection
Originally published in The Medical Letter – January 2008; 50:2

Raltegravir (*Isentress* – Merck), the first in a new class of oral HIV drugs called HIV-1 integrase strand transfer inhibitors (InSTI), has received accelerated FDA approval for use in combination therapy for treatment-experienced adults infected with HIV-1 strains resistant to multiple antiretroviral agents.[1]

Maraviroc (*Selzentry* – Pfizer), the first CCR5 (CC chemokine receptor 5) antagonist has received the same FDA approval but is restricted to use in adults with CCR5-tropic HIV-1 ("R5 virus"). A commercial assay is available for R5 tropism.

MECHANISM OF ACTION — HIV-1 integrase catalyzes the process that results in viral DNA insertion into the host cell genome. **Raltegravir** inhibits the enzyme's activity, preventing viral DNA from integrating with cellular DNA. It is active against HIV strains resistant to other antiretroviral drugs.

CCR5 is the major co-receptor involved in viral entry into the cell for CCR5-tropic HIV-1 strains; these strains predominate during the early stages of infection and remain dominant in 50-60% of late-stage disease.[1] **Maraviroc** binds to the CCR5 co-receptor, preventing the virus from entering the host cell. Like raltegravir, it is active against HIV strains resistant to other antiretroviral drugs.

CLINICAL STUDIES — Raltegravir – A dose-ranging study in 178 patients with treatment-refractory HIV-1 infection found that, compared to those taking a placebo plus optimized background therapy (OBT), more patients taking raltegravir 200-600 mg bid plus OBT had viral loads of <400 copies/mL (70-71% vs. 16%) and <50 copies/mL (56-67% vs. 13%) after 24 weeks.[2] These results were largely maintained through 48 weeks.[3]

Two New Drugs for HIV Infection

PHARMACOLOGY

	Raltegravir	Maraviroc
Drug class	InST inhibitor	CCR5 antagonist
Formulation	400-mg tablets	150-mg and 300-mg tablets
Route	Oral	Oral
Elimination half-life	9 hrs	14-18 hrs
Metabolism	Glucuronidation in liver	CYP3A4 and P-glycoprotein
Excretion	Urine: 32% (9% unchanged) Feces: 51%	Urine: ~20% (8% unchanged) Feces: ~76% (25% unchanged)

FDA approval of raltegravir was based on pooled interim 24-week results (see table on page 194) from two unpublished, identical, randomized double-blind trials (BENCHMRK 1 & 2) in a total of 699 patients infected with HIV-1. Patients with virus resistant to at least one drug from each of 3 antiretroviral drug classes[4] received OBT plus either raltegravir (400 mg twice daily) or placebo.

A 48-week study in 198 **treatment-naïve patients** infected with HIV-1 compared various doses of raltegravir (100-600 bid) with efavirenz 600 mg once/day, each combined with tenofovir and lamivudine. Raltegravir was similar in efficacy to efavirenz after 24 and 48 weeks, and produced more rapid declines in viral loads.[5]

Maraviroc – FDA approval of maraviroc was based on pooled interim 24-week results (see table on page 194) from two unpublished, identical, double-blind placebo-controlled studies (MOTIVATE 1 & 2) in a total of 1,076 patients infected with HIV-1 virus resistant to at least one drug from each of 3 classes. Patients receiving OBT plus maraviroc (150 or

300 mg once or twice daily, depending on their background therapy) improved more than those receiving placebo, and improvements were sustained through week 48.[6,7]

In a non-inferiority study, maraviroc 300 mg bid was compared to efavirenz 600 mg once/d in **treatment-naïve patients** infected with CCR5-tropic HIV-1 who were also receiving zidovudine/lamivudine. After 48 weeks, maraviroc was "non-inferior" to efavirenz in the percentage of patients achieving HIV-1 RNA <400 copies/mL (70.6% vs. 73.1%), but not for those with <50 copies/mL (65.3% vs. 69.3%).[8]

RESISTANCE — Viral resistance to **raltegravir**, apparently due to mutations in integrase, has occurred in patients not taking any other fully active drugs and was associated with clinical failure.[9]

Viral resistance to **maraviroc** due to emergence of HIV strains that use the CXCR4 ("X4 virus") instead of the CCR5 co-receptor to gain entry into the cell has been described.[10] A commercial assay is available (for about $2000) that can determine whether HIV-1 is R5, X4 or dual-tropic, but it is insensitive and may fail to detect the presence of small numbers of X4-tropic virus, which would proliferate and cause maraviroc to fail.

ADVERSE EFFECTS — The adverse effects of **raltegravir** have included diarrhea, nausea and headache and were comparable in incidence to those with placebo. Increases in serum creatine kinase, myopathy and rhabdomyolysis have occurred in clinical trials, but cause and effect are not clear.

Adverse effects that occurred more often with **maraviroc** than with placebo include cough, pyrexia, upper respiratory tract infection, rash, musculoskeletal symptoms, abdominal pain and postural dizziness. Hepatotoxicity has been reported, sometimes associated with a rash and eosinophilia. In clinical studies, cardiovascular events including

CLINICAL STUDIES

	BENCHMRK 1 & 2 (24-wk pooled results)* Raltegravir (400 mg bid + OBT)	Placebo + OBT
Mean change in HIV-1 RNA ($\log_{10}$ copies/mL)	-1.85	-0.84
% of patients with <400 copies/mL	75.5%	39.3%
% of patients with <50 copies/mL	62.6%	33.3%
Mean change in CD4 count (cells/mm³)	+89	+35

* Summarized in the package insert.
OBT = optimized background therapy

myocardial ischemia and/or infarction occurred in 1.3% of patients taking maraviroc compared to none with placebo. Increases in infection and malignancy are a theoretical concern because some immune cells have CCR5 receptors.

DRUG INTERACTIONS — Raltegravir is metabolized through uridine diphosphate glucuronosyltransferase (UGT) 1A1; caution should be used with coadministration of strong inducers of this enzyme such as rifampin or inhibitors such as the protease inhibitor atazanavir. Raltegravir is not an inducer, inhibitor or substrate of CYP3A4.

Maraviroc is a substrate of CYP3A and P-glycoprotein (P-gp); its metabolism may be affected by inducers or inhibitors of these enzymes/transporters.[11]

| MOTIVATE 1 & 2 (24-wk pooled results)* | |
Maraviroc (150-300 bid + OBT)	Placebo + OBT
-1.96	-0.99
61%	28%
45%	23%
+106	+57

DOSAGE AND COST — The dosage of **raltegravir** is 400 mg twice daily taken orally. Dosage adjustments are not necessary in patients with renal or mild to moderate hepatic dysfunction. The cost for 30 days treatment with *Isentress* is $972.[12]

Maraviroc is available in 150- and 300-mg tablets. The recommended dosage is 150 mg bid when given with strong CYP3A inhibitors, including protease inhibitors (except that the dose with the combination of tipranavir and ritonavir is 300 mg bid), and is 600 mg bid when given with CYP3A inducers such as efavirenz. A dose of 300 mg bid can be used with nevirapine, all NRTIs and enfuvirtide. The cost of *Selzentry* 150 or 300 mg bid is $1044 per month.[12]

CONCLUSION — **Raltegravir** *(Isentress),* the first integrase strand transfer inhibitor, taken with other active antiretroviral drugs is effective

Two New Drugs for HIV Infection

in patients infected with treatment-refractory HIV-1 infection. **Maraviroc** *(Selzentry),* the first CCR5 antagonist, is also effective in combination therapy for patients failing other antiretroviral drugs, but only about 50% of treatment-experienced patients will be eligible to take it.

1. P Dorr et al. Maraviroc (UK-427,857), a potent, orally bioavailable, and selective small-molecule inhibitor of chemokine receptor CCR5 with broad-spectrum anti-human immunodeficiency virus type 2 activity. Antimicrob Agents Chemother 2005; 49: 4721.

2. B Grinsztejn et al. Safety and efficacy of the HIV-1 integrase inhibitor raltegravir (MK-0518) in treatment-experienced patients with multidrug-resistant virus: a phase II randomized controlled trial. Lancet 2007; 369:1261.

3. B Grinsztejn et al. 48 week efficacy and safety of MK-0518, a novel HIV-1 integrase inhibitor, in patients with triple-class resistant virus. 47th ICAAC; Chicago, Illinois, September 17-20, 2007; abstract H-713.

4. Drugs for HIV infection. Treat Guidel Med Lett 2006; 4:67.

5. M Markowitz et al. Rapid and durable antiretroviral effect of the HIV-1 Integrase inhibitor raltegravir as part of combination therapy in treatment-naive patients with HIV-1 infection: results of a 48-week controlled study. J Acquir Immune Defic Syndr 2007; 46:125.

6. J Lalezari and H Mayer. The MOTIVATE 1 Study Team. Efficacy and safety of maraviroc in antiretroviral treatment-experienced patients infected with CCR5-tropic HIV-1: 48-week results of MOTIVATE 1. 47th ICAAC; Chicago, Illinois, September 17-20, 2007; Abstract H-718a.

7. G Fätkenheuer et al. Efficacy and safety of maraviroc plus optimized background therapy in viraemic, antiretroviral treatment-experienced patients infected with CCR5-tropic HIV-1 in Europe, Australia and North America (MOTIVATE 2): 48-week results. 11th European AIDS Conference; Madrid, Spain, October 24-27, 2007; Abstract PS3/5.

8. M Saag et al. A multicenter, randomized, double-blind, comparative trial of a novel CCR5 antagonist, maraviroc versus efavirenz, both in combination with Combivir (zidovudine [ZDV]/lamivudine [3TC]), for the treatment of antiretroviral naïve patients infected with R5 HIV 1: Week 48 results of the MERIT study. Special session: 4th IAS Conference on HIV Pathogenesis, Treatment and Prevention 2007: abstract WESS104.

9. DJ Hazuda et al. Resistance to the HIV-integrase inhibitor Raltegravir: analysis of protocol 005, a phase 2 study in patients with triple-class resistant HIV-1 infection. Program and abstracts of the XVI International HIV Drug Resistance Workshop, June 12-16, 2007, abstract 8. Available at www.natap.org/2007/Resiswksp/ResisWksp_37.htm.

10. M Westby. Emergence of CXCR4-using human immunodeficiency virus Type 1 (HIV-1) variants in a minority of HIV-1-infected patients following treatment with the CCR5 antagonist maraviroc is from a pretreatment CXCR4-using virus reservoir. J Virol 2006; 80:4909.

11. CYP3A and drug interactions. Med Lett Drugs Ther 2005; 47:54.

12. Price according to AWP listings in *Red Book Update*, January 2008.

DRUGS FOR
Non-HIV Viral Infections

Original publication date – July 2007

The drugs of choice for treatment of non-HIV viral infections with their dosages and cost are listed in the tables on the pages that follow. Some of the indications and dosages recommended here have not been approved by the FDA. Vaccines used in the prevention of viral infections are discussed in the "Adult Immunization" issue of *Treatment Guidelines*.[1]

DRUGS FOR HERPES SIMPLEX AND
VARICELLA-ZOSTER VIRUS

ACYCLOVIR (*Zovirax*, and others) — Available in topical, oral and intravenous (IV) formulations, acyclovir is used to treat herpes simplex virus (HSV) and varicella-zoster virus (VZV) infections. Topical acyclovir cream reduces the duration of herpes labialis (cold sores) by about half a day. Oral acyclovir is effective for primary orolabial, genital and anorectal HSV infection as well as for recurrent orolabial and genital HSV infections. Long-term oral suppression with acyclovir decreases the frequency of symptomatic genital HSV recurrences and asymptomatic viral shedding. Oral acyclovir begun within 24 hours after the onset of rash decreases the severity of primary varicella infection and can also be used to treat localized zoster. IV acyclovir is the drug of choice for treatment of HSV infections that are visceral, disseminated or

DRUGS FOR HERPES SIMPLEX VIRUS

Infection	Drug	Adult dosage[1]	Cost[2]
OROLABIAL			
Topical			
	Acyclovir – *Zovirax*	5% cream 5x/d x 4d	$46.86[3]
	Docosanol – *Abreva*[4]	10% cream 5x/d until healing	14.98[5]
	Penciclovir – *Denavir*	1% cream applied q2h while awake x 4d	36.59[6]
Oral			
	Acyclovir – generic	400 mg PO 5x/d q4h x 5d	48.25
	Zovirax		104.75
	Famciclovir – *Famvir*	1500 mg PO single dose	31.89
	Valacyclovir – *Valtrex*	2 g PO q12h x 1d	44.28
GENITAL			
First episode			
	Acyclovir – generic	400 mg PO tid or 200 mg	29.40
	Zovirax	PO 5x/d x 7-10d[7]	75.95
	Famciclovir[8] – *Famvir*	250 mg PO tid x 7-10d	111.13
	Valacyclovir – *Valtrex*	1 g PO bid x 7-10d	154.98
Episodic treatment of recurrences[9]			
	Acyclovir – generic	800 mg PO tid x 2d or	17.37
	Zovirax	400 mg PO tid x 3-5d[10]	37.71
	Famciclovir – *Famvir*	1 g PO bid x 1d[11]	42.52
	Valacyclovir – *Valtrex*	500 mg PO bid x 3d	35.40
Suppression of recurrences[12]			
	Acyclovir – generic	400 mg PO bid	115.80[13]
	Zovirax		251.40[13]
	Famciclovir – *Famvir*	250 mg PO bid	318.00[13]
	Valacyclovir – *Valtrex*	500 mg - 1 g PO 1x/d[14]	177.00[13]
MUCOCUTANEOUS IN IMMUNOCOMPROMISED PATIENTS			
	Acyclovir – generic IV	5 mg/kg IV q8h x 7-14d[15]	452.76
	generic PO or	400 mg PO 5x/d x 7-10d	67.55
	Zovirax PO		146.65

Continued on next page.

DRUGS FOR HERPES SIMPLEX VIRUS (continued)

Infection	Drug	Adult dosage[1]	Cost[2]
MUCOCUTANEOUS IN IMMUNOCOMPROMISED PATIENTS (continued)			
	Famciclovir – *Famvir*	500 mg PO bid x 7-10d	148.82
	Valacyclovir[8] – *Valtrex*	500 mg-1 g PO bid x 7-10d	82.60
ENCEPHALITIS			
	Acyclovir – generic	10-15 mg/kg IV q8h x 14-21d[16]	1,811.04
NEONATAL			
	Acyclovir – generic	10-20 mg/kg IV q8h x 14-21d	77.62[17]
KERATOCONJUNCTIVITIS[18]			
	Trifluridine – generic	1% ophth solution 1 drop q2h (max 9 drops/d)[19]	99.38[20]
	Viroptic		115.13[20]
ACYCLOVIR-RESISTANT			
Severe infection, immunocompromised			
	Foscarnet – generic	40 mg/kg IV q8h x 14-21d	1,323.00
	Foscavir		1,809.57

1. Dosage adjustment may be required for renal insufficiency.
2. Based on the lowest recommended dosage for a 70-kg patient, according to the most recent data (April 30, 2007) from retail pharmacies nationwide, available from Wolters Kluwer Health. For IV drugs, the cost of administration may increase the total cost. For generic drugs, average cost is given.
3. Based on purchase of 2-g tube.
4. Available without a prescription.
5. Based on purchase of 0.07 oz (2 g) tube on drugstore.com (June 1, 2007).
6. Based on purchase of 1.5-g tube containing 15 mg of penciclovir on drugstore.com (June 1, 2007).
7. For severe infection, IV acyclovir (5-10 mg/kg q8h for 5-7d) can be used.
8. Not approved by the FDA for this indication.
9. Antiviral therapy is variably effective and only if started early.
10. No published data are available to support 3 days' use.
11. For recurrent HSV in HIV-positive patients, 500 mg bid for 7d.
12. Some clinicians discontinue treatment for 1-2 mos/yr to assess the frequency of recurrences.
13. For 30 days' therapy.
14. 500 mg once/d in patients with <10 recurrences/yr and 500 mg bid or 1 g/d in patients with ≥10 recurrences/yr.
15. Pediatric dosage (<12 yrs of age) is 10 mg/kg IV q8h x 7-14d.
16. Pediatric dosage (3 mos-12 yrs of age) is 20 mg/kg IV q8h x 14-21d.
17. Based on a 3-kg infant.
18. An ophthalmic preparation of acyclovir is available in some countries. Treatment of HSV ocular infections should be supervised by an ophthalmologist; duration of therapy and dosage depend on response.
19. Once the cornea has re-epithelialized the dose can be decreased to 1 drop q4h x 7d.
20. Based on purchase of a 7.5-mL bottle.

involve the central nervous system (CNS) and for serious or disseminated VZV infections.

Adverse Effects – By any route of administration, acyclovir is generally well tolerated. Gastrointestinal (GI) disturbances and headache can occur. Given IV, the drug may cause phlebitis and inflammation at sites of infusion, or extravasation. IV acyclovir can also cause reversible renal dysfunction due to crystalline nephropathy; rapid infusion, dehydration, renal insufficiency and high dosage increase the risk. IV and, rarely, oral acyclovir have been associated with encephalopathy, including tremors, hallucinations, seizures and coma. Neutropenia and other signs of bone marrow toxicity have been reported rarely.

Pregnancy – Use of acyclovir during pregnancy has not been associated with an increased risk of congenital abnormalities, and many clinicians prescribe the drug for treatment of genital herpes during pregnancy. Suppression of recurrent genital herpes in pregnant women near term may reduce the need for cesarean sections to avoid neonatal herpes infection.

Resistance – Despite widespread use of acyclovir, the development of HSV resistance in immunocompetent subjects is uncommon (prevalence <1%). Resistant virus can be isolated, however, even from treatment-naïve subjects,[2] and should be considered when antiviral response is less than anticipated. Almost all acyclovir-resistant HSV occurs in immunocompromised patients treated with the drug; isolates are usually cross-resistant to famciclovir and valacyclovir. Resistant HSV infection in HIV-positive patients has been associated with progressive mucosal disease and, rarely, visceral involvement. Acyclovir-resistant VZV strains in HIV-positive patients have been associated with chronic cutaneous lesions and, rarely, invasive disease.

Infections with acyclovir-resistant HSV or VZV may respond to foscarnet or cidofovir, which are primarily used for treatment of cytomegalovirus (CMV) infection and are discussed on pages 206 and 207.

DRUGS FOR VARICELLA-ZOSTER VIRUS

Infection	Drug	Adult dosage[1]	Cost[2]
VARICELLA			
	Acyclovir – generic	20 mg/kg (800 mg max) PO	$74.00
	Zovirax	qid x 5d	165.80
HERPES ZOSTER			
	Valacyclovir – *Valtrex*	1 g PO tid x 7d	232.47
	Famciclovir – *Famvir*	500 mg PO tid x 7d	223.23
	Acyclovir – generic	800 mg PO 5x/d x 7-10d	129.50
	Zovirax		290.15
VARICELLA OR ZOSTER IN IMMUNOCOMPROMISED PATIENTS			
	Acyclovir – generic	10 mg/kg IV q8h x 7d[3]	514.50
ACYCLOVIR-RESISTANT ZOSTER			
	Foscarnet[4] – generic	40 mg/kg IV q8h x 10d	1,015.00
	Foscavir		1,292.55[5]

1. Dosage adjustment may be required for renal insufficiency.
2. Cost for the lowest recommended dosage for a 70-kg patient, based on the most recent data (April 30, 2007) from retail pharmacies nationwide available from Wolters Kluwer Health. For IV drugs, the cost of administration may increase the total cost. For generic drugs, average cost is given.
3. Pediatric dosage (≤12 yrs of age) is 20 mg/kg q8h x 7-10d.
4. Not approved by the FDA for this indication.
5. Cost based on AWP listings in *Red Book* 2007.

FAMCICLOVIR *(Famvir)* — Famciclovir, which is rapidly converted to penciclovir after oral administration, is an alternative to acyclovir. It is effective in treating first episodes and recurrences of genital HSV and for chronic suppression. Single-day, patient-initiated famciclovir reduced time to healing of herpes labialis (1 dose) and genital herpes lesions (2 doses) by about 2 days compared to placebo.[3,4] In immunocompromised patients with herpes zoster, famciclovir begun within 72 hours after onset of rash is effective in speeding the resolution of zoster-associated pain and shortening the duration of postherpetic neuralgia.

Resistance – HSV and VZV strains resistant to acyclovir are generally also resistant to famciclovir.

Adverse Effects – Famciclovir is generally well tolerated. Headache, nausea and diarrhea have been reported. Like acyclovir, famciclovir is classified as category B for use in pregnancy.

VALACYCLOVIR *(Valtrex)* — Valacyclovir is an L-valyl ester of acyclovir that is metabolized to acyclovir after oral administration, resulting in higher serum concentrations than with oral acyclovir. Acyclovir serum concentrations following high doses of oral valacyclovir resemble those following IV administration of acyclovir.

For herpes labialis, 1 day of oral valacyclovir therapy improves time to healing by 1 day and reduces duration of discomfort by half a day compared to placebo.[5] In first-episode or recurrent genital herpes, valacyclovir twice daily is as effective as acyclovir given 5 times a day. Valacyclovir 500 mg once daily is effective for suppression of genital HSV. Daily suppressive therapy was shown to reduce clinical and subclinical shedding by 64% and 58% respectively.[6] One 8-month study of discordant heterosexual couples found that suppressive valacyclovir taken by the infected partner reduced the risk of HSV transmission to the susceptible partner by about half.[7] A higher dose (500 mg twice daily or 1 g once daily) may be needed for suppression in patients with frequent recurrences. One study suggested that valacyclovir is superior to famciclovir for virologic suppression of recurrent genital herpes.[8] Suppressive therapy with valacyclovir 500 mg twice daily was shown in one small study to decrease HIV shedding and viral load in HSV-HIV coinfected women with an average CD4 count of about 450 cells/mm^3 who were not being treated with HAART; the long-term effects on outcomes are not clear.[9]

Adverse Effects – Valacyclovir is generally well tolerated; adverse effects are similar to those with acyclovir. GI disturbance, headache, rash, CNS effects such as hallucinations and confusion, and nephrotoxicity can occur. Thrombotic thrombocytopenic purpura/hemolytic uremic syndrome has been reported in some severely immunocompromised patients taking high doses (8 g/day). Like acyclovir, valacyclovir is classified as category B for use in pregnancy.

Resistance – Isolates resistant to acyclovir are also resistant to valacyclovir.

OTHER TOPICAL DRUGS — Penciclovir *(Denavir)* – Topical penciclovir 1% cream applied every 2 hours while awake decreases the healing time of recurrent orolabial herpes by about 0.7 days in immunocompetent adults.[10]

Docosanol *(Abreva)* – Topical docosanol cream, available without a prescription, started within 12 hours of prodromal symptoms, decreases healing time by about half a day in recurrent orolabial herpes. Application site reaction, rash and pruritus are common adverse effects.

Trifluridine (*Viroptic*, and others) – Trifluridine is a nucleoside analog active against herpes viruses, including acyclovir-resistant strains. Marketed as an ophthalmic preparation, it is approved for treatment of HSV keratoconjunctivitis and recurrent epithelial keratitis. It is also active against vaccinia virus and has been used to treat accidental ocular infection following smallpox vaccination.[11]

DRUGS FOR CYTOMEGALOVIRUS

GANCICLOVIR (*Cytovene*, and others) — IV ganciclovir is FDA-approved for both induction and maintenance treatment of cytomegalovirus (CMV) retinitis in immunocompromised patients and for prevention of CMV infection in transplant recipients. It is also used to treat CMV infections in other sites (colon, esophagus, lungs, etc.) and for preemptive treatment of immunosuppressed patients with CMV anti-

DRUGS FOR CYTOMEGALOVIRUS

	Drug	Adult dosage[1]	Cost[2]
CYTOMEGALOVIRUS (CMV)[3]			
	Valganciclovir – *Valcyte*	900 mg PO bid x 21d followed by 900 mg once/d	$3,097.92 2,212.80[4]
or	Ganciclovir – *Cytovene*	5 mg/kg IV q12h x 14-21d followed by 5 mg/kg IV once/d	1,087.80
		or 6 mg/kg IV 5x/wk	932.40[4]
	generic	or 1 g PO tid[5]	1,377.60[4]
	Vitrasert implant[6]	4.5 mg intraocularly q5-8 mos	5,400.00[7]
or	Foscarnet – generic *Foscavir*	60 mg/kg IV q8h or 90 mg/kg IV q12h x 14-21d followed by 90-120 mg/kg IV once/d[9]	2,131.50[8] 2,714.36[8,10]
or	Cidofovir – *Vistide*	5 mg/kg IV once/wk x 2 then 5 mg/kg IV q2wks[11]	1,553.91[8]

1. Dosage adjustment may be required for renal insufficiency.
2. Cost for the lowest recommended dosage for a 70-kg patient, based on most recent data (April 30, 2007) from retail pharmacies nationwide available from Wolters Kluwer Health. For generic drugs, average cost is given. For IV drugs, the cost of administration may exceed the total cost.
3. Chronic suppression is recommended in AIDS and in other highly immunocompromised patients with retinitis. Both oral ganciclovir (1g tid) and valganciclovir (900 mg once/d) are approved for prevention of CMV disease in solid organ transplant recipients.
4. Based on 4 weeks' maintenance therapy.
5. Lower doses of ganciclovir have been used to minimize leukopenia in renal transplant patients with renal insufficiency who are also taking azathioprine *(Imuran)* or mycophenolate mofetil *(CellCept)* (SM Flechner et al. Transplantation 1998; 66:1682).
6. Systemic therapy is recommended to prevent CMV disease in the contralateral eye and other organ systems.
7. Cost of one implant based on AWP listings in *Red Book* 2007.
8. Cost of induction treatment. The cost of 4 weeks' maintenance therapy at the lowest recommended dosage is the same.
9. Higher doses (120 mg/kg/d) may be more effective but less well tolerated.
10. Based on AWP listings in *Red Book* 2007.
11. To minimize renal toxicity patients should receive 1 L 0.9% saline over 1-2 hrs prior to a 1-hour cidofovir infusion; they should also receive oral probenicid 2 g 3 hours prior to infusion of cidofovir and 1 g 2 and 8 hrs after the infusion. Patients who can tolerate additional fluid should receive a second 1 L of 0.9% saline, started immediately after the cidofovir infusion. Not recommended for patients with serum creatinine >1.5 mg/dL, creatinine clearance ≤55 mL/min or proteinuria ≥100 mg/dL (2+ by dipstick). Dose reduction to 3 mg/kg is recommended for serum creatinine 0.3-0.4 mg/dL above baseline.

genemia or viremia. Oral ganciclovir is less effective than IV due to lower bioavailability. It has largely been replaced by valganciclovir.

Prophylactic oral ganciclovir, or IV ganciclovir followed by either oral ganciclovir or high-dose oral acyclovir, reduces the risk of CMV in patients who have had liver transplantation, including seronegative recipients of seropositive donors.

An intraocular implant that releases ganciclovir (*Vitrasert* – Bausch & Lomb) has been more effective than IV ganciclovir for CMV retinitis, but is not effective systemically.

Adverse Effects – In animals, ganciclovir is teratogenic, carcinogenic and mutagenic, and causes aspermatogenesis. It is classified as category C for use in pregnancy, and men treated with the drug should use barrier contraception during treatment and for at least 90 days afterward. Granulocytopenia, anemia and thrombocytopenia, which are usually reversible, are more common with the IV than with the oral formulation. Severe myelosuppression may occur more frequently when the drug is given concurrently with zidovudine (AZT; *Retrovir,* and others), azathioprine (*Imuran,* and others) or mycophenolate mofetil *(CellCept).* Granulocyte-colony-stimulating factors (GM-CSF; G-CSF) have been used to treat ganciclovir-induced neutropenia. Other adverse effects of systemic ganciclovir include fever, rash, phlebitis, confusion, abnormal liver function, renal dysfunction, headache, GI toxicity and, rarely, psychiatric disturbances and seizures. Intravitreal ganciclovir implants have been associated with vitreous hemorrhage and retinal detachments.

Resistance – Ganciclovir resistance may be associated with persistent viremia and progressive disease. Ganciclovir-resistant CMV can emerge and cause late morbidity when the drug is used for prophylaxis in solid-organ transplant recipients taking highly potent immunosuppressive drugs.[12] CMV strains resistant to ganciclovir *in vitro* may be susceptible to foscarnet or cidofovir.

VALGANCICLOVIR *(Valcyte)* — Valganciclovir, an oral prodrug of ganciclovir, achieves plasma concentrations similar to those with IV administration of ganciclovir; it has largely replaced oral ganciclovir. Valganciclovir is as effective as IV ganciclovir for induction and mainte-nance therapy of CMV retinitis in patients with AIDS and has replaced both IV and oral ganciclovir for treatment of patients with CMV retinitis whose lesions are peripheral and not immediately sight threatening. Valganciclovir once daily is as effective as oral ganciclovir taken 3 times a day for prevention of CMV disease in mismatched (Donor [D]+, Recipient [R]-) solid organ transplant recipients.[13] Both prophylactic and preemptive therapy (treatment for "CMV DNAemia" before devel-opment of disease) have been shown to be beneficial in those at risk of CMV disease (D+R-, D+R+, D-R+).[14] Valganciclovir is not FDA-approved for use in liver transplant recipients due to data (summarized in the package insert) showing increased tissue-invasive CMV with valgan-ciclovir compared to ganciclovir (14% vs. 3%) in these patients.

Adverse Effects – Adverse effects are similar to those of IV ganciclovir.

Resistance – Isolates that are resistant to ganciclovir are also resistant to valganciclovir.

FOSCARNET (*Foscavir*, **and others**) — IV foscarnet is an alternative to ganciclovir and valganciclovir for treatment of CMV infection. It is approved for use in CMV retinitis in patients with AIDS, including pro-gressive disease due to ganciclovir-resistant strains, and for treatment of acyclovir-resistant HSV or VZV infections. Foscarnet is more expensive and generally less well tolerated than ganciclovir, and requires controlled infusion rates and large volumes of fluid. In allogeneic stem cell trans-plant recipients who develop CMV infection, treatment with foscarnet is as effective as IV ganciclovir and causes less hematologic toxicity.[15]

Adverse Effects – Renal dysfunction often develops during treatment with foscarnet and is usually reversible, but renal failure requiring dialysis may occur. Renal toxicity is increased in patients receiving other nephrotoxic drugs; adequate hydration may decrease the risk. Nausea, vomiting, anemia, fatigue, headache, genital ulceration, CNS disturbances, hypo- and (rarely) hypercalcemia, hypo- and hyperphosphatemia, hypo-kalemia and hypomagnesemia have also occurred. Foscarnet given with zidovudine may increase the risk of anemia. The risk of severe hypocalcemia, sometimes fatal, is increased by concurrent use of IV pentamidine (*Pentam*, and others). It causes chromosomal damage *in vitro* and *in vivo*. Rapid infusion of the drug has been associated with seizures and arrhythmias. Foscarnet is classified as category C for use during pregnancy.

Resistance – HSV, VZV and CMV strains resistant to foscarnet can emerge during treatment. Combined use of foscarnet and ganciclovir may benefit some patients, but CMV strains resistant to both ganciclovir and foscarnet have been reported.

CIDOFOVIR *(Vistide)* — IV cidofovir is used for treatment of CMV retinitis in AIDS patients who are failing ganciclovir or foscarnet therapy. Given once weekly for 2 weeks and then once every 2 weeks for maintenance therapy, cidofovir can delay progression of CMV retinitis in patients with AIDS. Cidofovir has been used to treat other CMV infections (pneumonitis, gastroenteritis), acyclovir- or foscarnet-resistant HSV infections, certain forms of human papillomavirus disease, and invasive adenoviral and BK virus infections in transplant populations.

Adverse Effects – About 25% of patients discontinue cidofovir because of adverse effects such as nephrotoxicity, neutropenia and metabolic acidosis. To decrease the risk of nephrotoxicity, IV 0.9% saline and oral probenecid must be given with each cidofovir dose. Cidofovir is contraindicated in patients taking other nephrotoxic agents. Iritis, uveitis or ocular hypotony can also occur. Adverse effects are more common in patients simultaneously taking antiretroviral drugs. The drug is carcinogenic, teratogenic and causes hypospermia in animals. It is classified as category C for use in pregnancy.

DRUGS FOR INFLUENZA A AND B

Drug[1]	Adult Dosage[2]	
	Prophylaxis	Treatment
Oseltamivir – Tamiflu[4]	75 mg PO 1x/d[5]	75 mg PO bid[5]
Zanamivir – Relenza[6]	2x 5 mg oral inhalations 1x/d	2x 5 mg oral inhalations bid

1. Antiviral drugs may interfere with the efficacy of *FluMist*, the live-attenuated intranasal vaccine (Med Lett Drugs Ther 2006; 48:81); they should be stopped at least 48 hours before and should not be started for ≥2 weeks after *FluMist* administration. Inactivated vaccines *(Fluarix, Fluvirin, Fluzone, FluLaval)* are not affected by antiviral drug therapy.
2. For prophylaxis of exposures in institutions, the drug should be taken for at least 2 weeks, and must be continued for 1 week after the end of the outbreak. For postexposure prophylaxis in households, shorter courses (10 days) may be effective. For treatment of infection, the duration is usually 5 days.

Resistance – Most ganciclovir-resistant CMV isolates remain sensitive to cidofovir, but cross-resistance can occur. Acyclovir-resistant HSV or VZV frequently are susceptible to cidofovir.

FOMIVIRSEN *(Vitravene)* — Fomivirsen, an antisense oligonucleotide, was FDA-approved for intravitreal treatment of CMV retinitis in HIV-infected patients who cannot tolerate or have not responded to other drugs.[16] It is no longer commercially available in the US.

DRUGS FOR INFLUENZA

OSELTAMIVIR *(Tamiflu)* — This oral neuraminidase inhibitor is a prodrug that is rapidly converted to the active antiviral during absorption. Started within 48 hours of symptom onset, it can decrease the severity and duration of symptoms caused by either influenza A or B in

Pediatric Dosage[2]		
Prophylaxis	Treatment	Cost[3]
≥1 yr:	**≥1 yr:**	
≤15 kg: 30 mg PO 1x/d[5]	≤15 kg: 30 mg PO bid[5]	$80.20
16-23 kg: 45 mg PO 1x/d[5]	16-23 kg: 45 mg PO bid[5]	
24-40 kg: 60 mg PO 1x/d[5]	24-40 kg: 60 mg PO bid[5]	
>40 kg: 75 mg PO 1x/d[5]	>40 kg: 75 mg PO bid[5]	
≥5 yrs: 2x 5 mg oral	**≥7 yrs:** 2x 5 mg oral	
inhalations 1x/d	inhalations bid	64.20

3. Cost for 5 days' treatment at adult dosage, according to the most recent data (April 30, 2007) from retail pharmacies nationwide available from Wolters Kluwer Health.
4. Available as capsules (75 mg) or a powder for oral suspension (60 mg/5 mL; 25 mL bottle). Approved for treatment and prophylaxis of influenza in patients ≥1 year old.
5. In patients with CrCl between 10-30 mL/min, doses should be given every other day for prophylaxis and once/d for treatment.
6. Available as a packet containing 5 rotadisks; each rotadisk contains 4 blisters of drug (5 mg each blister). Approved for treatment of children ≥7 years old and prophylaxis of children ≥5 years.

both children and adults. In retrospective pooled analyses, treatment of proven influenza infection has been reported to lower the incidence of influenza-related lower respiratory tract complications.[17,18] Taken prophylactically, oseltamivir has been effective in preventing clinical influenza.[19] Prophylaxis is indicated to control institutional influenza outbreaks and protect high-risk patients immunized after or <2 weeks before an epidemic has begun. The drug can also be used as prophylaxis for immunodeficient patients who may respond poorly to influenza vaccine, and in unvaccinated persons who are at high risk for influenza or are caring for high-risk patients.

Oseltamivir has been effective against clinical isolates of avian influenza and is the drug of choice for prophylaxis and treatment of H5N1 disease.[20]

Adverse Effects – Nausea, vomiting and headache are the most common adverse effects of oseltamivir. Taking the drug with food decreases the incidence of nausea. In juvenile rats, very high doses of oseltamivir (about 250 times the recommended pediatric dose) have been associated with deaths and unexpectedly high concentrations in the brain, possibly related to an immature blood-brain barrier. Oseltamivir has been used in infants, but is FDA-approved only for patients 1 year and older.

Pregnancy – Both oseltamivir and zanamivir are classified as category C for use during pregnancy.

Resistance – During treatment, resistant variants emerge in about 1% of immunocompetent adults and in about 9% of children. No person-to-person transmission of resistant variants has been documented to date. Higher levels of resistance have been described during oseltamivir therapy of H5N1 infection.[21]

ZANAMIVIR *(Relenza)* — Started within 2 days after onset of symptoms, this orally inhaled neuraminidase inhibitor can shorten the duration of illness and may decrease the incidence of lower respiratory complications. It is FDA-approved for treatment of acute uncomplicated influenza A or B in patients ≥7 years of age. Once-daily inhaled zanamivir is approved for prophylaxis of influenza in patients ≥5 years of age. Zanamivir has been effective against some avian strains of influenza in animal studies and should be effective for prophylaxis and treatment of H5N1 disease, but human data are lacking.[20]

Adverse Effects – Nasal and throat discomfort and cough can occur. Bronchospasm, sometimes severe, has been reported uncommonly in patients with reactive airway disease; zanamivir should be avoided in such patients. It has rarely caused bronchospasm in previously healthy persons with influenza.

Pregnancy – Zanamivir is classified as category C for use during pregnancy.

Resistance – Zanamivir is active against amantadine/rimantadine-resistant influenza A and some oseltamivir-resistant strains. Zanamivir resistance has been described in an immunocompromised patient.

AMANTADINE (*Symmetrel*, and others) and RIMANTADINE (*Flumadine*, and others) — Treatment with oral amantadine or rimantadine begun within 48 hours after the onset of illness can decrease the duration of fever and symptoms by about 1 day. Whether these drugs decrease influenza-related complications or are effective in treating severe influenza pneumonia is unknown. Neither amantadine nor rimantadine is effective against influenza B virus.

Amantadine and rimantadine have been 70-90% effective in preventing influenza A when started before exposure.[22] In recent years, however, widespread resistance of influenza A to amantadine and rimantadine has occurred, and these drugs are therefore not currently recommended for prophylaxis or treatment of influenza in the US.[23]

Adverse Effects – Amantadine may cause anorexia, nausea, peripheral edema and, particularly in the elderly, minor CNS effects such as nervousness, anxiety, insomnia, lethargy, difficulty concentrating, and lightheadedness. These effects usually diminish after the first week of use and rapidly disappear after the drug is stopped. Serious CNS effects (confusion, hallucinations, seizures) can occur, especially with old age, renal insufficiency, seizure disorders, concomitant CNS stimulant or anticholinergic drug therapy and underlying psychiatric illness. Amantadine is excreted mainly in urine; the dose must be reduced for creatinine clearance below 50 mL/min.

Rimantadine has GI adverse effects similar to those of amantadine, but a lower risk of CNS effects. It is extensively metabolized by the liver before renal excretion, so dosage reductions are not needed until the creatinine clearance falls below 10 mL/min.

Pregnancy – Both amantadine and rimantadine are teratogenic in animals and contraindicated during pregnancy.

Resistance – Influenza A viruses cross-resistant to both amantadine and rimantadine can emerge when either drug is used for treatment or prophylaxis of influenza. Viruses resistant to amantadine and rimantadine are transmissible from person to person and retain their pathogenicity. They are almost always still susceptible to oseltamivir and zanamivir. Resistance to amantadine and rimantadine has occurred in human isolates of avian H5N1 influenza virus.[24]

DRUGS FOR HEPATITIS B AND C

INTERFERON ALFA — Interferon alfa is available as alfacon-1 *(Infergen)*, alfa-n3 *(Alferon N)*, alfa-2a *(Roferon-A)*, alfa-2b *(Intron A)*, pegylated alfa-2b *(PEG-Intron)*, and pegylated alfa-2a *(Pegasys)*.

In about one third of patients with chronic **hepatitis B**, treatment with interferon alfa-2b leads to loss of HBeAg, return to normal aminotransferase activity, sustained histological improvement and, in adults, a lower risk of progressive liver disease. AIDS patients coinfected with hepatitis B virus (HBV), however, generally respond poorly to interferon. Hepatitis D (hepatitis delta virus), which occurs only in patients infected with HBV, may respond to treatment with high doses of interferon alfa, but relapse is common.

The efficacy of peginterferon alfa-2a is similar to or slightly better than that of conventional interferon.[25] Compared to lamivudine, it has been associated with higher rates of sustained response in patients with HBeAg-negative chronic hepatitis B[26] and in HBeAg-positive patients.[27] Peginterferon alfa-2b monotherapy has been effective for patients with

HBeAg-positive chronic hepatitis B; addition of lamivudine was not superior to monotherapy.[28]

Peginterferon plus ribavirin is the treatment of choice for chronic **hepatitis C**; it provides sustained viral responses (SVRs) in 54-63% of patients. In one report, most of the responses were durable for years after treatment.[29] When used as monotherapy, peginterferons once weekly are more effective than standard interferon 3 times a week, producing SVRs in 30-40%. The combination of peginterferon plus ribavirin is more effective than combinations of standard interferons and ribavirin in patients coinfected with HIV and hepatitis C virus (HCV).[30-32] In a retrospective study, use of interferon appeared to decrease the risk of hepatocellular carcinoma in patients with chronic HCV infection, especially among patients with sustained responses.[33,34] In one study, interferon alfa-2b treatment of acute hepatitis C prevented chronic infection in most patients.[35]

Adverse Effects – Intramuscular or subcutaneous injection of interferon is commonly associated with an influenza-like syndrome, especially during the first week of therapy. High-dose or chronic therapy may be limited by bone marrow suppression, profound fatigue, myalgia, weight loss, rash, cough, increased susceptibility to bacterial infections, psychiatric syndromes including depression, anxiety, psychosis, mania, agitation and neurocognitive impairment, increased aminotransferase activity, alopecia, hypo- or hyperthyroidism, tinnitus, reversible hearing loss, auto-antibody formation, retinopathy, pneumonitis and possibly cardiotoxicity. Injection-site reactions and dose-related neutropenia and thrombocytopenia have been more common with pegylated interferon. Autoimmune chronic hepatitis and other autoimmune diseases like thyroiditis may be induced or exacerbated by treatment with interferon.

Granulocyte-colony stimulating factors and erythropoietin *(Procrit, Epogen)* have been used to treat interferon-induced bone marrow suppression. Depression caused by interferon alfa might be treatable with an anti-

DRUGS FOR HEPATITIS B AND C

Drug	Adult dosage[1]	Cost[2]
HEPATITIS B VIRUS (HBV)		
Chronic		
Lamivudine[3] – *Epivir HBV*	100 mg PO 1x/d x 1-3 yrs[4,5]	$3,281.35
Interferon alfa-2b – *Intron A*	5 million units/d or 10 million units 3x/wk SC or IM x 4 mos[6]	8,143.20
Peginterferon alfa-2a – *Pegasys*	180 mcg once/wk SC x 48 wks	21,913.44
Adefovir – *Hepsera*	10 mg PO 1x/d x 1-3 yrs[4]	8,537.35
Entecavir – *Baraclude*	0.5 mg/d PO x 1-3 yrs[4,7]	9,212.60
Telbivudine – *Tyzeka*	600 mg/d PO x 1-3 yrs[4]	7,066.40
HEPATITIS C VIRUS (HCV)		
Chronic		
Peginterferon alfa-2b – *PEG-Intron*	1.5 mcg/kg once/wk SC x 48 wks[8]	20,831.04
plus ribavirin – generic *Rebetol*	800-1200 mg PO/d x 48 wks[8]	8,534.40 / 13,964.16
or Peginterferon alfa-2a – *Pegasys*	180 mcg once/wk SC x 48 wks[8]	21,913.44
plus ribavirin – generic *Copegus*	800-1200 mg PO/d x 48 wks[8]	8,534.40 / 12,888.96
Acute		
Interferon alfa-2b[9] – *Intron A*	5 million units/d x 3 wks, then 3x/wk x 20 wks	1,241.07 / 3,545.90

1. Dosage adjustment may be required for renal insufficiency.
2. Cost for the lowest recommended dosage for a 70-kg patient, according to the most recent data (April 30, 2007) from retail pharmacies nationwide available from Wolters Kluwer Health. For generic drugs, average cost is given.
3. In patients coinfected with HIV, use of lamivudine to treat HBV may result in loss of its usefulness in treating the HIV because patients with active HIV replication rapidly develop resistance to lamivudine monotherapy. *Epivir HBV*, which is formulated in a lower dose, cannot be substituted for lamivudine *(Epivir)* in HIV treatment regimens.
4. Optimal duration of therapy is uncertain. Some experts recommend that treatment continue for 6 mos after anti-HBe serocon-version and negative or stable HBV DNA levels are achieved (EB Keeffe et al. Clin Gastroenterol Hepatol 2004; 2:87).
5. Pediatric dose is 3 mg/kg/d (maximum 100 mg/dose).

Continued on next page.

DRUGS FOR HEPATITIS B AND C (continued)

6. Pediatric dosage is 3 million units/m^2 3x/wk SC for first wk, then 6 million units/m^2 (maximum 10 million units) 3x/wk for 16 to 24 wks.
7. Dose for nucleoside-naïve patients. The recommended dosage for patients who are refractory to lamivudine is 1 mg/d (same price as 0.5 mg/d).
8. Shorter courses (12 rather than 48 wks) and lower ribavirin doses (800 rather than 1000 or 1200 mg/d) appear to be effective for HCV genotypes 2 and 3 but not genotype 1, which is the most common in North America (SJ Hadziyannis et al. Ann Intern Med 2004; 140:346; A Mangia et al. N Engl J Med 2005; 352:2609).
9. Not approved by the FDA for this indication.

depressant without stopping the interferon; some Medical Letter consultants initiate antidepressant therapy prior to initiating interferon. Interferons are classified as category C for use in pregnancy, but are often used together with ribavirin, which is contraindicated for use in pregnancy.

RIBAVIRIN (*Copegus, Rebetol*, and others) — Combination treatment of HCV with peginterferon alfa and oral ribavirin has produced higher sustained response rates than peginterferon alone and is now considered the regimen of choice for chronic HCV. Patients relapsing after interferon monotherapy may still respond to the combination. Ribavirin is not effective as monotherapy for HCV.

Adverse Effects – Systemic ribavirin has been associated with hemolytic anemia. Oral ribavirin plus interferon appears to cause a higher incidence of cough, pruritus and rash than interferon alone. Acute deterioration of respiratory function has been reported with use of ribavirin aerosol *(Virazole)* in infants and in adults with bronchospastic lung disease. The drug should be used with caution in patients coinfected with HIV who are taking zidovudine because of the risk of severe anemia.

Pregnancy – Ribavirin is teratogenic and embryotoxic in animals, and is contraindicated in pregnancy. Pregnant women should not directly care for patients receiving ribavirin aerosol. Patients exposed to the drug should not conceive children during treatment or for 6 months after stopping it.

LAMIVUDINE (3TC; *Epivir HBV*) — This oral antiretroviral nucleoside analog used to treat HIV[36] is also FDA-approved in a lower-dose formulation for treatment of chronic HBV infection. A trial in Asian patients with chronic HBV infection treated for 2 years found that 52% taking lamivudine 100 mg daily had sustained suppression of HBV DNA, 50% had normalization of aminotransferase activity, and seroconversion to anti-HBeAg occurred in 27%.[37] In patients with cirrhosis or advanced fibrosis, treatment for up to 42 months reduces by about half the risk of clinical progression and development of hepatocellular cancer.[38] Lamivudine is also active in chronically infected children aged ≥2 years, with 55% showing sustained normalization of aminotransferase levels, 61% DNA suppression, and 22% anti-HBe seroconversion after 1 year of therapy.[39] Lamivudine appears to reduce the risk of HBV reinfection in liver transplant recipients. Combination therapy with lamivudine and peginterferon alfa-2b, but not standard interferon alfa, may lead to higher response rates than lamivudine monotherapy. In one study, however, the combination of peginterferon alfa-2b and lamivudine was no better than peginterferon alfa-2b alone.[28]

Adverse Effects — Lamivudine is generally well tolerated. Headache, nausea and dizziness are rare. Pancreatitis has been reported in adults and children coinfected with HIV. It is classified as category C for use during pregnancy. Severe exacerbations of hepatitis B including fatal liver failure have resulted from sudden discontinuation of lamivudine therapy.

Resistance — Resistance emerges in 14-32% of HBV-infected patients receiving lamivudine for one year and increases to 69% at 5 years.[40] Resistant variants have been associated with hepatitis flares, rebound viremia and progressive liver disease.

HIV Coinfection — Resistance is more common in patients coinfected with HIV. To minimize resistance, patients who need treatment for both infections should take 2 antiretrovirals that are also active against HBV. Coinfected patients who need treatment for HBV but not HIV should not receive monotherapy with HBV drugs that are also active against HIV, such as lamivudine, emtricitabine or tenofovir. Adefovir may be considered, however, since the theoretical risk of induction of resistance to nucleoside reverse transcriptase inhibitors has not been observed *in vivo*.

ADEFOVIR DIPIVOXIL *(Hepsera)* — This phosphonate nucleotide analog inhibits replication of HBV, including variants resistant to lamivudine. It also has activity against HIV. Adefovir treatment of HBeAg-positive or -negative chronic hepatitis B is associated with marked reductions in HBV DNA levels, aminotransferase normalization in 48-72% of patients, and histologic improvements in 53-64% at 48 weeks.[41,42] More prolonged therapy results in higher rates of response; anti-HBeAg seroconversion occurs in 23% by 72 weeks. Chronic treatment with adefovir for up to 5 years maintained virologic suppression with associated histologic improvement and no increase in toxicity.[43] The antiviral effects of adefovir are similar in lamivudine-resistant HBV infections.[44] Some experts recommend adefovir over lamivudine for long-term treatment of HBeAg-negative or cirrhotic patients because of the high risk of emergence of lamivudine resistance.

Adverse Effects – Doses of adefovir used for HBV infection are generally well tolerated, but may be associated with asthenia, headache, diarrhea and abdominal pain. Higher than recommended doses (30-60 mg/d) and pre-existing renal impairment are risk factors for azotemia and renal tubular dysfunction. Hepatitis flares may occur after the drug is stopped. Adefovir is classified as category C for use in pregnancy.

Resistance – Adefovir-resistant variants emerge at a low frequency (3.9% of patients after 3 years of use and 20% after 5 years)[43] and have been associated with a rebound in HBV DNA levels; these variants may remain susceptible to lamivudine. Primary resistance has been reported.[45]

ENTECAVIR *(Baraclude)* — Entecavir, a deoxyguanosine analog, is more potent than lamivudine and retains some activity against lamivudine-resistant HBV variants.[46] It may have some activity against HIV. Well-absorbed after oral administration, its prolonged plasma half-life (128-149 hours) allows once-daily dosing. Compared with lamivudine, entecavir appears to be more efficacious in reducing hepatitis B DNA levels and normalizing serum aminotransferases, as well as in improving histologic abnormalities.[47] Higher doses are indicated in lamivudine-resistant infections.

Adverse Effects – Entecavir is generally well tolerated. Adverse effects reported during therapy include headache, fatigue, dizziness, nausea, abdominal pain, rhinitis, fever, diarrhea, cough and myalgia. It is classified as category C for use in pregnancy.

Resistance – HBV isolates from lamivudine-refractory patients failing entecavir therapy remained susceptible to adefovir *in vitro*. Entecavir monotherapy probably should not be used in HIV-HBV coinfected patients who need HBV but not HIV treatment (see discussion of HIV coinfection on page 216).

TELBIVUDINE *(Tyzeka)* — Telbivudine, a synthetic thymidine analog, is approved for the treatment of chronic HBV infection.[48] It is not active against HIV. In comparative trials against lamivudine, telbivudine demonstrated greater virologic response at week 52 (60% vs. 40% of subjects HBV DNA-negative).

Adverse Effects – Headache, nausea and vomiting are common with telbivudine. Severe acute exacerbations of hepatitis B have been reported in patients who have discontinued anti-HBV therapy. Myopathy, manifested by muscle aches and/or weakness with increased CPK has been reported rarely. Lactic acidosis and severe hepatomegaly, sometimes fatal, with steatosis have occurred with other nucleoside analogues, but have not yet been reported with telbivudine. It is classified as category B for use in pregnancy.

Resistance – After 2 years of treatment, 21.6% of HBeAg-positive and 8.6% of HBeAg-negative telbivudine recipients had a rebound of HBV DNA that was associated with resistance mutations. Lamivudine-resistant HBV strains have a high level of cross resistance to telbivudine and reduced susceptibility to entecavir, but generally remain susceptible to adefovir. Some adefovir-resistant strains remain susceptible to telbivudine.

TENOFOVIR *(Viread)* **AND EMTRICITABINE** *(Emtriva)* — Although neither drug is approved for treatment of HBV, a combination of tenofovir/emtricitabine *(Truvada)* is commonly used to treat HIV/HBV coinfection. Tenofovir is structurally similar to adefovir; emtricitabine is the 5-fluorinated derivative of lamivudine.

Adverse Effects – Both tenofovir and emtricitabine are generally well tolerated. Tenofovir can cause renal toxicity, and emtricitabine can cause hyperpigmentation. Both drugs are classified as category B for use in pregnancy.

DRUGS FOR PAPILLOMAVIRUS, RESPIRATORY SYNCYTIAL VIRUS, AND OTHER VIRUSES

IMIQUIMOD *(Aldara)* — This immunomodulator is FDA-approved for topical treatment of external and perianal genital warts, which are caused by human papillomavirus (HPV). Gradual clearance of warts occurs in about 50% of patients over an average of 8-10 weeks. Recurrences are less common than after ablative therapies.

Adverse Effects – Application site reactions (irritation, pruritus, flaking, erosion) are generally mild to moderate in intensity and resolve within 2 weeks of cessation. Pigment changes may persist. Systemic adverse effects including fatigue and influenza-like illness have been reported.

DRUGS FOR HPV AND RSV

Drug	Adult dosage	Cost[1]
PAPILLOMAVIRUS - ANOGENITAL WARTS[2]		
Imiquimod – *Aldara*[3]	3x/wk (wash off 6-10 hrs after application) x 16 wks max	$256.56[4]
Podofilox 0.5% – generic *Condylox*[3]	2x/d x 3d, 4 days rest, then repeated up to 4x	84.84[5] 111.34[5]
RESPIRATORY SYNCYTIAL VIRUS (RSV)[6]		
Ribavirin – *Virazole*	aerosol treatment 12-18 hrs/d x 3-7d[7]	5,103.84[8]

1. Cost according to the most recent data (April 30, 2007) from retail pharamacies nationwide available from Wolters Kluwer Health.
2. Trichloroacetic acid, bichloroacetic acid, podophyllin and liquid nitrogen are also often used in doctors' offices to treat genital warts.
3. Pregnancy category C.
4. Cost of a box containing 12 250-mg packets.
5. Cost of a 3.5-mL tube of podofilox 0.5% solution.
6. Immunoprophylaxis with IM palivizumab *(Synagis)*, a monoclonal antibody given by monthly injection, can prevent illness in children <24 mos old with chronic lung disease, in infants who were premature (≤35 wks gestation), and in some children ≤24 mos with congenital heart disease (Committee on Infectious Diseases in LK Pickering eds, *2003 Red Book: Report of the Committee on Infectious Diseases* 26th ed, Evanston, Ill: American Academy of Pediatrics 2003, page 523).
7. Requires respiratory therapy monitoring for administration and a special aerosol-generating device *(Spag-2* – Viratek) that delivers an aerosol containing 190 mcg/L at a rate of 12.5 L/min.
8. Cost of 3 days' treatment using one 6-g vial/d, based on AWP listings in *Red Book* 2007.

PODOFILOX *(Condylox)* — Also known as podophyllotoxin, podofilox is the main cytotoxic ingredient of podophyllin, a resin used for many years for topical treatment of warts. The exact mechanism of action is unknown. Podofilox 0.5% solution or gel is similar in effectiveness to imiquimod but may have more adverse effects.[49] Systemic adverse reactions have not been reported. Local adverse effects of the drug such as pain, burning, inflammation, and erosion occur in more than 50% of patients.

TRICHLOROACETIC ACID, PODOPHYLLIN AND CRYO-THERAPY — Trichloroacetic acid, podophyllin and cryotherapy (with liquid nitrogen or a cryoprobe) remain the most widely used treatments for external genital warts, but the response rate is only 60-70%, and at least 20-30% of responders will have a recurrence.

RIBAVIRIN *(Virazole)* — An aerosal formulation of ribavirin, a synthetic nucleoside, may decrease morbidity in some children hospitalized with respiratory syncytial virus (RSV) bronchiolitis and pneumonia,[50] but because of its potential adverse effects it is not generally recommended for such use. Pregnant women should not directly care for patients receiving ribavirin aerosol. (For adverse effects and use in pregnancy, see page 215.)

Other viruses — IV ribavirin appears to decrease mortality in Lassa fever and in hantavirus hemorrhagic fever with renal syndrome. *In vitro*, high concentrations inhibit West Nile virus, but clinical data are lacking. There are case reports of systemic ribavirin use with some success in cases of LaCrosse encephalitis, Nipah virus encephalitis, and Congo-Crimean hemorrhagic fever, but it is ineffective in SARS and hantavirus cardiopulmonary syndrome.[51]

CIDOFOVIR — IV and topical cidofovir (3% cream, once daily)[52] have been reported to produce resolution of molluscum contagiosum in immunosuppressed patients.[53] Cidofovir has also been used for adenovirus infection in allogeneic stem cell transplant recipients.[54] *In vitro*, cidofovir is active against vaccinia, variola, and other pox viruses and has been effective in animal models of lethal infection with these viruses.[55] (For adverse effects, see page 207.)

1. Adult immunization. Treat Guidel Med Lett 2006; 4:47
2. D Malvy et al. A retrospective, case-control study of acyclovir resistance in herpes simplex virus. Clin Infect Dis 2005; 41:320.

3. SL Spruance et al. Single-dose, patient-initiated famciclovir: a randomized, double-blind, placebo-controlled trial for episodic treatment of herpes labialis. J Am Acad Dermatol 2006; 55:47.

4. FY Aoki et al. Single-day, patient-initiated famciclovir therapy for recurrent genital herpes: a randomized, double-blind, placebo-controlled trial. Clin Infect Dis 2006; 42:8.

5. SL Spruance et al. High-dose, short-duration, early valacyclovir therapy for episodic treatment of cold sores: results of two randomized, placebo-controlled, multicenter studies. Antimicrob Agents Chemother 2003; 47:1072.

6. KH Fife et al. Effect of valacyclovir on viral shedding in immunocompetent patients with recurrent herpes simplex virus 2 genital herpes: a US-based randomized, double-blind, placebo-controlled clinical trial. Mayo Clin Proc 2006; 81:1321.

7. L Corey et al. Once-daily valacyclovir to reduce the risk of transmission of genital herpes. N Engl J Med 2004; 350:11.

8. A Wald et al. Comparative efficacy of famciclovir and valacyclovir for suppression of recurrent genital herpes and viral shedding. Sex Trans Dis 2006; 33:529.

9. N Nagot et al. Reduction of HIV-1 RNA levels with therapy to suppress herpes simplex virus. N Engl J Med 2007; 356:790.

10. SL Spruance et al. Penciclovir cream for the treatment of herpes simplex labialis. A randomized, multicenter, double-blind, placebo-controlled trial. Topical Penciclovir Collaborative Study Group. JAMA 1997; 277:1374.

11. JS Pepose et al. Ocular complications of smallpox vaccination. Am J Ophthalmol 2003; 136:343.

12. AP Limaye et al. Emergence of ganciclovir-resistant cytomegalovirus disease among recipients of solid-organ transplants. Lancet 2000; 356:645.

13. C Paya et al. Efficacy and safety of valganciclovir vs. oral ganciclovir for prevention of cytomegalovirus disease in solid organ transplant recipients. Am J Transplant 2004; 4:611.

14. JA Khoury et al. Prophylactic versus preemptive oral valganciclovir for the management of cytomegalovirus infection in adult renal transplant recipients. Am J Transplant 2006; 6:2134.

15. P Reusser et al. Randomized multicenter trial of foscarnet versus ganciclovir for preemptive therapy of cytomegalovirus infection after allogeneic stem cell transplantation. Blood 2002; 99:1159.

16. CM Perry and JA Balfour. Fomivirsen. Drugs 1999; 57:375.

17. L Kaiser et al. Impact of zanamivir on antibiotic use for respiratory events following acute influenza in adolescents and adults. Arch Intern Med 2000; 160:3234.

18. L Kaiser et al. Impact of oseltamivir treatment on influenza-related lower respiratory tract complications and hospitalizations. Arch Intern Med 2003; 163:1667.

19. Antiviral drugs prophylaxis and treatment of influenza. Med Lett Drugs Ther 2006; 48:87.

20. HJ Schunemann et al. WHO Rapid Advice Guidelines for pharmacological management of sporadic human infection with avian influenza A (H5N1) virus. Lancet Infect Dis 2007; 7:21.

21. MD de Jong et al. Oseltamivir resistance during treatment of influenza A (H5N1) infection. N Engl J Med 2005; 353:2667.

22. RB Couch. Prevention and treatment of influenza. N Engl J Med 2000; 343:1778.

23. Antiviral drugs for prophylaxis and treatment of influenza. Med Lett Drugs Ther 2006; 48:87.

24. TH Tran et al. Avian influenza A (H5N1) in 10 patients in Vietnam. N Engl J Med 2004; 350:1179.

25. WG Cooksley et al. Peginterferon alpha-2a (40 kDa): an advance in the treatment of hepatitis B e antigen-positive chronic hepatitis B. J Viral Hepat 2003; 10:298.

26. P Marcellin et al. Peginterferon alfa-2a alone, lamivudine alone, and the two in combination in patients with HBeAg-negative chronic hepatitis B. N Engl J Med 2004; 351:1206.

27. GK Lau et al. Peginterferon alfa-2a, lamivudine, and the combination for HBeAg-positive chronic hepatitis B. N Engl J Med 2005; 352:2682.

28. HL Janssen et al. Pegylated interferon alfa-2b alone or in combination with lamivudine for HBeAg-positive chronic hepatitis B: a randomised trial. Lancet 2005; 365:123.

29. MG Swain et al. Sustained virologic response (SVR) resulting from treatment with peginterferon alfa-2a (40 KD) (Pegasys) alone or in combination with ribavirin (Copegus) is durable and constitutes a cure: an ongoing 5-year follow-up (abstract). Digestive Disease Week; May 21, 2007; Washington DC.

30. FJ Torriani et al. Peginterferon alfa-2a plus ribavirin for chronic hepatitis C virus infection in HIV-infected patients. N Engl J Med 2004; 351:438.

31. RT Chung et al. Peginterferon alfa-2a plus ribavirin versus interferon alfa-2a plus ribavirin for chronic hepatitis C in HIV-coinfected persons. N Engl J Med 2004; 351:451.

32. F Carrat et al. Pegylated interferon alfa-2b vs standard interferon alfa-2b, plus ribavirin, for chronic hepatitis C in HIV-infected patients: a randomized controlled trial. JAMA 2004; 292:2839.

33. Y Shiratori et al. Antiviral therapy for cirrhotic hepatitis C: association with reduced hepatocellular carcinoma development and improved survival. Ann Intern Med 2005; 142:105.

34. H Yoshida et al. Interferon therapy reduces the risk for hepatocellular carcinoma: national surveillance program of cirrhotic and noncirrhotic patients with chronic hepatitis C in Japan. IHIT Study Group. Inhibition of Hepatocarcinogenesis by Interferon Therapy. Ann Intern Med 1999; 131:174.

35. E Jaeckel et al. Treatment of acute hepatitis C with interferon alfa-2b. N Engl J Med 2001; 345:1452.

36. Drugs for HIV infection. Treat Guidel Med Lett 2006; 4:67.

37. YF Liaw et al. Effects of extended lamivudine therapy in Asian patients with chronic hepatitis B. Asia Hepatitis Lamivudine Study Group. Gastroenterology 2000; 119:172.

38. YF Liaw et al. Lamivudine for patients with chronic hepatitis B and advanced liver disease. N Engl J Med 2004; 351:1521.

39. MM Jonas et al. Clinical trial of lamivudine in children with chronic hepatitis B. N Engl J Med 2002; 346:1706.

40. EB Keeffe et al. A treatment algorithm for the management of chronic hepatitis B virus infection in the United States. Clin Gastroenterol Hepatol 2004; 2:87.

41. SJ Hadziyannis et al. Adefovir dipivoxil for the treatment of hepatitis B e antigen-negative chronic hepatitis B. N Engl J Med 2003; 348:800.

Drugs for Non-HIV Viral Infections

42. P Marcellin et al. Adefovir dipivoxil for the treatment of hepatitis B e antigen-positive chronic hepatitis B. N Engl J Med 2003; 348:808.
43. SJ Hadziyannis et al. Long-term therapy with adefovir dipivoxil for HBeAg-negative chronic hepatitis B for up to 5 years. Gastroenterology 2006; 131:1743.
44. MG Peters et al. Adefovir dipivoxil alone or in combination with lamivudine in patients with lamivudine-resistant chronic hepatitis B. Gastroenterology 2004; 126:91.
45. O Schildgen et al. Variant of hepatitis B virus with primary resistance to adefovir. N Engl J Med 2006; 354:1807.
46. Entecavir *(Baraclude)* for chronic hepatitis B. Med Lett Drugs Ther 2005; 47:48.
47. TT Chang et al. A comparison of entecavir and lamivudine for HBeAg-positive chronic hepatitis B. N Engl J Med 2006; 354:1001.
48. Telbivudine *(Tyzeka)* for chronic hepatitis B. Med Lett Drugs Ther 2007; 49:11.
49. J Yan et al. Meta-analysis of 5% imiquimod and 0.5% podophyllotoxin in the treatment of condylomata acuminata. Dermatology 2006; 213:218.
50. American Academy of Pediatrics Committee on Infectious Diseases eds, Report of the Committee on Infectious Diseases 26th ed, Evanston, Ill: American Academy of Pediatrics, 2003; page 524.
51. GJ Mertz et al. Placebo-controlled, double-blind trial of intravenous ribavirin for the treatment of hantavirus cardiopulmonary syndrome in North America. Clin Infect Dis 2004; 39:1307.
52. The cream is not marketed commercially, but may be available from some compounding pharmacies.
53. E De Clercq. Clinical potential of the acyclic nucleoside phosphonates cidofovir, adefovir, and tenofovir in treatment of DNA virus and retrovirus infections. Clin Microbiol Rev 2003; 16:569.
54. P Ljungman et al. Cidofovir for adenovirus infections after allogeneic hematopoietic stem cell transplantation: a survey by the Infectious Diseases Working Party of the European Group for Blood and Marrow Transplantation. Bone Marrow Transplant 2003; 31:481.
55. M Bray and CJ Roy. Antiviral prophylaxis of smallpox. J Antimicrob Chemother 2004; 54:1.

DRUGS FOR
Parasitic Infections

Original publication date – Supplement 2007

With increasing travel, immigration, use of immunosuppressive drugs and the spread of AIDS, physicians anywhere may see infections caused by parasites. The table on page 226 lists first-choice and alternative drugs for most parasitic infections. The table on page 272 summarizes the known prenatal risks of antiparasitic drugs. The brand names and manufacturers of the drugs are listed on page 277.

DRUGS FOR PARASITIC INFECTIONS

Infection		Drug
***ACANTHAMOEBA* keratitis**		
Drug of choice:		See footnote 1
AMEBIASIS *(Entamoeba histolytica)*		
asymptomatic		
Drug of choice:		Iodoquinol[2]
	OR	Paromomycin[3]
	OR	Diloxanide furoate[4]*
mild to moderate intestinal disease		
Drug of choice:[5]		Metronidazole
	OR	Tinidazole[6]
		either followed by
		Iodoquinol[2]
	OR	Paromomycin[3]
severe intestinal and extraintestinal disease		
Drug of choice:		Metronidazole
	OR	Tinidazole[6]
		either followed by
		Iodoquinol[2]
	OR	Paromomycin[3]

* Availability problems. See table on page 277.
1. Topical 0.02% chlorhexidine and polyhexamethylene biguanide (PHMB, 0.02%), either alone or in combination, have been used successfully in a large number of patients. Treatment with either chlorhexidine or PHMB is often combined with propamidine isethionate *(Brolene)* or hexamidine *(Desmodine)*. None of these drugs is commercially available or approved for use in the US, but they can be obtained from compounding pharmacies (see footnote 2). Leiter's Park Avenue Pharmacy, San Jose, CA (800-292-6773; www.leiterrx.com) is a compounding pharmacy that specializes in ophthalmic drugs. Propamidine is available over the counter in the UK and Australia. Hexamidine is available in France. The combination of chlorhexidine, natamycin (pimaricin) and debridement also has been successful (K Kitagawa et al, Jpn J Ophthalmol 2003; 47:616). Debridement is most useful during the stage of corneal epithelial infection. Most cysts are resistant to neomycin; its use is no longer recommended. Azole antifungal drugs (ketoconazole, itraconazole) have been used as oral or topical adjuncts (FL Shuster and GS Visvesvara, Drug Resist Update 2004; 7:41). Use of corticosteroids is controversial (K Hammersmith, Curr Opinions Ophthal 2006; 17:327; ST Awwad et al, Eye Contact Lens 2007; 33:1).
2. Iodoquinol should be taken after meals.
3. Paromomycin should be taken with a meal.

Adult dosage	Pediatric dosage
650 mg PO tid x 20d	30-40 mg/kg/d (max 2g) PO in 3 doses x 20d
25-35 mg/kg/d PO in 3 doses x 7d	25-35 mg/kg/d PO in 3 doses x 7d
500 mg PO tid x 10d	20 mg/kg/d PO in 3 doses x 10d
500-750 mg PO tid x 7-10d	35-50 mg/kg/d PO in 3 doses x 7-10d
2 g once PO daily x 3d	≥3yrs: 50 mg/kg/d (max 2g) PO in 1 dose x 3d
650 mg PO tid x 20d	30-40 mg/kg/d (max 2g) PO in 3 doses x 20d
25-35 mg/kg/d PO in 3 doses x 7d	25-35 mg/kg/d PO in 3 doses x 7d
750 mg PO tid x 7-10d	35-50 mg/kg/d PO in 3 doses x 7-10d
2 g once PO daily x 5d	≥3yrs: 50 mg/kg/d (max 2g) PO in 1 dose x 3d
650 mg PO tid x 20d	30-40 mg/kg/d (max 2g) PO in 3 doses x 20d
25-35 mg/kg/d PO in 3 doses x 7d	25-35 mg/kg/d PO in 3 doses x 7d

4. Not available commercially. It may be obtained through compounding pharmacies such as Panorama Compounding Pharmacy, 6744 Balboa Blvd, Van Nuys, CA 91406 (800-247-9767) or Medical Center Pharmacy, New Haven, CT (203-688-6816). Other compounding pharmacies may be found through the National Association of Compounding Pharmacies (800-687-7850) or the Professional Compounding Centers of America (800-331-2498, www.pccarx.com).

5. Nitazoxanide may be effective against a variety of protozoan and helminth infections (DA Bobak, Curr Infect Dis Rep 2006; 8:91; E Diaz et al, Am J Trop Med Hyg 2003; 68:384). It was effective against mild to moderate amebiasis, 500 mg bid x 3d, in a recent study (JF Rossignol et al, Trans R Soc Trop Med Hyg 2007 Oct; 101:1025 E pub 2007 July 20). It is FDA-approved only for treatment of diarrhea caused by *Giardia* or *Cryptosporidium* (Med Lett Drugs Ther 2003; 45:29). Nitazoxanide is available in 500-mg tablets and an oral suspension; it should be taken with food.

6. A nitroimidazole similar to metronidazole, tinidazole appears to be as effective as metronidazole and better tolerated (Med Lett Drugs Ther 2004; 46:70). It should be taken with food to minimize GI adverse effects. For children and patients unable to take tablets, a pharmacist can crush the tablets and mix them with cherry syrup (*Humco*, and others). The syrup suspension is good for 7 days at room temperature and must be shaken before use (HB Fung and TL Doan et al, Clin Ther 2005; 27:1859). Ornidazole, a similar drug, is also used outside the US.

Continued on next page.

DRUGS FOR PARASITIC INFECTIONS (continued)

Infection	Drug
AMEBIC MENINGOENCEPHALITIS, primary and granulomatous	
Naegleria	
Drug of choice:	Amphotericin B[7,8]
Acanthamoeba	
Drug of choice:	See footnote 9
Balamuthia mandrillaris	
Drug of choice:	See footnote 10
Sappinia diploidea	
Drug of choice:	See footnote 11

*   Availability problems. See table on page 277.
7.   Not FDA-approved for this indication.
8.   Although A *Naegleria fowleri* infection was treated successfully in a 9-year old girl with combination of amphotericin B and miconazole both intravenous and intrathecal, plus oral rifampin (JS Seidel et al NEJM 1982;306:346). Amphotericin B and miconazole appear to have a synergistic effect, but Medical Letter consultants believe the rifampin probably had no additional effect (GS Visvesvara et al, FEMS Immunol Med Microbiol 2007; 50:1). Parenteral miconazole is no longer available in the US. Azithromycin has been used successfully in combination therapy to treat *Balmuthia* infection, but was changed to clarithromycin because of toxicity concerns and for better penetration into the cerebrospinal fluid. *In vitro*, azithromycin is more active than clarithromycin against *Naegleria*, so may be a better choice combined with amphotericin B for treatment of *Naegleria* (TR Deetz et al, Clin Infect Dis 2003; 37:1304; FL Schuster and GS Visvesvara, Drug Resistance Updates 2004; 7:41). Combinations of amphotericin B, ornidazole and rifampin (R Jain et al, Neurol Indian 2002; 50:470) and amphotericin B fluconazole and rifampin have also been used (J Vargas-Zepeda et al, Arch Med Research 2005;36:83). Case reports of other successful therapy have been published (FL Schuster and GS Visvesvara, Int J Parasitol 2004; 34:1001).
9.   Several patients with granulomatous amebic encephalitis (GAE) have been successfully treated with combinations of pentamidine, sulfadiazine, flucytosine, and either fluconazole or itraconazole (GS Visvesvara et al, FEMS Immunol Med Microbiol 2007; 50:1, epub Apr 11). GAE in an AIDS patient was treated successfully with sulfadiazine, pyrimethamine and fluconazole combined with surgical resection of the CNS lesion (M Seijo Martinez et al, J Clin Microbiol 2000; 38:3892). Chronic *Acanthamoeba* meningitis was successfully treated in 2 children with a combination of oral trimethoprim/sulfamethoxazole, rifampin and ketoconazole (T Singhal et al, Pediatr Infect Dis J 2001; 20:623). Disseminated cutaneous infection in an immunocompromised patient was treated successfully with IV pentamidine, topical chlorhexidine and 2% ketoconazole cream, followed by oral itraconazole (CA Slater et al, N Engl J Med 1994; 331:85) and with voriconazole and amphotericin B lipid complex (R Walia et al, Transplant Infect Dis 2007; 9:51). Other reports of successful therapy have been described (FL Schuster and GS Visvesvara, Drug Resistance Updates 2004; 7:41). Susceptibility testing of *Acanthamoeba* isolates has shown differences in drug sensitivity between species and even among strains of a single species; antimicrobial susceptibility testing is advisable (FL Schuster and GS Visvesvara, Int J Parasitiol 2004; 34:1001).

Adult dosage	Pediatric dosage
1.5 mg/kg/d IV in 2 doses x 3d, then 1 mg/kg/d x 6d plus 1.5 mg/d intrathecally x 2d, then 1 mg/d every other day x 8d	1.5 mg/kg/d IV in 2 doses x 3d, then 1 mg/kg/d x 6d plus 1.5 mg/d intrathecally x 2d, then 1 mg/d every other day x 8d

10. *B. mandrillaris* is a free-living ameba that causes subacute to fatal granulomatous amebic encephalitis (GAE) and cutaneous disease. Two cases of *Balamuthia* encephalitis have been successfully treated with flucytosine, pentamidine, fluconazole and sulfadiazine plus either azithromycin or clarithromycin (phenothiazines were also used) combined with surgical resection of the CNS lesion (TR Deetz et al, Clin Infect Dis 2003; 37:1304). Another case was successfully treated following open biopsy with pentamidine, fluconazole, sulfadiazine and clarithromycin (S Jung et al, Arch Pathol Lab Med 2004; 128:466).
11. A free-living ameba once thought not to be pathogenic to humans. *S. diploidea* has been successfully treated with azithromycin, pentamidine, itraconazole and flucytosine combined with surgical resection of the CNS lesion (BB Gelman et al, J Neuropathol Exp Neurol 2003; 62:990).

Continued on next page.

DRUGS FOR PARASITIC INFECTIONS (continued)

Infection		Drug
ANCYLOSTOMA caninum (Eosinophilic enterocolitis)		
Drug of choice:		Albendazole[7,12]
	OR	Mebendazole
	OR	Pyrantel pamoate[7,13*]
	OR	Endoscopic removal
Ancylostoma duodenale, see HOOKWORM		
ANGIOSTRONGYLIASIS *(Angiostrongylus cantonensis,* *Angiostrongylus costaricensis)*		
Drug of choice:		See footnote 14
ANISAKIASIS *(Anisakis* spp.)		
Treatment of choice:[15]		Surgical or endoscopic removal
ASCARIASIS *(Ascaris lumbricoides,* roundworm)		
Drug of choice:[5]		Albendazole[7,12]
	OR	Mebendazole
	OR	Ivermectin[7,16]
BABESIOSIS *(Babesia microti)*		
Drug of choice:[17]		Clindamycin[7,18]
		plus quinine[7,19]
	OR	Atovaquone[7,20]
		plus azithromycin[7]

* Availability problems. See table on page 277.
12. Albendazole must be taken with food; a fatty meal increases oral bioavailability.
13. Pyrantel pamoate suspension can be mixed with milk or fruit juice.
14. *A. cantonensis* causes predominantly neurotropic disease. *A. costaricensis* causes gastrointestinal disease. Most patients infected with either species have a self-limited course and recover completely. Analgesics, corticosteroids and careful removal of CSF at frequent intervals can relieve symptoms from increased intracranial pressure (V Lo Re III and SJ Gluckman, Am J Med 2003; 114:217). Treatment of *A. cantonensis* is controversial and varies across endemic areas. No antihelminthic drug is proven to be effective and some patients have worsened with therapy (TJ Slom et al, N Engl J Med 2002; 346:668). Mebendazole and a corticosteroid, however, appear to shorten the course of infection (H-C Tsai et al, Am J Med 2001; 111:109; V Chotmongkol et al, Am J Trop Med Hyg 2006; 74:1122). Albendazole has also relieved symptoms of angiostrongyliasis (XG Chen et al, Emerg Infect Dis 2005; 11:1645).
15. A Repiso Ortega et al, Gastroenterol Hepatol 2003; 26:341. Successful treatment of *Anisakiasis* with albendazole 400 mg PO bid x 3-5d has been reported, but the diagnosis was presumptive (DA Moore et al, Lancet 2002; 360:54; E Pacios et al, Clin Infect Dis 2005; 41:1825).

Adult dosage	Pediatric dosage
400 mg PO once	400 mg PO once
100 mg PO bid x 3d	100 mg PO bid x 3d
11 mg/kg (max 1g) PO x 3d	11 mg/kg (max 1g) PO x 3d
400 mg PO once	400 mg PO once
100 mg bid PO x 3d or 500 mg once	100 mg PO bid x 3d or 500 mg once
150-200 mcg/kg PO once	150-200 mcg/kg PO once
1.2 g bid IV or 600 mg tid PO x 7-10d	20-40 mg/kg/d PO in 3 doses x 7-10d
650 mg PO tid x 7-10d	30 mg/kg/d PO in 3 doses x 7-10d
750 mg PO bid x 7-10d	20 mg/kg/d PO in 2 doses x 7-10d
600 mg PO daily x 7-10d	12 mg/kg/d PO x 7-10d

16 Safety of ivermectin in young children (<15 kg) and pregnant women remains to be established. Ivermectin should be taken on an empty stomach with water.
17. Exchange transfusion has been used in severely ill patients and those with high (>10%) parasitemia (VI Powell and K Grima, Transfus Med Rev 2002; 16:239). In patients who were not severely ill, combination therapy with atovaquone and azithromycin was as effective as clindamycin and quinine and may have been better tolerated (PJ Krause et al, N Engl J Med 2000; 343:1454). Longer treatment courses may be needed in immunosuppressed patients and those with asplenia. Patients are commonly co-infected with Lyme disease (Med Lett Drugs Ther 2007; 49:49; AC Steere et al, Clin Infect Dis 2003; 36:1078).
18. Oral clindamycin should be taken with a full glass of water to minimize esophageal ulceration.
19. Quinine should be taken with or after a meal to decrease gastrointestinal adverse effects.
20. Atovaquone is available in an oral suspension that should be taken with a meal to increase absorption.

Continued on next page.

DRUGS FOR PARASITIC INFECTIONS (continued)

Infection	Drug
Balamuthia mandrillaris, see AMEBIC MENINGOENCEPHALITIS, PRIMARY	
BALANTIDIASIS *(Balantidium coli)*	
Drug of choice:	Tetracycline[7,21]
Alternative:	Metronidazole[7]
OR	Iodoquinol[2,7]
BAYLISASCARIASIS *(Baylisascaris procyonis)*	
Drug of choice:	See footnote 22
BLASTOCYSTIS hominis infection	
Drug of choice:	See footnote 23
CAPILLARIASIS *(Capillaria philippinensis)*	
Drug of choice:	Mebendazole[7]
Alternative:	Albendazole[7,12]
Chagas' disease, see TRYPANOSOMIASIS	
Clonorchis sinensis, see FLUKE infection	
CRYPTOSPORIDIOSIS *(Cryptosporidium)*	
Non-HIV infected	
Drug of choice:	Nitazoxanide[5]
HIV infected	
Drug of choice:	See footnote 24

*   Availability problems. See table on page 277.
21. Use of tetracyclines is contraindicated in pregnancy and in children <8 years old. Tetracycline should be taken 1 hour before or 2 hours after meals and/or dairy products.
22. No drug has been demonstrated to be effective. Albendazole 25 mg/kg/d PO x 20d started as soon as possible (up to 3d after possible infection) might prevent clinical disease and is recommended for children with known exposure (ingestion of raccoon stool or contaminated soil) (WJ Murray and KR Kazacos, Clin Infect Dis 2004; 39:1484). Mebendazole, levamisole or ivermectin could be tried if albendazole is not available. Steroid therapy may be helpful, especially in eye and CNS infections (PJ Gavin et al, Clin Microbiol Rev 2005; 18:703). Ocular baylisascariasis has been treated successfully using laser photocoagulation therapy to destroy the intraretinal larvae (CA Garcia et al, Eye 2004; 18:624).
23. Clinical significance of these organisms is controversial; metronidazole 750 mg PO tid x 10d, iodoquinol 650 mg PO tid x 20d or trimethoprim/sulfamethoxazole 1 DS tab PO bid x 7d have been reported to be effective (DJ Stenzel and PFL Borenam, Clin Microbiol Rev 1996; 9:563; UZ Ok et al, Am J Gastroenterol 1999; 94:3245). Metronidazole resistance may be common in some areas (K Haresh et al, Trop Med Int Health 1999; 4:274). Nitazoxanide has been effective in clearing organism and improving symptoms (E Diaz et al, Am J Trop Med Hyg 2003; 68:384; JF Rossignol, Clin Gastroenterol Hepatol 2005; 18:703).

Adult dosage	Pediatric dosage
500 mg PO qid x 10d	40 mg/kg/d (max 2 g) PO in 4 doses x 10d
750 mg PO tid x 5d	35-50 mg/kg/d PO in 3 doses x 5d
650 mg PO tid x 20d	30-40 mg/kg/d (max 2 g) PO in 3 doses x 20d
200 mg PO bid x 20d	200 mg PO bid x 20d
400 mg PO daily x 10d	400 mg PO daily x 10d
500 mg PO bid x 3d	1-3yrs: 100 mg PO bid x 3d
	4-11yrs: 200 mg PO bid x 3d
	>12yrs: 500 mg PO q12h x 3d

24. No drug has proven efficacy against cryptosporidiosis in advanced AIDS (I Abubakar et al, Cochrane Database Syst Rev 2007; 1:CD004932). Treatment with HAART is the mainstay of therapy. Nitazoxanide (JF Rossignol, Aliment Pharmacol Ther 2006; 24:807), paromomycin (P Maggi et al, Clin Infect Dis 2000; 33:1609), or a combination of paromomycin and azithromycin (NH Smith et al, J Infect Dis 1998; 178:900) may be tried to decrease diarrhea and recalcitrant malabsorption of antimicrobial drugs, which can occur with chronic cryptosporidiosis.

Continued on next page.

DRUGS FOR PARASITIC INFECTIONS (continued)

Infection		Drug
CUTANEOUS LARVA MIGRANS (creeping eruption, dog and cat hookworm)		
Drug of choice:[25]		Albendazole[7,12]
	OR	Ivermectin[7,16]
CYCLOSPORIASIS (*Cyclospora cayetanensis*)		
Drug of choice:[26]		Trimethoprim/ sulfamethoxazole[7]
CYSTICERCOSIS, see TAPEWORM infection		
DIENTAMOEBA fragilis infection[27]		
Drug of choice:		Iodoquinol[2,7]
	OR	Paromomycin[3,7]
	OR	Tetracycline[7,21]
	OR	Metronidazole[7]
Diphyllobothrium latum, see TAPEWORM infection		
DRACUNCULUS medinensis (guinea worm) infection		
Drug of choice:		See footnote 28
Echinococcus, see TAPEWORM infection		
Entamoeba histolytica, see AMEBIASIS		
ENTEROBIUS vermicularis (pinworm) infection		
Drug of choice:[29]		Mebendazole
	OR	Pyrantel pamoate[13]*
	OR	Albendazole[7,12]
Fasciola hepatica, see FLUKE infection		

*   Availability problems. See table on page 277.
25. G Albanese et al, Int J Dermatol 2001; 40:67; D Malvy et al, J Travel Med 2006; 13:244.
26. HIV-infected patients may need higher dosage and long-term maintenance. Successful use of nita-zoxanide (see also footnote 5) has been reported in one patient with sulfa allergy (SM Zimmer et al, Clin Infect Dis 2007; 44:466).
27. A Norberg et al, Clin Microbiol Infect 2003; 9:65; O Vandenberg et al, Int J Infect Dis 2006; 10:255.

Adult dosage	Pediatric dosage
400 mg PO daily x 3d	400 mg PO daily x 3d
200 mcg/kg PO daily x 1-2d	200 mcg/kg PO daily x 1-2d
TMP 160 mg/SMX	TMP 5 mg/kg/SMX
800 mg (1 DS tab) PO bid x 7-10d	25 mg/kg/d PO in 2 doses x 7-10d
650 mg PO tid x 20d	30-40 mg/kg/d (max 2g) PO in 3 doses x 20d
25-35 mg/kg/d PO in 3 doses x 7d	25-35 mg/kg/d PO in 3 doses x 7d
500 mg PO qid x 10d	40 mg/kg/d (max 2g) PO in 4 doses x 10d
500-750 mg PO tid x 10d	35-50 mg/kg/d PO in 3 doses x 10d
100 mg PO once; repeat in 2wks	100 mg PO once; repeat in 2wks
11 mg/kg base PO once (max 1 g); repeat in 2wks	11 mg/kg base PO once (max 1 g); repeat in 2wks
400 mg PO once; repeat in 2wks	400 mg PO once; repeat in 2wks

28. No drug is curative against *Dracunculus*. A program for monitoring local sources of drinking water to eliminate transmission has dramatically decreased the number of cases worldwide (M Barry, N Engl J Med 2007; 356:2561). The treatment of choice is slow extraction of worm combined with wound care and pain management (C Greenaway, CMAJ 2004; 170:495).
29. Since family members are usually infected, treatment of the entire household is recommended.

Continued on next page.

DRUGS FOR PARASITIC INFECTIONS (continued)

Infection	Drug
FILARIASIS[30]	
Wuchereria bancrofti, Brugia malayi, Brugia timori	
Drug of choice:[31]	Diethylcarbamazine*
Loa loa	
Drug of choice:[34]	Diethylcarbamazine*
Mansonella ozzardi	
Drug of choice:	See footnote 35
Mansonella perstans	
Drug of choice:	Albendazole[7,12]
OR	Mebendazole[7]
Mansonella streptocerca	
Drug of choice:[36]	Diethylcarbamazine*
OR	Ivermectin[7,16]
Tropical Pulmonary Eosinophilia (TPE)[37]	
Drug of choice:	Diethylcarbamazine*
Onchocerca volvulus (River blindness)	
Drug of choice:	Ivermectin[16,38]

---

*   Availability problems. See table on page 277.

30. Antihistamines or corticosteroids may be required to decrease allergic reactions to components of disintegrating microfilariae that result from treatment, especially in infection caused by *Loa loa*. Endosymbiotic *Wolbachia* bacteria may have a role in filarial development and host response, and may represent a potential target for therapy. Addition of doxycycline 100 or 200 mg/d PO x 6-8wks in lymphatic filariasis and onchocerciasis has resulted in substantial loss of *Wolbachia* and decrease in both micro- and macrofilariae (MJ Taylor et al, Lancet 2005; 365:2116; AY Debrah et al, Plos Pathog 2006; e92:0829); but use of tetracyclines is contraindicated in pregnancy and in children <8 yrs old.

31. Most symptoms are caused by adult worm. A single-dose combination of albendazole (400 mg PO) with either ivermectin (200 mcg/kg PO) or diethylcarbamazine (6 mg/kg PO) is effective for reduction or suppression of *W. bancrofti* microfilaria, but the albendazole/ivermectin combination does not kill all the adult worms (D Addiss et al, Cochrane Database Syst Rev 2004; CD003753).

32. For patients with microfilaria in the blood, Medical Letter consultants start with a lower dosage and scale up: d1: 50 mg; d2: 50 mg tid; d3: 100 mg tid; d4-14: 6 mg/kg in 3 doses (for *Loa Loa* d4-14: 9 mg/kg in 3 doses). Multi-dose regimens have been shown to provide more rapid reduction in microfilaria than single-dose diethylcarbamazine, but microfilaria levels are similar 6-12 months after treatment (LD Andrade et al, Trans R Soc Trop Med Hyg 1995; 89:319; PE Simonsen et al, Am J Trop Med Hyg 1995; 53:267). A single dose of 6 mg/kg is used in endemic areas for mass treatment (J Figueredo-Silva et al, Trans R Soc Trop Med Hyg 1996; 90:192; J Noroes et al, Trans R Soc Trop Med Hyg 1997; 91:78).

33. Diethylcarbamazine should not be used for treatment of *Onchocerca volvulus* due to the risk of increased ocular side effects including blindness associated with rapid killing of the worms. It should be used cautiously in geographic regions where *O. volvulus* coexists with other filariae. Diethylcarbamazine is contraindicated during pregnancy. See also footnote 38.

Adult dosage	Pediatric dosage
6 mg/kg/d PO in 3 doses x 12d[32,33]	6 mg/kg/d PO in 3 doses x 12d[32,33]
6 mg/kg/d PO in 3 doses x 12d[32,33]	6 mg/kg/d PO in 3 doses x 12d[32,33]
400 mg PO bid x 10d 100 mg PO bid x 30d	400 mg PO bid x 10d 100 mg PO bid x 30d
6 mg/kg/d PO x 12d[33] 150 mcg/kg PO once	6 mg/kg/d PO x 12d[33] 150 mcg/kg PO once
6 mg/kg/d in 3 doses x 12-21d[33]	6 mg/kg/d in 3 doses x 12-21d[33]
150 mcg/kg PO once, repeated every 6-12mos until asymptomatic	150 mcg/kg PO once, repeated every 6-12mos until asymptomatic

34. In heavy infections with *Loa loa*, rapid killing of microfilariae can provoke encephalopathy. Apheresis has been reported to be effective in lowering microfilarial counts in patients heavily infected with *Loa loa* (EA Ottesen, Infect Dis Clin North Am 1993; 7:619). Albendazole may be useful for treatment of loiasis when diethylcarbamazine is ineffective or cannot be used, but repeated courses may be necessary (AD Klion et al, Clin Infect Dis 1999; 29:680; TE Tabi et al, Am J Trop Med Hyg 2004; 71:211). Ivermectin has also been used to reduce microfilaremia, but albendazole is preferred because of its slower onset of action and lower risk of precipitating encephalopathy (AD Klion et al, J Infect Dis 1993; 168:202; M Kombila et al, Am J Trop Med Hyg 1998; 58:458). Diethylcarbamazine, 300 mg PO once/wk, has been recommended for prevention of loiasis (TB Nutman et al, N Engl J Med 1988; 319:752).
35. Diethylcarbamazine has no effect. A single dose of ivermectin 200 mcg/kg PO reduces microfilaria densities and provides both short- and long-term reductions in *M. ozzardi* microfilaremia (AA Gonzalez et al, W Indian Med J 1999; 48:231).
36. Diethylcarbamazine is potentially curative due to activity against both adult worms and microfilariae. Ivermectin is active only against microfilariae.
37. AK Boggild et al, Clin Infect Dis 2004; 39:1123. Relapses occur and can be treated with a repeated course of diethylcarbamazine.
38. Diethylcarbamazine should not be used for treatment of this disease because rapid killing of the worms can lead to blindness. Periodic treatment with ivermectin (every 3-12 months), 150 mcg/kg PO, can prevent blindness due to ocular onchocerciasis (DN Udall, Clin Infect Dis 2007; 44:53). Skin reactions after ivermectin treatment are often reported in persons with high microfilarial skin densities. Ivermectin has been inadvertently given to pregnant women during mass treatment programs; the rates of congenital abnormalities were similar in treated and untreated women. Because of the high risk of blindness from onchocerciasis, the use of ivermectin after the first trimester is considered acceptable according to the WHO. Doxycycline (100 mg/day PO for 6 weeks), followed by a single 150 mcg/kg PO dose of ivermectin, resulted in up to 19 months of amicrofilaridermia and 100% elimination of *Wolbachia* species (A Hoerauf et al, Lancet 2001; 357:1415).

Continued on next page.

DRUGS FOR PARASITIC INFECTIONS (continued)

Infection	Drug
FLUKE, hermaphroditic, infection	
Clonorchis sinensis (Chinese liver fluke)	
Drug of choice:	Praziquantel[39]
OR	Albendazole[7,12]
Fasciola hepatica (sheep liver fluke)	
Drug of choice:[40]	Triclabendazole[*]
Alternative:	Bithionol[*]
OR	Nitazoxanide[5,7]
Fasciolopsis buski, Heterophyes heterophyes, Metagonimus yokogawai (intestinal flukes)	
Drug of choice:	Praziquantel[7,39]
Metorchis conjunctus (North American liver fluke)	
Drug of choice:	Praziquantel[7,39]
Nanophyetus salmincola	
Drug of choice:	Praziquantel[7,39]
Opisthorchis viverrini (Southeast Asian liver fluke)	
Drug of choice:	Praziquantel[39]
Paragonimus westermani (lung fluke)	
Drug of choice:	Praziquantel[7,39]
Alternative:[42]	Bithionol[*]

* Availability problems. See table on page 277.

39. Praziquantel should be taken with liquids during a meal.

40. Unlike infections with other flukes, *Fasciola hepatica* infections may not respond to praziquantel. Triclabendazole (*Egaten* - Novartis) appears to be safe and effective, but data are limited (DY Aksoy et al, Clin Microbiol Infect 2005; 11:859). It is available from Victoria Pharmacy, Zurich, Switzerland (www.pharmaworld.com; 41-1-211-24-32) and should be given with food for better absorption. Nitazoxanide also appears to have efficacy in treating fascioliasis in adults and in children (L Favennec et al, Aliment Pharmacol Ther 2003; 17:265; JF Rossignol et al, Trans R Soc Trop Med Hyg 1998; 92:103; SM Kabil et al, Curr Ther Res 2000; 61:339).

Adult dosage	Pediatric dosage
75 mg/kg/d PO in 3 doses x 2d	75 mg/kg/d PO in 3 doses x 2d
10 mg/kg/d PO x 7d	10 mg/kg/d PO x 7d
10 mg/kg PO once or twice[41]	10 mg/kg PO once or twice[41]
30-50 mg/kg on alternate days	30-50 mg/kg on alternate days
x 10-15 doses	x 10-15 doses
500 mg PO bid x 7d	1-3yrs: 100 mg PO q12h x 7d
	4-11yrs: 200 mg PO q12h x 7d
	>12yrs: 500 mg PO q12h x 7d
75 mg/kg/d PO in 3 doses x 1d	75 mg/kg/d PO in 3 doses x 1d
75 mg/kg/d PO in 3 doses x 1d	75 mg/kg/d PO in 3 doses x 1d
60 mg/kg/d PO in 3 doses x 1d	60 mg/kg/d PO in 3 doses x 1d
75 mg/kg/d PO in 3 doses x 2d	75 mg/kg/d PO in 3 doses x 2d
75 mg/kg/d PO in 3 doses x 2d	75 mg/kg/d PO in 3 doses x 2d
30-50 mg/kg on alternate days	30-50 mg/kg on alternate days
x 10-15 doses	x 10-15 doses

41. J Keiser et al, Expert Opin Investig Drugs 2005; 14:1513.
42. Triclabendazole may be effective in a dosage of 5 mg/kg PO once/d x 3d or 10 mg/kg PO bid x 1d (M Calvopiña et al, Trans R Soc Trop Med Hyg 1998; 92:566). See footnote 40 for availability.

Continued on next page.

DRUGS FOR PARASITIC INFECTIONS (continued)

Infection		Drug
GIARDIASIS (*Giardia duodenalis*)		
Drug of choice:		Metronidazole[7]
	OR	Tinidazole[6]
	OR	Nitazoxanide[5]
Alternative:[43]		Paromomycin[3,7,44]
	OR	Furazolidone[*]
	OR	Quinacrine[4,45*]
GNATHOSTOMIASIS (*Gnathostoma spinigerum*) [46]		
Treatment of choice:		Albendazole[7,12]
	OR	Ivermectin[7,16]
		either
	±	Surgical removal
GONGYLONEMIASIS (*Gongylonema* sp.) [47]		
Treatment of choice:		Surgical removal
	OR	Albendazole[7,12]
HOOKWORM infection (*Ancylostoma duodenale, Necator americanus*)		
Drug of choice:		Albendazole[7,12]
	OR	Mebendazole
	OR	Pyrantel pamoate[7,13*]
Hydatid cyst, see TAPEWORM infection		
Hymenolepis nana, see TAPEWORM infection		
ISOSPORIASIS (*Isospora belli*)		
Drug of choice:[48]		Trimethoprim/sulfamethoxazole[7]

---

* Availability problems. See table on page 277.
43. Another alternative is albendazole 400 mg/d PO x 5d in adults and 10 mg/kg/d PO x 5d in children (K Yereli et al, Clin Microbiol Infect 2004; 10:527; O Karabay et al, World J Gastroenterol 2004; 10:1215). Combination treatment with standard doses of metronidazole and quinacrine x 3wks has been effective for a small number of refractory infections (TE Nash et al, Clin Infect Dis 2001; 33:22). In one study, nitazoxanide was used successfully in high doses to treat a case of *Giardia* resistant to metronidazole and albendazole (P Abboud et al, Clin Infect Dis 2001; 32:1792).
44. Poorly absorbed; may be useful for treatment of giardiasis in pregnancy.
45. Quinacrine should be taken with liquids after a meal.

Adult dosage	Pediatric dosage
250 mg PO tid x 5-7d	15 mg/kg/d PO in 3 doses x 5-7d
2 g PO once	50 mg/kg PO once (max 2 g)
500 mg PO bid x 3d	1-3yrs: 100 mg PO q12h x 3d
	4-11yrs: 200 mg PO q12h x 3d
	>12yrs: 500 mg PO q12h x 3d
25-35 mg/kg/d PO in 3 doses x 5-10d	25-35 mg/kg/d PO in 3 doses x 5-10d
100 mg PO qid x 7-10d	6 mg/kg/d PO in 4 doses x 7-10d
100 mg PO tid x 5d	2 mg/kg/d PO in 3 doses x 5d (max 300 mg/d)
400 mg PO bid x 21d	400 mg PO bid x 21d
200 mcg/kg/d PO x 2d	200 mcg/kg/d PO x 2d
400 mg/d PO x 3d	400 mg/d PO x 3d
400 mg PO once	400 mg PO once
100 mg PO bid x 3d or 500 mg once	100 mg PO bid x 3d or 500 mg once
11 mg/kg (max 1g) PO x 3d	11 mg/kg (max 1g) PO x 3d
TMP 160 mg/SMX 800 mg (1 DS tab) PO bid x 10d	TMP 5 mg/kg/d/SMX 25 mg/kg/d PO in 2 doses x 10d

46. P Nontasut et al, Southeast Asian J Trop Med Pub Health 2005; 36:650; M de Gorgolas et al, J Travel Med 2003; 10:358. All patients should be treated with medication whether surgery is attempted or not.
47. ME Wilson et al, Clin Infect Dis 2001; 32:1378; G Molavi et al, J Helminth 2006; 80:425.
48. Usually a self-limited illness in immunocompetent patients. Immunosuppressed patients may need higher doses, longer duration (TMP/SMX qid x 10d, followed by bid x 3wks) and long-term maintenance. In sulfonamide-sensitive patients, pyrimethamine 50-75 mg daily in divided doses (plus leucovorin 10-25 mg/d) has been effective.

Continued on next page.

DRUGS FOR PARASITIC INFECTIONS (continued)

Infection		Drug
LEISHMANIA		
Visceral[49,50]		
Drug of choice:		Liposomal amphotericin B[51]
	OR	Sodium stibogluconate*
	OR	Miltefosine[53]*
Alternative:		Meglumine antimonate*
	OR	Amphotericin B[7]
	OR	Paromomycin[7,13,54]*

---

* Availability problems. See table on page 277.

49. To maximize effectiveness and minimize toxicity, the choice of drug, dosage, and duration of therapy should be individualized based on the region of disease acquisition, a likely infecting species, and host factors such as immune status (BL Herwaldt, Lancet 1999; 354:1191). Some of the listed drugs and regimens are effective only against certain *Leishmania* species/strains and only in certain areas of the world (J Arevalo et al, Clin Infect Dis 2007; 195:1846). Medical Letter consultants recommend consultation with physicians experienced in management of this disease.

50. Visceral infection is most commonly due to the Old World species *L. donovani* (kala-azar) and *L. infantum* and the New World species *L. chagasi*.

51. Liposomal amphotericin B *(AmBisome)* is the only lipid formulation of amphotericin B FDA-approved for treatment of visceral leishmania, largely based on clinical trials in patients infected with *L. infantum* (A Meyerhoff, Clin Infect Dis 1999; 28:42). Two other amphotericin B lipid formulations, amphotericin B lipid complex *(Abelcet)* and amphotericin B cholesteryl sulfate *(Amphotec)* have been used, but are considered investigational for this condition and may not be as effective (C Bern et al, Clin Infect Dis 2006; 43:917).

52. The FDA-approved dosage regimen for immunocompromised patients (e.g., HIV infected) is 4 mg/kg/d IV on days 1-5, 10, 17, 24, 31 and 38. The relapse rate is high; maintenance therapy (secondary prevention) may be indicated, but there is no consensus as to dosage or duration.

Adult dosage	Pediatric dosage
3 mg/kg/d IV d 1-5, 14 and 21[52]	3 mg/kg/d IV d 1-5, 14 and 21[52]
20 mg Sb/kg/d IV or IM x 28d	20 mg Sb/kg/d IV or IM x 28d
2.5 mg/kg/d PO (max 150 mg/d) x 28d	2.5 mg/kg/d PO (max 150 mg/d) x 28d
20 mg Sb/kg/d IV or IM x 28d	20 mg Sb/kg/d IV or IM x 28d
1 mg/kg IV daily x 15-20d or every second day for up to 8 wks	1 mg/kg IV daily x 15-20d or every second day for up to 8 wks
15 mg/kg/d IM x 21d	15 mg/kd/d IM x 21d

53. Effective for both antimony-sensitive and -resistant *L. donovani* (Indian); miltefosine *(Impavido)* is manufactured in 10- or 50-mg capsules by Zentaris (Frankfurt, Germany at info@zentaris.com) and is available through consultation with the CDC. The drug is contraindicated in pregnancy; a negative pregnancy test before drug initiation and effective contraception during and for 2 months after treatment is recommended (H Murray et al, Lancet 2005; 366:1561). In a placebo-controlled trial in patients ≥12 years old, oral miltefosine 2.5 mg/kg/d x 28d was also effective for treatment of cutaneous leishmaniasis due to *L.(V.) panamensis* in Colombia, but not *L.(V.) braziliensis* or *L. mexicana* in Guatemala (J Soto et al, Clin Infect Dis 2004; 38:1266). "Motion sickness," nausea, headache and increased creatinine are the most frequent adverse effects (J Soto and P Soto, Expert Rev Anti Infect Ther 2006; 4:177).

54. Paromomycin IM has been effective against leishmania in India; it has not yet been tested in South America or the Mediterranean and there is insufficient data to support its use in pregnancy (S Sundar et al, N Engl J Med 2007; 356:2371). Topical paromomycin should be used only in geographic regions where cutaneous leishmaniasis species have low potential for mucosal spread. A formulation of 15% paromomycin/12% methylbenzethonium chloride *(Leshcutan)* in soft white paraffin for topical use has been reported to be partially effective against cutaneous leishmaniasis due to *L. major* in Israel and *L. mexicana* and *L. (V.) braziliensis* in Guatemala, where mucosal spread is very rare (BA Arana et al, Am J Trop Med Hyg 2001; 65:466). The methylbenzethonium is irritating to the skin; lesions may worsen before they improve.

Continued on next page.

DRUGS FOR PARASITIC INFECTIONS (continued)

Infection		Drug
LEISHMANIA (continued)		
Cutaneous[49,55]		
Drugs of choice:		Sodium stibogluconate*
	OR	Meglumine antimonate*
	OR	Miltefosine[53]*
Alternative:[56]		Paromomycin[7,13,54]*
	OR	Pentamidine[7]
Mucosal[49,58]		
Drug of choice:		Sodium stibogluconate*
	OR	Meglumine antimonate*
	OR	Amphotericin B[7]
	OR	Miltefosine[53]*
LICE infestation *(Pediculus humanus, P. capitis, Phthirus pubis)*[59]		
Drug of choice:		0.5% Malathion[60]
	OR	1% Permethrin[61]
Alternative:		Pyrethrins with piperonyl butoxide[61]
	OR	Ivermectin[7,16,62]

Loa loa, see FILARIASIS

---

*   Availability problems. See table on page 277.

55. Cutaneous infection is most commonly due to the Old World species *L. major* and *L. tropica* and the New World species *L. mexicana, L. (Viannia) braziliensis,* and others.

56. Although azole drugs (fluconazole, ketoconazole, itraconazole) have been used to treat cutaneous disease, they are not reliably effective and have no efficacy against mucosal disease (AJ Magill, Infect Dis Clin North Am 2005; 19:241). For treatment of *L. major* cutaneous lesions, a study in Saudi Arabia found that oral fluconazole, 200 mg once/d x 6wks appeared to speed healing (AA Alrajhi et al, N Engl J Med 2002; 346:891). Thermotherapy may be an option for cutaneous *L. tropica* infection (R Reithinger et al, Clin Infect Dis 2005; 40:1148). A device that generates focused and controlled heating of the skin has been approved by the FDA for this indication (*ThermoMed* – ThermoSurgery Technologies Inc., Phoenix, AZ, 602-264-7300; www.thermosurgery.com).

57. At this dosage pentamidine has been effective in Colombia predominantly against *L. (V.) panamensis* (J Soto-Mancipe et al, Clin Infect Dis 1993; 16:417; J Soto et al, Am J Trop Med Hyg 1994; 50:107). Activity against other species is not well established.

58. Mucosal infection is most commonly due to the New World species *L. (V.) braziliensis, L. (V.) panamensis,* or *L. (V.) guyanensis.*

Adult dosage	Pediatric dosage
20 mg Sb/kg/d IV or IM x 20d	20 mg Sb/kg/d IV or IM x 20d
20 mg Sb/kg/d IV or IM x 20d	20 mg Sb/kg/d IV or IM x 20d
2.5 mg/kg/d PO (max 150 mg/d) x 28d	2.5 mg/kg/d PO (max 150 mg/d) x 28d
Topically 2x/d x 10-20d	Topically 2x/d x 10-20d
2-3 mg/kg IV or IM daily or every second day x 4-7 doses[57]	2-3 mg/kg IV or IM daily or every second day x 4-7 doses[57]
20 mg Sb/kg/d IV or IM x 28d	20 mg Sb/kg/d IV or IM x 28d
20 mg Sb/kg/d IV or IM x 28d	20 mg Sb/kg/d IV or IM x 28d
0.5-1 mg/kg IV daily or every second day for up to 8wks	0.5-1 mg/kg IV daily or every second day for up to 8wks
2.5 mg/kg/d PO (max 150 mg/d) x 28d	2.5 mg/kg/d PO (max 150 mg/d) x 28d
Topically	Topically
Topically	Topically
Topically	Topically
200 mcg/kg PO	≥15kg: 200 mcg/kg PO

59. Pediculocides should not be used for infestations of the eyelashes. Such infestations are treated with petrolatum ointment applied 2-4x/d x 8-10d. Oral TMP/SMX has also been used (TL Meinking and D Taplin, Curr Probl Dermatol 1996; 24:157). For pubic lice, treat with 5% permethrin or ivermectin as for scabies (see page 260). TMP/SMX has also been effective when used together with permethrin for head lice (RB Hipolito et al, Pediatrics 2001; 107:E30).
60. Malathion is both ovicidal and pediculocidal; 2 applications at least 7 days apart are generally necessary to kill all lice and nits.
61. Permethrin and pyrethrin are pediculocidal; retreatment in 7-10d is needed to eradicate the infestation. Some lice are resistant to pyrethrins and permethrin (TL Meinking et al, Arch Dermatol 2002; 138:220).
62. Ivermectin is pediculocidal, but more than one dose is generally necessary to eradicate the infestation (KN Jones and JC English 3rd, Clin Infect Dis 2003; 36:1355). The number of doses and interval between doses has not been established, but in one study of body lice, 3 doses administered at 7-day intervals were effective (C Fouault et al, J Infect Dis 2006; 193:474).

Continued on next page.

DRUGS FOR PARASITIC INFECTIONS (continued)

Infection	Drug

MALARIA, Treatment of *(Plasmodium falciparum,*[63] *P. vivax,*[64] *P. ovale, and P. malariae*[65]*)*

ORAL[66]

P. falciparum or unidentified species acquired in areas of chloroquine-resistant *P. falciparum*[63]

Drug of choice:[67]   Atovaquone/proguanil[68]

                    OR   Quinine sulfate
                          plus
                          doxycycline[7,21,71]
                          or plus
                          tetracycline[7,21]
                          or plus
                          clindamycin[7,18,72]

---

*   Availability problems. See table on page 277.
63. Chloroquine-resistant *P. falciparum* occurs in all malarious areas except Central America (including Panama north and west of the Canal Zone), Mexico, Haiti, the Dominican Republic, Paraguay, northern Argentina, North and South Korea, Georgia, Armenia, most of rural China and some countries in the Middle East (chloroquine resistance has been reported in Yemen, Oman, Saudi Arabia and Iran). For treatment of multiple-drug-resistant *P. falciparum* in Southeast Asia, especially Thailand, where mefloquine resistance is frequent, atovaquone/proguanil, quinine plus either doxycycline or clindamycin, or artemether/lumefantrine may be used.
64. *P. vivax* with decreased susceptibility to chloroquine is a significant problem in Papua-New Guinea and Indonesia. There are also a few reports of resistance from Myanmar, India, the Solomon Islands, Vanuatu, Guyana, Brazil, Colombia and Peru (JK Baird et al, Curr Infect Dis Rep 2007; 9:39).
65. Chloroquine-resistant *P. malariae* has been reported from Sumatra (JD Maguire et al, Lancet 2002; 360:58).
66. Uncomplicated or mild malaria may be treated with oral drugs. Severe malaria (e.g. impaired consciousness, parasitemia >5%, shock, etc.) should be treated with parenteral drugs (KS Griffin et al, JAMA 2007; 297:2264).
67. Primaquine is given for prevention of relapse after infection with *P. vivax* or *P. ovale.* Some experts also prescribe primaquine phosphate 30 mg base/d (0.6 mg base/kg/d for children) for 14d after departure from areas where these species are endemic (Presumptive Anti-Relapse Therapy [PART], "terminal prophylaxis"). Since this is not always effective as prophylaxis (E Schwartz et al, N Engl J Med 2003; 349:1510), others prefer to rely on surveillance to detect cases when they occur, particularly when exposure was limited or doubtful. See also footnote 79.

Adult dosage	Pediatric dosage
2 adult tabs bid[69] or 4 adult tabs once/d x 3d	<5kg: not indicated
	5-8kg: 2 peds tabs once/d x 3d
	9-10kg: 3 peds tabs once/d x 3d
	11-20kg: 1 adult tab once/d x 3d
	21-30kg: 2 adult tabs once/d x 3d
	31-40kg: 3 adult tabs once/d x 3d
	>40kg: 4 adult tabs once/d x 3d
650 mg q8h x 3 **or** 7d[70]	30 mg/kg/d in 3 doses x 3 **or** 7d[70]
100 mg bid x 7d	4 mg/kg/d in 2 doses x 7d
250 mg qid x 7d	6.25 mg/kg/d in 4 doses x 7d
20 mg/kg/d in 3 doses x 7d[73]	20 mg/kg/d in 3 doses x 7d

68. Atovaquone/proguanil is available as a fixed-dose combination tablet: adult tablets (*Malarone*; 250 mg atovaquone/100 mg proguanil) and pediatric tablets (*Malarone Pediatric*; 62.5 mg atovaquone/25 mg proguanil). To enhance absorption and reduce nausea and vomiting, it should be taken with food or a milky drink. Safety in pregnancy is unknown; outcomes were normal in 24 women treated with the combination in the 2nd and 3rd trimester (R McGready et al, Eur J Clin Pharmacol 2003; 59:545). The drug should not be given to patients with severe renal impairment (creatinine clearance <30mL/min). There have been isolated case reports of resistance in *P. falciparum* in Africa, but Medical Letter consultants do not believe there is a high risk for acquisition of *Malarone*-resistant disease (E Schwartz et al, Clin Infect Dis 2003; 37:450; A Farnert et al, BMJ 2003; 326:628; S Kuhn et al, Am J Trop Med Hyg 2005; 72:407; CT Happi et al, Malaria Journal 2006; 5:82).
69. Although approved for once-daily dosing, Medical Letter consultants usually divide the dose in two to decrease nausea and vomiting.
70. Available in the US in a 324-mg capsule; 2 capsules suffice for adult dosage. In Southeast Asia, relative resistance to quinine has increased and treatment should be continued for 7d. Quinine should be taken with or after meals to decrease gastrointestinal adverse effects.
71. Doxycycline should be taken with adequate water to avoid esophageal irritation. It can be taken with food to minimize gastrointestinal adverse effects.
72. For use in pregnancy and in children <8 yrs.

Continued on next page.

DRUGS FOR PARASITIC INFECTIONS (continued)

Infection	Drug
MALARIA, Treatment of (continued)	
Alternative:[67]	Mefloquine[74,75]
	OR Artemether/lumefantrine[76,77]*
	OR Artesunate[76]* **plus** see footnote 78

---

* Availability problems. See table on page 277.

73. B Lell and PG Kremsner, Antimicrob Agents Chemother 2002; 46:2315; M Ramharter et al, Clin Infect Dis 2005; 40:1777.

74. At this dosage, adverse effects include nausea, vomiting, diarrhea and dizziness. Disturbed sense of balance, toxic psychosis and seizures can also occur. Mefloquine should not be used for treatment of malaria in pregnancy unless there is no other treatment option because of increased risk for stillbirth (F Nosten et al, Clin Infect Dis 1999; 28:808). It should be avoided for treatment of malaria in persons with active depression or with a history of psychosis or seizures and should be used with caution in persons with any psychiatric illness. Mefloquine can be given to patients taking β-blockers if they do not have an underlying arrhythmia; it should not be used in patients with conduction abnormalities. Mefloquine should not be given together with quinine or quinidine, and caution is required in using quinine or quinidine to treat patients with malaria who have taken mefloquine for prophylaxis. Mefloquine should not be taken on an empty stomach; it should be taken with at least 8 oz of water.

75. *P. falciparum* with resistance to mefloquine is a significant problem in the malarious areas of Thailand and in areas of Myanmar and Cambodia that border on Thailand. It has also been reported on the borders between Myanmar and China, Laos and Myanmar, and in Southern Vietnam. In the US, a 250-mg tablet of mefloquine contains 228 mg mefloquine base. Outside the US, each 275-mg tablet contains 250 mg base.

76. The artemisinin-derivatives, artemether and artesunate, are both frequently used globally in combination regimens to treat malaria. Both are available in oral, parenteral and rectal formulations, but manufacturing standards are not consistent (HA Karunajeewa et al, JAMA 2007; 297:2381; EA Ashley and NJ White, Curr Opin Infect Dis 2005; 18:531). In the US, only the IV formulation of artesunate is available; it can be obtained through the CDC under an IND for patients with severe disease who do not have timely access, cannot tolerate, or fail to respond to IV quinidine (www.cdc.gov/malaria/features/artesunate_now_available.htm). To avoid development of resistance, monotherapy should be avoided (PE Duffy and CH Sibley, Lancet 2005; 366:1908). In animal studies artemisinins have been embryotoxic and caused low incidence of teratogenicity; no adverse pregnancy outcome has been observed in limited studies in humans. (S Dellicour et al, Malaria Journal 2007; 6:15).

Adult dosage	Pediatric dosage
750 mg followed 12 hrs later by 500 mg	15 mg/kg followed 12 hrs later by 10 mg/kg
6 doses over 3d (4 tabs/dose at 0, 8, 24, 36, 48 and 60 hours)	6 doses over 3d at same intervals as adults; <15kg: 1 tab/dose 15-25kg: 2 tabs/dose 25-35kg: 3 tabs/dose >35kg: 4 tabs/dose
4 mg/kg/d x 3d	4 mg/kg/d x 3d

77. Artemether/lumefantrine is available as a fixed-dose combination tablet (*Coartem* in countries with endemic malaria, *Riamet* in Europe and countries without endemic malaria); each tablet contains 20 mg artemether and 120 mg lumefantrine (M van Vugt et al, Am J Trop Med Hyg 1999; 60:936). In animal studies artemisinins have been embryotoxic and caused low incidence of teratogenicity; no adverse pregnancy outcome has been observed in limited human studies (S Dellicour et al, Malaria Journal 2007; 6:15). The tablets should be taken with food. Artemether/lumefantrine should not be used in patients with cardiac arrhythmias, bradycardia, severe cardiac disease or QT prolongation. Concomitant use of drugs that prolong the QT interval or are metabolized by CYP2D6 is contraindicated.

78. Adults treated with artesunate should also receive oral treatment doses of either atovaquone/proguanil, doxycycline, clindamycin or mefloquine; children should take either atovaquone/proguanil, clindamycin or mefloquine (F Nosten et al, Lancet 2000; 356:297; M van Vugt, Clin Infect Dis 2002; 35:1498; F Smithuis et al, Trans R Soc Trop Med Hyg 2004; 98:182). If artesunate is given IV, oral medication should be started when the patient is able to tolerate it (SEAQUAMAT group, Lancet 2005; 366:717).

Continued on next page.

DRUGS FOR PARASITIC INFECTIONS (continued)

Infection	Drug
MALARIA, Treatment of (continued)	
P. vivax acquired in areas of chloroquine-resistant *P. vivax*[64]	
Drug of choice:[67]	Mefloquine[74]
	OR Atovaquone/proguanil[68]
	either followed by
	primaquine phosphate[79]
Alternative:[67]	Chloroquine phosphate[80]
	OR Quinine sulfate
	plus
	doxycycline[7,21,71]
	either followed by
	primaquine phosphate[79]
All *Plasmodium* species except chloroquine-resistant *P. falciparum*[63] and chloroquine-resistant *P. vivax*[64]	
Drug of choice:[67]	Chloroquine phosphate[80]

---

*   Availability problems. See table on page 277.

79. Primaquine phosphate can cause hemolytic anemia, especially in patients whose red cells are deficient in G-6-PD. This deficiency is most common in African, Asian and Mediterranean peoples. Patients should be screened for G-6-PD deficiency before treatment. Primaquine should not be used during pregnancy. It should be taken with food to minimize nausea and abdominal pain. Primaquine-tolerant *P. vivax* can be found globally. Relapses of primaquine-resistant strains may be retreated with 30 mg (base) x 28d.

Adult dosage	Pediatric dosage
750 mg PO followed 12 hrs later by 500 mg	15 mg/kg PO followed 12 hrs later by 10 mg/kg
2 adult tabs bid[69] or 4 adult tabs once/d x 3d	<5kg: not indicated
	5-8kg: 2 peds tabs once/d x 3d
	9-10kg: 3 peds tabs once/d x 3d
	11-20kg: 1 adult tab once/d x 3d
	21-30kg: 2 adult tabs once/d x 3d
	31-40kg: 3 adult tabs once/d x 3d
	>40kg: 4 adult tabs once/d x 3d
30 mg base/d PO x 14d	0.6 mg/kg/d PO x 14d
25 mg base/kg PO in 3 doses over 48 hrs[81]	25 mg base/kg PO in 3 doses over 48 hrs[81]
650 mg PO q8h x 3-7d[70]	30 mg/kg/d PO in 3 doses x 3-7d[70]
100 mg PO bid x 7d	4 mg/kg/d PO in 2 doses x 7d
30 mg base/d PO x 14d	0.6 mg/kg/d PO x 14d
1 g (600 mg base) PO, then 500 mg (300 mg base) 6 hrs later, then 500mg (300 mg base) at 24 and 48 hrs[81]	10 mg base/kg (max 600 mg base) PO, then 5 mg base/kg 6 hrs later, then 5 mg base/kg at 24 and 48 hrs[81]

80. Chloroquine should be taken with food to decrease gastrointestinal adverse effects. If chloroquine phosphate is not available, hydroxychloroquine sulfate is as effective; 400 mg of hydroxychloroquine sulfate is equivalent to 500 mg of chloroquine phosphate.
81. Chloroquine combined with primaquine was effective in 85% of patients with P. vivax resistant to chloroquine and could be a reasonable choice in areas where other alternatives are not available (JK Baird et al, J Infect Dis 1995; 171:1678).

Continued on next page.

DRUGS FOR PARASITIC INFECTIONS (continued)

Infection	Drug
MALARIA, Treatment of (continued) **PARENTERAL**[66] All *Plasmodium* species (Chloroquine-sensitive and resistant) Drug of choice:[67,82]	Quinidine gluconate[83]
OR	Quinine dihydrochloride[83*]
OR	Artesunate[76*]
	plus see footnote 78
MALARIA, Prevention of[84] All *Plasmodium* species in chloroquine-sensitive areas[63,64,65] Drug of choice:[67,85]	Chloroquine phosphate[80,86]

---

* Availability problems. See table on page 277.
82. Exchange transfusion is controversial, but has been helpful for some patients with high-density (>10%) parasitemia, altered mental status, pulmonary edema or renal complications (VI Powell and K Grima, Transfus Med Rev 2002; 16:239; MS Riddle et al, Clin Infect Dis 2002; 34:1192).
83. Continuous EKG, blood pressure and glucose monitoring are recommended, especially in pregnant women and young children. For problems with quinidine availability, call the manufacturer (Eli Lilly, 800-821-0538) or the CDC Malaria Hotline (770-488-7788). Quinidine may have greater antimalarial activity than quinine. The loading dose should be decreased or omitted in patients who have received quinine or mefloquine. If more than 48 hours of parenteral treatment is required, the quinine or quinidine dose should be reduced by 30-50%.

Adult dosage	Pediatric dosage
10 mg/kg IV loading dose (max 600 mg) in normal saline over 1-2 hrs, followed by continuous infusion of 0.02 mg/kg/min until PO therapy can be started 20 mg/kg IV loading dose in 5% dextrose over 4 hrs, followed by 10 mg/kg over 2-4 hrs q8h (max 1800 mg/d) until PO therapy can be started 2.4 mg/kg/dose IV x 3d at 0, 12, 24, 48 and 72 hrs	10 mg/kg IV loading dose (max 600 mg) in normal saline over 1-2 hrs, followed by continuous infusion of 0.02 mg/kg/min until PO therapy can be started 20 mg/kg IV loading dose in 5% dextrose over 4 hrs, followed by 10 mg/kg over 2-4 hrs q8h (max 1800 mg/d) until PO therapy can be started 2.4 mg/kg/dose IV x 3d at 0, 12, 24, 48 and 72 hrs
500 mg (300 mg base) PO once/wk[87]	5 mg/kg base PO once/wk, up to adult dose of 300 mg base[87]

84. No drug guarantees protection against malaria. Travelers should be advised to seek medical attention if fever develops after they return. Insect repellents, insecticide-impregnated bed nets and proper clothing are important adjuncts for malaria prophylaxis (Med Lett Drugs Ther 2005; 47:100). Malaria in pregnancy is particularly serious for both mother and fetus; prophylaxis is indicated if exposure cannot be avoided.
85. Alternatives for patients who are unable to take chloroquine include atovaquone/proguanil, mefloquine, doxycycline or primaquine dosed as for chloroquine-resistant areas.
86. Has been used extensively and safely for prophylaxis in pregnancy.
87. Beginning 1-2wks before travel and continuing weekly for the duration of stay and for 4wks after leaving.

Continued on next page.

DRUGS FOR PARASITIC INFECTIONS (continued)

Infection	Drug
MALARIA, Prevention of[84] (continued)	
All *Plasmodium* species in chloroquine-resistant areas[63,64,65]	
Drug of choice:[67]	Atovaquone/proguanil[68]
	OR Doxycycline[7,21,71]
	OR Mefloquine[74,75,90]
Alternative:[92]	Primaquine phosphate[7,79]
MALARIA, Prevention of relapses: *P. vivax* and *P. ovale*[67]	
Drug of choice:	Primaquine phosphate[79]

*   Availability problems. See table on page 277.

88.   Beginning 1-2d before travel and continuing for the duration of stay and for 1wk after leaving. In one study of malaria prophylaxis, atovaquone/proguanil was better tolerated than mefloquine in non-immune travelers (D Overbosch et al, Clin Infect Dis 2001; 33:1015). The protective efficacy of *Malarone* against *P. vivax* is variable ranging from 84% in Indonesian New Guinea (J Ling et al, Clin Infect Dis 2002; 35:825) to 100% in Colombia (J Soto et al, Am J Trop Med Hyg 2006; 75:430). Some Medical Letter consultants prefer alternate drugs if traveling to areas where *P. vivax* predominates.

89.   Beginning 1-2d before travel and continuing for the duration of stay and for 4wks after leaving. Use of tetracyclines is contraindicated in pregnancy and in children <8 years old. Doxycycline can cause gastrointestinal disturbances, vaginal moniliasis and photosensitivity reactions.

90.   Mefloquine has not been approved for use during pregnancy. However, it has been reported to be safe for prophylactic use during the second and third trimester of pregnancy and possibly during early pregnancy as well (CDC Health Information for International Travel, 2008, page 228; BL Smoak et al, J Infect Dis 1997; 176:831). For pediatric doses <½ tablet, it is advisable to have a pharmacist crush the tablet, estimate doses by weighing, and package them in gelatin capsules. There is no data for use in children <5 kg, but based on dosages in other weight groups, a dose of 5 mg/kg can be used. Not recommended for use in travelers with active depression or with a history of psychosis or seizures and should be used with caution in persons with psychiatric illness. Mefloquine can be given to patients taking β-blockers if they do not have an underlying arrhythmia; it should not be used in patients with conduction abnormalities.

Adult dosage	Pediatric dosage
1 adult tab/d[88]	5-8kg: ½ peds tab/d[68,88]
	9-10kg: ¾ peds tab/d[68,88]
	11-20kg: 1 peds tab/d[68,88]
	21-30kg: 2 peds tabs/d[68,88]
	31-40kg: 3 peds tabs/d[68,88]
	>40kg: 1 adult tab/d[68,88]
100 mg PO daily[89]	2 mg/kg/d PO, up to 100 mg/d[89]
250 mg PO once/wk[91]	5-10kg: $1/_8$ tab once/wk[91]
	11-20kg: ¼ tab once/wk[91]
	21-30kg: ½ tab once/wk[91]
	31-45kg: ¾ tab once/wk[91]
	>45kg: 1 tab once/wk[91]
30 mg base PO daily[93]	0.6 mg/kg base PO daily[93]
30 mg base/d PO x 14d	0.6 mg base/kg/d PO x 14d

91. Beginning 1-2wks before travel and continuing weekly for the duration of stay and for 4wks after leaving. Most adverse events occur within 3 doses. Some Medical Letter consultants favor starting mefloquine 3 weeks prior to travel and monitoring the patient for adverse events, this allows time to change to an alternative regimen if mefloquine is not tolerated.
92. The combination of weekly chloroquine (300 mg base) and daily proguanil (200 mg) is recommended by the World Health Organization (www.WHO.int) for use in selected areas; this combination is no longer recommended by the CDC. Proguanil (*Paludrine* – AstraZeneca, United Kingdom) is not available alone in the US but is widely available in Canada and Europe. Prophylaxis is recommended during exposure and for 4 weeks afterwards. Proguanil has been used in pregnancy without evidence of toxicity (PA Phillips-Howard and D Wood, Drug Saf 1996; 14:131).
93 Studies have shown that daily primaquine beginning 1d before departure and continued until 3-7d after leaving the malarious area provides effective prophylaxis against chloroquine-resistant *P. falciparum* (JK Baird et al, Clin Infect Dis 2003; 37:1659). Some studies have shown less efficacy against *P. vivax*. Nausea and abdominal pain can be diminished by taking with food.

Continued on next page.

DRUGS FOR PARASITIC INFECTIONS (continued)

Infection	Drug
MALARIA, Self-Presumptive Treatment[94]	
Drug of Choice:	Atovaquone/proguanil[7,68]
	OR Quinine sulfate **plus** doxycycline[7,21,71]
	OR Artesunate[76]* **plus** see footnote 78

MICROSPORIDIOSIS	
Ocular (Encephalitozoon hellem, E.cuniculi, Vittaforma corneae [Nosema corneum])	
Drug of choice:	Albendazole[7,12] **plus** fumagillin[95]*
Intestinal (E. bieneusi, E. [Septata] intestinalis) **E. bieneusi**	
Drug of choice:	Fumagillin[96]*
E. intestinalis	
Drug of choice:	Albendazole[7,12]
Disseminated (E. hellem, E. cuniculi, E. intestinalis, Pleistophora sp., Trachipleistophora sp. and Brachiola vesicularum)	
Drug of choice:[97]	Albendazole[7,12]*

* Availability problems. See table on page 277.
94. A traveler can be given a course of medication for presumptive self-treatment of febrile illness. The drug given for self-treatment should be different from that used for prophylaxis. This approach should be used only in very rare circumstances when a traveler would not be able to get medical care promptly.
95. CM Chan et al, Ophthalmology 2003; 110:1420. Ocular lesions due to *E. hellem* in HIV-infected patients have responded to fumagillin eyedrops prepared from *Fumidil-B* (bicyclohexyl ammonium fumagillin) used to control a microsporidial disease of honey bees (MJ Garvey et al, Ann Pharmacother 1995; 29:872), available from Leiter's Park Avenue Pharmacy (see footnote 1). For lesions due to *V. corneae*, topical therapy is generally not effective and keratoplasty may be required (RM Davis et al, Ophthalmology 1990; 97:953).

Adult dosage	Pediatric dosage
4 adult tabs once/d x 3d[69]	<5kg: not indicated 5-8kg: 2 peds tabs once/d x 3d 9-10kg: 3 peds tabs once/d x 3d 11-20kg: 1 adult tab once/d x 3d 21-30kg: 2 adult tabs once/d x 3d 31-40kg: 3 adult tabs once/d x 3d >40kg: 4 adult tabs once/d x 3d[69]
650 mg PO q8h x 3 or 7d[70]	30 mg/kg/d PO in 3 doses x 3 or 7d[70]
100 mg PO bid x 7d	4 mg/kg/d PO in 2 doses x 7d
4 mg/kg/d PO x 3d	4 mg/kg/d PO x 3d
400 mg PO bid	
20 mg PO tid x 14d	
400 mg PO bid x 21d	
400 mg PO bid	

96. Oral fumagillin (*Flisint* – Sanofi-Aventis, France) has been effective in treating *E. bieneusi* (J-M Molina et al, N Engl J Med 2002; 346:1963), but has been associated with thrombocytopenia and neutropenia. Highly active antiretroviral therapy (HAART) may lead to microbiologic and clinical response in HIV-infected patients with microsporidial diarrhea. Octreotide *(Sandostatin)* has provided symptomatic relief in some patients with large-volume diarrhea.

97. J-M Molina et al, J Infect Dis 1995; 171:245. There is no established treatment for *Pleistophora*. For disseminated disease due to *Trachipleistophora* or *Brachiola*, itraconazole 400 mg PO once/d plus albendazole may also be tried (CM Coyle et al, N Engl J Med 2004; 351:42).

Continued on next page.

DRUGS FOR PARASITIC INFECTIONS (continued)

Infection	Drug
Mites, see SCABIES	
MONILIFORMIS *moniliformis* infection	
Drug of choice:	Pyrantel pamoate[7,13*]
Naegleria **species**, see AMEBIC MENINGOENCEPHALITIS, PRIMARY	
Necator americanus, see HOOKWORM infection	
OESOPHAGOSTOMUM *bifurcum*	
Drug of choice:	See footnote 98
Onchocerca volvulus, see FILARIASIS	
Opisthorchis viverrini, see FLUKE infection	
Paragonimus westermani, see FLUKE infection	
Pediculus capitis, humanus, Phthirus pubis, see LICE	
Pinworm, see ENTEROBIUS	
PNEUMOCYSTIS JIROVECI (formerly *carinii*) pneumonia (PCP)[99]	
Drug of choice:	Trimethoprim/sulfamethoxazole
Alternative:	Primaquine[7,79]
	plus clindamycin[7,18]
	OR Trimethoprim[7]
	plus dapsone[7]
	OR Pentamidine
	OR Atovaquone

---

* Availability problems. See table on page 277.
98. Albendazole or pyrantel pamoate may be effective (JB Ziem et al, Ann Trop Med Parasitol 2004; 98:385).

Adult dosage	Pediatric dosage
11 mg/kg PO once, repeat twice, 2wks apart	11 mg/kg PO once, repeat twice, 2wks apart
TMP 15 mg/SMX 75 mg/kg/d, PO or IV in 3 or 4 doses x 21d	TMP 15 mg/SMX 75 mg/kg/d, PO or IV in 3 or 4 doses x 21d
30 mg base PO daily x 21d	0.3 mg/kg base PO daily x 21d
600 mg IV q6h x 21d, or 300-450 mg PO q6h x 21d	15-25 mg/kg IV q6h x 21d, or 10 mg/kg PO q6h x 21d
5 mg/kg PO tid x 21d	5 mg/kg PO tid x 21d
100 mg daily x 21d	2 mg/kg/d PO x 21d
3-4 mg/kg IV daily x 21d	3-4 mg/kg IV daily x 21d
750 mg PO bid x 21d	1-3mos: 30 mg/kg/d PO x 21d
	4-24mos: 45 mg/kg/d PO x 21d
	>24mos: 30 mg/d PO x 21d

99. Pneumocystis has been reclassified as a fungus. In severe disease with room air $PO_2 \leq 70$ mmHg or Aa gradient ≥ 35 mmHg, prednisone should also be used (S Gagnon et al, N Engl J Med 1990; 323:1444; E Caumes et al, Clin Infect Dis 1994; 18:319).

Continued on next page.

DRUGS FOR PARASITIC INFECTIONS (continued)

Infection	Drug
PNEUMOCYSTIS JIROVECI (continued) **Primary and secondary prophylaxis**[100] Drug of Choice:	Trimethoprim/sulfamethoxazole
Alternative:	Dapsone[7]
OR	Dapsone[7] **plus** pyrimethamine[101]
OR	Pentamidine
OR	Atovaquone[7,20]

River Blindness, see FILARIASIS	
Roundworm, see ASCARIASIS	
Sappinia diploidea, See AMEBIC MENINGOENCEPHALITIS, PRIMARY	
SCABIES *(Sarcoptes scabiei)* Drug of choice: Alternative:[103]	5% Permethrin Ivermectin[7,16,104] 10% Crotamiton

*   Availability problems. See table on page 277.
100. Primary/secondary prophylaxis in patients with HIV can be discontinued after CD4 count increases to >200 x 10^6/L for >3mos.
101. Plus leucovorin 25 mg with each dose of pyrimethamine. Pyrimethamine should be taken with food to minimize gastrointestinal adverse effects.
102. Treatment may need to be repeated in 10-14 days. A second ivermectin dose taken 2 weeks later increases the cure rate to 95%, which is equivalent to that of 5% permethrin (V Usha et al, J Am Acad Dermatol 2000; 42:236; O Chosidow, N Engl J Med 2006; 354:1718; J Heukelbach and H Feldmeier, Lancet 2006; 367:1767).

Adult dosage	Pediatric dosage

1 tab (single or double strength) daily
  or 1 DS tab PO 3d/wk
50 mg PO bid or 100 mg PO daily
	TMP 150 mg/SMX 750 mg/m²/d
	  PO in 2 doses 3d/wk
	2 mg/kg/d (max 100 mg) PO or
	  4 mg/kg (max 200 mg) PO each wk

50 mg PO daily or 200 mg PO each wk
50 mg PO or 75 mg PO each wk
300 mg aerosol inhaled monthly via
  Respirgard II nebulizer
1500 mg PO daily
	≥5yrs: 300 mg inhaled monthly via
	  Respirgard II nebulizer
	1-3mos: 30 mg/kg/d PO
	4-24mos: 45 mg/kg/d PO
	>24mos: 30 mg/kg/d PO

Topically once[102] 200 mcg/kg PO once[102] Topically once/d x 2	Topically once[102] 200 mcg/kg PO once[102] Topically once/d PO x 2

103. Lindane (γ-benzene hexachloride) should be reserved for treatment of patients who fail to respond to other drugs. The FDA has recommended it not be used for immunocompromised patients, young children, the elderly, pregnant and breast-feeding women, and patients weighing <50 kg.

104. Ivermectin, either alone or in combination with a topical scabicide, is the drug of choice for crusted scabies in immunocompromised patients (P del Giudice, Curr Opin Infect Dis 2004; 15:123).

Continued on next page.

DRUGS FOR PARASITIC INFECTIONS (continued)

Infection	Drug
SCHISTOSOMIASIS (*Bilharziasis*)	
S. haematobium	
Drug of choice:	Praziquantel[39]
S. japonicum	
Drug of choice:	Praziquantel[39]
S. mansoni	
Drug of choice:	Praziquantel[39]
Alternative:	Oxamniquine[105]*
S. mekongi	
Drug of choice:	Praziquantel[39]
Sleeping sickness, see TRYPANOSOMIASIS	
STRONGYLOIDIASIS (*Strongyloides stercoralis*)	
Drug of choice:[107]	Ivermectin[16]
Alternative:	Albendazole[7,12]
TAPEWORM infection	
— **Adult** (intestinal stage)	
***Diphyllobothrium latum* (fish), *Taenia saginata* (beef), *Taenia solium* (pork), *Dipylidium caninum* (dog)**	
Drug of choice:	Praziquantel[7,39]
Alternative:	Niclosamide[108]*
***Hymenolepis nana* (dwarf tapeworm)**	
Drug of choice:	Praziquantel[7,39]
Alternative:	Nitazoxanide[5,7]

---

*   Availability problems. See table on page 277.
105. Oxamniquine, which is not available in the US, is generally not as effective as praziquantel. It has been useful, however, in some areas in which praziquantel is less effective (ML Ferrari et al, Bull World Health Organ 2003; 81:190; A Harder, Parasitol Res 2002; 88:395). Oxamniquine is contraindicated in pregnancy. It should be taken after food.
106. In East Africa, the dose should be increased to 30 mg/kg, and in Egypt and South Africa to 30 mg/kg/d x 2d. Some experts recommend 40-60 mg/kg over 2-3d in all of Africa (KC Shekhar, Drugs 1991; 42:379).
107. In immunocompromised patients or disseminated disease, it may be necessary to prolong or repeat therapy, or to use other agents. Veterinary parenteral and enema formulations of ivermectin have been used in severely ill patients with hyperinfection who were unable to take or reliably absorb oral medications (J Orem et al, Clin Infect Dis 2003; 37:152; PE Tarr Am J Trop Med Hyg 2003; 68:453; FM Marty et al, Clin Infect Dis 2005; 41:e5). In disseminated strongyloidiasis, combination therapy with albendazole and ivermectin has been suggested (S Lim et al, CMAJ 2004; 171:479).

Adult dosage	Pediatric dosage
40 mg/kg/d PO in 2 doses x 1d	40 mg/kg/d PO in 2 doses x 1d
60 mg/kg/d PO in 3 doses x 1d	60 mg/kg/d PO in 3 doses x 1d
40 mg/kg/d PO in 2 doses x 1d	40 mg/kg/d PO in 2 doses x 1d
15 mg/kg PO once[106]	20 mg/kg/d PO in 2 doses x 1d[106]
60 mg/kg/d PO in 3 doses x 1d	60 mg/kg/d PO in 3 doses x 1d
200 mcg/kg/d PO x 2d	200 mcg/kg/d PO x 2d
400 mg PO bid x 7d	400 mg PO bid x 7d
5-10 mg/kg PO once	5-10 mg/kg PO once
2 g PO once	50 mg/kg PO once
25 mg/kg PO once	25 mg/kg PO once
500 mg PO once/d or bid x 3d[109]	1-3yrs: 100 mg PO bid x 3d[109]
	4-11yrs: 200 mg PO bid x 3d[109]

108. Niclosamide must be chewed thoroughly before swallowing and washed down with water.
109. JO Juan et al, Trans R Soc Trop Med Hyg 2002; 96:193; JC Chero et al, Trans R Soc Trop Med Hyg 2007; 101:203; E Diaz et al, Am J Trop Med Hyg 2003; 68:384.

Continued on next page.

DRUGS FOR PARASITIC INFECTIONS (continued)

Infection	Drug
TAPEWORM infection (continued)	
— **Larval** (tissue stage)	
Echinococcus granulosus (hydatid cyst)	
Drug of choice:[110]	Albendazole[12]
Echinococcus multilocularis	
Treatment of choice:	See footnote 111
Taenia solium *(Cysticercosis)*	
Treatment of choice:	See footnote 112
Alternative:	Albendazole[12]
	OR Praziquantel[7,39]

Toxocariasis, see VISCERAL LARVA MIGRANS

---

*   Availability problems. See table on page 277.

110. Patients may benefit from surgical resection or percutaneous drainage of cysts. Praziquantel is useful preoperatively or in case of spillage of cyst contents during surgery. Percutaneous aspiration-injection-reaspiration (PAIR) with ultrasound guidance plus albendazole therapy has been effective for management of hepatic hydatid cyst disease (RA Smego, Jr. et al, Clin Infect Dis 2003; 37:1073; S Nepalia et al, J Assoc Physicians India 2006; 54:458; E Zerem and R Jusufovic Surg Endosc 2006; 20:1543).

111. Surgical excision is the only reliable means of cure. Reports have suggested that in nonresectable cases use of albendazole (400 mg bid) can stabilize and sometimes cure infection (P Craig, Curr Opin Infect Dis 2003; 16:437; O Lidove et al, Am J Med 2005; 118:195).

112. Initial therapy for patients with inflamed parenchymal cysticercosis should focus on symptomatic treatment with anti-seizure medication (LS Yancey et al, Curr Infect Dis Rep 2005; 7:39; AH del Brutto et al, Ann Intern Med 2006; 145:43). Patients with live parenchymal cysts who have seizures should be treated with albendazole together with steroids (dexamethasone 6 mg/d or prednisone 40-60 mg/d) and an anti-seizure medication (HH Garcia et al, N Engl J Med 2004; 350:249). Patients with subarachnoid cysts or giant cysts in the fissures should be treated for at least 30d (JV Proaño et al, N Engl J Med 2001; 345:879). Surgical intervention (especially neuroendoscopic removal) or CSF diversion followed by albendazole and steroids is indicated for obstructive hydocephalus. Arachnoiditis, vasculitis or cerebral edema is treated with prednisone 60 mg/d or dexamethasone 4-6 mg/d together with albendazole or praziquantel (AC White, Jr., Annu Rev Med 2000; 51:187). Any cysticercocidal drug may cause irreparable damage when used to treat ocular or spinal cysts, even when corticosteroids are used. An ophthalmic exam should always precede treatment to rule out intraocular cysts.

Adult dosage	Pediatric dosage
400 mg PO bid x 1-6mos	15 mg/kg/d (max 800 mg) x 1-6mos
400 mg PO bid x 8-30d; can be repeated as necessary	15 mg/kg/d (max 800 mg) PO in 2 doses x 8-30d; can be repeated as necessary
100 mg/kg/d PO in 3 doses x 1 day then 50 mg/kg/d in 3 doses x 29 days	100 mg/kg/d PO in 3 doses x 1 day then 50 mg/kg/d in 3 doses x 29 days

Continued on next page.

DRUGS FOR PARASITIC INFECTIONS (continued)

Infection	Drug
TOXOPLASMOSIS *(Toxoplasma gondii)*	
Drug of choice:[113]	Pyrimethamine[114]
	plus
	sulfadiazine[116]
TRICHINELLOSIS *(Trichinella spiralis)*	
Drug of choice:	Steroids for severe symptoms
	plus
	Albendazole[7,12]
Alternative:	Mebendazole[7]
TRICHOMONIASIS *(Trichomonas vaginalis)*	
Drug of choice:[117]	Metronidazole
OR	Tinidazole[6]
TRICHOSTRONGYLUS infection	
Drug of choice:	Pyrantel pamoate[7,13]*
Alternative:	Mebendazole[7]
OR	Albendazole[7,12]

* Availability problems. See table on page 277.

113. To treat CNS toxoplasmosis in HIV-infected patients, some clinicians have used pyrimethamine 50-100 mg/d (after a loading dose of 200 mg) with sulfadiazine and, when sulfonamide sensitivity developed, have given clindamycin 1.8-2.4 g/d in divided doses instead of the sulfonamide. Treatment is usually given for at least 4-6 weeks. Atovaquone (1500 mg PO bid) plus pyrimethamine (200 mg loading dose, followed by 75 mg/d PO) for 6 weeks appears to be an effective alternative in sulfa-intolerant patients (K Chirgwin et al, Clin Infect Dis 2002; 34:1243). Atovaquone must be taken with a meal to enhance absorption. Treatment is followed by chronic suppression with lower dosage regimens of the same drugs. For primary prophylaxis in HIV patients with <100 x 10^6/L CD4 cells, either trimethoprim-sulfamethoxazole, pyrimethamine with dapsone, or atovaquone with or without pyrimethamine can be used. Primary or secondary prophylaxis may be discontinued when the CD4 count increases to >200 x 10^6/L for >3mos (MMWR Morb Mortal Wkly Rep 2004; 53 [RR15]:1). In ocular toxoplasmosis with macular involvement, corticosteroids are recommended in addition to antiparasitic therapy for an anti-inflammatory effect. In one randomized single-blind study, trimethoprim/sulfamethoxazole was reported to be as effective as pyrimethamine/sulfadiazine for treatment of ocular toxoplasmosis (M Soheilian et al, Ophthalmology 2005; 112:1876). Women who develop toxoplasmosis during the first trimester of pregnancy should be treated with spiramycin (3-4 g/d). After the first trimester, if there is no documented transmission to the fetus, spiramycin can be continued until term. If transmission has occurred *in utero*, therapy with pyrimethamine and sulfadiazine should be started (JG Montoya and O Liesenfeld, Lancet 2004; 363:1965). Pyrimethamine is a potential teratogen and should be used only after the first trimester.

Adult dosage	Pediatric dosage
25-100 mg/d PO x 3-4wks	2 mg/kg/d PO x 2d, then 1 mg/kg/d (max 25 mg/d) x 4wks[115]
1-1.5 g PO qid x 3-4wks	100-200 mg/kg/d PO x 3-4wks
400 mg PO bid x 8-14d	400 mg PO bid x 8-14d
200-400 mg PO tid x 3d, then 400-500 mg tid x 10d	200-400 mg PO tid x 3d, then 400-500 mg tid x 10d
2 g PO once or 500 mg bid x 7d	15 mg/kg/d PO in 3 doses x 7d
2 g PO once	50 mg/kg once (max 2 g)
11 mg/kg base PO once (max 1 g)	11 mg/kg PO once (max 1 g)
100 mg PO bid x 3d	100 mg PO bid x 3d
400 mg PO once	400 mg PO once

114. Plus leucovorin 10-25 mg with each dose of pyrimethamine. Pyrimethamine should be taken with food to minimize gastrointestinal adverse effects.
115. Congenitally infected newborns should be treated with pyrimethamine every 2 or 3 days and a sulfonamide daily for about one year (JS Remington and G Desmonts in JS Remington and JO Klein, eds, *Infectious Disease of the Fetus and Newborn Infant*, 6th ed, Philadelphia:Saunders, 2006, page 1038).
116. Sulfadiazine should be taken on an empty stomach with adequate water.
117. Sexual partners should be treated simultaneously with same dosage. Metronidazole-resistant strains have been reported and can be treated with higher doses of metronidazole (2-4 g/d x 7-14d) or with tinidazole (MMWR Morb Mortal Wkly Rep 2006; 55 [RR11]:1).

Continued on next page.

DRUGS FOR PARASITIC INFECTIONS (continued)

Infection	Drug
TRICHURIASIS (*Trichuris trichiura*, whipworm)	
Drug of choice:	Mebendazole
Alternative:	Albendazole[7,12]
OR	Ivermectin[7,16]
TRYPANOSOMIASIS[118]	
T. cruzi (American trypanosomiasis, Chagas' disease)	
Drug of choice:	Nifurtimox*
OR	Benznidazole[119]*
T. brucei gambiense (West African trypanosomiasis, sleeping sickness)	
hemolymphatic stage	
Drug of choice:[120]	Pentamidine[7]
Alternative:	Suramin*
Late disease with CNS involvement	
Drug of Choice:	Eflornithine[121]*
OR	Melarsoprol[122]

---

* Availability problems. See table on page 277.
118. MP Barrett et al, Lancet 2003; 362:1469. Treatment of chronic or indeterminate Chagas' disease with benznidazole has been associated with reduced progression and increased negative seroconversion (R Viotti et al, Ann Intern Med 2006; 144:724).
119. Benznidazole should be taken with meals to minimize gastrointestinal adverse effects. It is contraindicated during pregnancy.
120. Pentamidine and suramin have equal efficacy, but pentamidine is better tolerated.
121. Eflornithine is highly effective in *T.b. gambiense*, but not in *T.b. rhodesiense* infections. In one study of treatment of CNS disease due to *T.b. gambiense*, there were fewer serious complications with eflornithine than with melarsoprol (F Chappuis et al, Clin Infect Dis 2005; 41:748). Eflornithine is available in limited supply only from the WHO and the CDC. It is contraindicated during pregnancy.

Adult dosage	Pediatric dosage
100 mg PO bid x 3d or 500 mg once	100 mg PO bid x 3d or 500 mg once
400 mg PO x 3d	400 mg PO x 3d
200 mcg/kg PO daily x 3d	200 mcg/kg/d PO x 3d
8-10 mg/kg/d PO in 3-4 doses x 90-120d	1-10yrs: 15-20 mg/kg/d PO in 4 doses x 90-120d
	11-16yrs: 12.5-15 mg/kg/d in 4 doses x 90-120d
5-7 mg/kg/d PO in 2 doses x 30-90d	≤12yrs: 10 mg/kg/d PO in 2 doses x 30-90d
	>12 yrs: 5-7 mg/kg/d in 2 doses x 30-90d
4 mg/kg/d IM x 7d	4 mg/kg/d IM x 7d
100-200 mg (test dose) IV, then 1 g IV on days 1,3,7,14 and 21	20 mg/kg on d 1,3,7,14 and 21
400 mg/kg/d IV in 4 doses x 14d	400 mg/kg/d IV in 4 doses x 14d
2.2 mg/kg/d IV x 10d	2.2 mg/kg/d IV x 10d

122. E Schmid et al, J Infect Dis 2005; 191:1922. Corticosteroids have been used to prevent arsenical encephalopathy (J Pepin et al, Trans R Soc Trop Med Hyg 1995; 89:92). Up to 20% of patients with *T.b.gambiense* fail to respond to melarsoprol (MP Barrett, Lancet 1999; 353:1113). In one study, a combination of low-dose melarsoprol (1.2 mg/kg/d IV) and nifurtimox (7.5 mg/kg PO bid) x 10d was more effective than standard-dose melarsoprol alone (S Bisser et al, J Infect Dis 2007; 195:322).

Continued on next page.

DRUGS FOR PARASITIC INFECTIONS (continued)

Infection	Drug
TRYPANOSOMIASIS[118] (continued)	
T. b. rhodesiense (East African trypanosomiasis, sleeping sickness)	
hemolymphatic stage	
Drug of choice:	Suramin*
Late disease with CNS involvement	
Drug of choice:	Melarsoprol[122]
VISCERAL LARVA MIGRANS[123] *(Toxocariasis)*	
Drug of choice:	Albendazole[7,12]
OR	Mebendazole[7]
Whipworm, see TRICHURIASIS	
Wuchereria bancrofti, see FILARIASIS	

* Availability problems. See table on page 277.
123. Optimum duration of therapy is not known; some Medical Letter consultants would treat x 20d. For severe symptoms or eye involvement, corticosteroids can be used in addition (D Despommier, Clin Microbiol Rev 2003; 16:265).

Adult dosage	Pediatric dosage
100-200 mg (test dose) IV, then 1 g IV on days 1,3,7,14 and 21	20 mg/kg on d 1,3,7,14 and 21
2-3.6 mg/kg/d IV x 3d; after 7d 3.6 mg/kg/d x 3d; repeat again after 7d	2-3.6 mg/kg/d x 3d; after 7d 3.6 mg/kg/d x 3d; repeat again after 7d
400 mg PO bid x 5d 100-200 mg PO bid x 5d	400 mg PO bid x 5d 100-200 mg PO bid x 5d

SAFETY OF ANTIPARASITIC DRUGS IN PREGNANCY

Drug	Toxicity in Pregnancy	Recommendations
Albendazole *(Albenza)*		
	Teratogenic and embryotoxic in animals	Caution*
Amphotericin B *(Fungizone*, and others)		
	None known	Caution*
Amphotericin B liposomal *(AmBisome)*		
	None known	Caution*
Artemether/lumefantrine *(Coartem, Riamet)*[1]		
	Embryocidal and teratogenic in animals	Caution*
Artesunate[1]		
	Embryocidal and teratogenic in animals	Caution*
Atovaquone *(Mepron)*		
	Maternal and fetal toxicity in animals	Caution*
Atovaquone/proguanil *(Malarone)*[2]		
	Maternal and fetal toxicity in animals	Caution*
Azithromycin *(Zithromax*, and others)		
	None known	Probably safe
Benznidazole *(Rochagan)*		
	Unknown	Contraindicated
Chloroquine *(Aralen*, and others)		
	None known with doses recommended for malaria prophylaxis	Probably safe in low doses
Clarithromycin *(Biaxin*, and others)		
	Teratogenic in animals	Contraindicated
Clindamycin *(Cleocin*, and others)		
	None known	Caution*
Crotamiton *(Eurax)*		
	Unknown	Caution*

Continued on next page.

SAFETY OF ANTIPARASITIC DRUGS IN PREGNANCY (continued)

Drug	Toxicity in Pregnancy	Recommendations
Dapsone		
	None known; carcinogenic in rats and mice; hemolytic reactions in neonates	Caution*, especially at term
Diethylcarbamazine (DEC; *Hetrazan*)		
	Not known; abortifacient in one study in rabbits	Contraindicated
Diloxanide *(Furamide)*		
	Safety not established	Caution*
Doxycycline (*Vibramycin*, and others)		
	Tooth discoloration and dysplasia, inhibition of bone growth in fetus; hepatic toxicity and azotemia with IV use in pregnant patients with decreased renal function or with overdosage	Contraindicated
Eflornithine *(Ornidyl)*		
	Embryocidal in animals	Contraindicated
Fluconazole (*Diflucan*, and others)		
	Teratogenic	Contraindicated for high dose; caution* for single dose
Flucytosine *(Ancoban)*		
	Teratogenic in rats	Contraindicated
Furazolidone *(Furoxone)*		
	None known; carcinogenic in rodents; hemolysis with G-6-PD deficiency in newborn	Caution*; contraindicated at term
Hydroxychloroquine *(Plaquenil)*		
	None known with doses recommended for malaria prophylaxis	Probably safe in low doses
Itraconazole (*Sporanox*, and others)		
	Teratogenic and embryotoxic in rats	Caution*

Continued on next page.

SAFETY OF ANTIPARASITIC DRUGS IN PREGNANCY (continued)

Drug	Toxicity in Pregnancy	Recommendations
Iodoquinol (*Yodoxin*, and others)		
	Unknown	Caution*
Ivermectin (*Stromectol*)		
	Teratogenic in animals	Contraindicated
Ketoconazole (*Nizoral*, and others)		
	Teratogenic and embryotoxic in rats	Contraindicated; topical probably safe
Lindane		
	Absorbed from the skin; potential CNS toxicity in fetus	Contraindicated
Malathion, topical (*Ovide*)		
	None known	Probably safe
Mebendazole (*Vermox*)		
	Teratogenic and embryotoxic in rats	Caution*
Mefloquine (*Lariam*)[3]		
	Teratogenic in animals	Caution*
Meglumine (*Glucantine*)		
	Not known	Caution*
Metronidazole (*Flagyl*, and others)		
	None known – carcinogenic in rats and mice	Caution*
Miconazole (*Monistat i.v.*)		
	None known	Caution*
Miltefosine (*Impavido*)		
	Teratogenic in rats and induces abortions in animals	Contraindicated; effective contraception must be used for 2 months after the last dose
Niclosamide (*Niclocide*)		
	Not absorbed; no known toxicity in fetus	Probably safe
Nitazoxanide (*Alinia*)		
	None known	Caution*
Oxamniquine (*Vansil*)		
	Embryocidal in animals	Contraindicated

Continued on next page.

SAFETY OF ANTIPARASITIC DRUGS IN PREGNANCY (continued)

Drug	Toxicity in Pregnancy	Recommendations
Paromomycin (Humatin)		
	Poorly absorbed; toxicity in fetus unknown	Oral capsules probably safe
Pentamidine (Pentam 300, NebuPent, and others)		
	Safety not established	Caution*
Permethrin (Nix, and others)		
	Poorly absorbed; no known toxicity in fetus	Probably safe
Praziquantel (Biltricide)		
	Not known	Probably safe
Primaquine		
	Hemolysis in G-6-PD deficiency	Contraindicated
Pyrantel pamoate (Antiminth, and others)		
	Absorbed in small amounts; no known toxicity in fetus	Probably safe
Pyrethrins and piperonyl butoxide (RID, and others)		
	Poorly absorbed; no known toxicity in fetus	Probably safe
Pyrimethamine (Daraprim)[4]		
	Teratogenic in animals	Caution*; contraindicated during 1st trimester
Quinacrine (Atabrine)		
	Safety not established	Caution*
Quinidine		
	Large doses can cause abortion	Probably safe
Quinine (Qualaquin)		
	Large doses can cause abortion; auditory nerve hypoplasia, deafness in fetus; visual changes, limb anomalies, visceral defects also reported	Caution*
Sodium stibogluconate (Pentostam)		
	Not known	Caution*

Continued on next page.

SAFETY OF ANTIPARASITIC DRUGS IN PREGNANCY (continued)

Drug	Toxicity in Pregnancy	Recommendations
Sulfonamides		
	Teratogenic in some animal studies; hemolysis in newborn with G-6-PD deficiency; increased risk of kernicterus in newborn	Caution*; contraindicated at term
Suramin sodium *(Germanin)*		
	Teratogenic in mice	Caution*
Tetracycline *(Sumycin,* and others)		
	Tooth discoloration and dysplasia, inhibition of bone growth in fetus; hepatic toxicity and azotemia with IV use in pregnant patients with decreased renal function or with overdosage	Contraindicated
Tinidazole *(Tindamax)*		
	Increased fetal mortality in rats	Caution*
Trimethoprim *(Proloprim,* and others)		
	Folate antagonism; teratogenic in rats	Caution*
Trimethoprim-sulfamethoxazole *(Bactrim,* and others)		
	Same as sulfonamides and trimethoprim	Caution*; contraindicated at term

*Use only for strong clinical indication in absence of suitable alternative.
1. See also footnote 76 on page 248.
2. See also footnote 68 on page 247.
3. See also footnotes 74 on page 248 and 90 on page 254.
4. See also footnote 113 on page 266.

MANUFACTURERS OF DRUGS USED TO TREAT PARASITIC INFECTIONS

albendazole – *Albenza* (GlaxoSmithKline)

Albenza (GlaxoSmithKline) – albendazole

Alinia (Romark) – nitazoxanide

AmBisome (Gilead) – amphotericin B, liposomal

amphotericin B – *Fungizone* (Apothecon), others

amphotericin B, liposomal – *AmBisome* (Gilead)

Ancobon (Valeant) – flucytosine

§ *Antiminth* (Pfizer) – pyrantel pamoate

• *Aralen* (Sanofi) – chloroquine HCl and chloroquine phosphate

§ artemether – *Artenam* (Arenco, Belgium)

§ artemether/lumefantrine – *Coartem, Riamet* (Novartis)

§ *Artenam* (Arenco, Belgium) – artemether

§ artesunate – (Guilin No. 1 Factory, People's Republic of China)

atovaquone – *Mepron* (GlaxoSmithKline)

atovaquone/proguanil – *Malarone* (GlaxoSmithKline)

azithromycin – *Zithromax* (Pfizer), others

• *Bactrim* (Roche) – TMP/Sulfa

§ benznidazole – *Rochagan* (Brazil)

• *Biaxin* (Abbott) – clarithromycin

§ *Biltricide* (Bayer) – praziquantel

† bithionol – *Bitin* (Tanabe, Japan)

† *Bitin* (Tanabe, Japan) – bithionol

§ *Brolene* (Aventis, Canada) – propamidine isethionate

chloroquine HCl and chloroquine phosphate – *Aralen* (Sanofi), others

clarithromycin – *Biaxin* (Abbott), others

• *Cleocin* (Pfizer) – clindamycin

clindamycin – *Cleocin* (Pfizer), others

Coartem (Novartis) – artemether/lumefantrine

crotamiton – *Eurax* (Westwood-Squibb)

dapsone – (Jacobus)

§ *Daraprim* (GlaxoSmithKline) – pyrimethamine USP

† diethylcarbamazine citrate (DEC) – *Hetrazan*

• *Diflucan* (Pfizer) – fluconazole

§ diloxanide furoate – *Furamide* (Boots, United Kingdom)

doxycycline – *Vibramycin* (Pfizer), others

† eflornithine (Difluoromethylornithine, DFMO) – *Ornidyl* (Aventis)

§ *Egaten* (Novartis) – triclabendazole

Elimite (Allergan) – permethrin

Ergamisol (Janssen) – levamisole

Eurax (Westwood-Squibb) – crotamiton

• *Flagyl* (Pfizer) – metronidazole

§ *Flisint* (Sanofi-Aventis, France) – fumagillin

Continued on next page.

MANUFACTURERS OF DRUGS USED TO TREAT PARASITIC INFECTIONS (continued)

fluconazole – *Diflucan* (Pfizer), others

flucytosine – *Ancobon* (Valeant)

§ fumagillin – *Flisint* (Sanofi-Aventis, France)

• *Fungizone* (Apothecon) – amphotericin

§ *Furamide* (Boots, United Kingdom) – diloxanide furoate

§ furazolidone – *Furozone* (Roberts)

§ *Furozone* (Roberts) – furazolidone

† *Germanin* (Bayer, Germany) – suramin sodium

§ *Glucantime* (Aventis, France) – meglumine antimonate

† *Hetrazan* – diethylcarbamazine citrate (DEC)

Humatin (Monarch) – paromomycin

§ *Impavido* (Zentaris, Germany) – miltefosine

iodoquinol – *Yodoxin* (Glenwood), others

itraconazole – *Sporanox* (Janssen-Ortho), others

ivermectin – *Stromectol* (Merck)

ketoconazole – *Nizoral* (Janssen), others

† *Lampit* (Bayer, Germany) – nifurtimox

Lariam (Roche) – mefloquine

§ *Leshcutan* (Teva, Israel) – topical paromomycin

levamisole – *Ergamisol* (Janssen)

lumefantrine/artemether – *Coartem, Riamet* (Novartis)

Malarone (GlaxoSmithKline) – atovaquone/proguanil

malathion – *Ovide* (Medicis)

mebendazole – *Vermox* (McNeil), others

mefloquine – *Lariam* (Roche)

§ meglumine antimonate – *Glucantime* (Aventis, France)

† melarsoprol – *Mel-B*

† *Mel-B* – melarsoprol

Mepron (GlaxoSmithKline) – atovaquone

metronidazole – *Flagyl* (Pfizer), others

§ miconazole – *Monistat i.v.*

§ miltefosine – *Impavido* (Zentaris, Germany)

§ *Monistat i.v.* – miconazole

NebuPent (Fujisawa) – pentamidine isethionate

Neutrexin (US Bioscience) – trimetrexate

§ niclosamide – *Yomesan* (Bayer, Germany)

† nifurtimox – *Lampit* (Bayer, Germany)

nitazoxanide – *Alinia* (Romark)

• *Nizoral* (Janssen) – ketoconazole

Nix (GlaxoSmithKline) – permethrin

§ ornidazole – *Tiberal* (Roche, France)

† *Ornidyl* (Aventis) – eflornithine (Difluoromethylornithine, DFMO)

Continued on next page.

MANUFACTURERS OF DRUGS USED TO TREAT PARASITIC INFECTIONS (continued)

Ovide (Medicis) – malathion

§ oxamniquine – *Vansil* (Pfizer)

§ *Paludrine* (AstraZeneca, United Kingdom) – proguanil

paromomycin – *Humatin* (Monarch); *Leshcutan* (Teva, Israel; (topical formulation not available in US)

Pentam 300 (Fujisawa) – pentamidine isethionate

pentamidine isethionate – *Pentam 300* (Fujisawa), *NebuPent* (Fujisawa)

† *Pentostam* (GlaxoSmithKline, United Kingdom) – sodium stibogluconate

permethrin – *Nix* (GlaxoSmithKline), *Elimite* (Allergan)

§ praziquantel – *Biltricide* (Bayer)

primaquine phosphate USP

§ proguanil – *Paludrine* (AstraZeneca, United Kingdom)

proguanil/atovaquone – *Malarone* (GlaxoSmithKline)

§ propamidine isethionate – *Brolene* (Aventis, Canada)

§ pyrantel pamoate – *Antiminth* (Pfizer)

pyrethrins and piperonyl butoxide – *RID* (Pfizer), others

§ pyrimethamine USP – *Daraprim* (GlaxoSmithKline)

Qualaquin – quinine sulfate (Mutual Pharmaceutical Co/ AR Scientific)

* quinidine gluconate (Eli Lilly)

§ quinine dihydrochloride

quinine sulfate – *Qualaquin* (Mutual Pharmaceutical Co/ AR Scientific)

Riamet (Novartis) – artemether/lumefantrine

• *RID* (Pfizer) – pyrethrins and piperonyl butoxide

• *Rifadin* (Aventis) – rifampin

rifampin – *Rifadin* (Aventis), others

§ *Rochagan* (Brazil) – benznidazole

* *Rovamycine* (Aventis) – spiramycin

† sodium stibogluconate – *Pentostam* (GlaxoSmithKline, United Kingdom)

* spiramycin – *Rovamycine* (Aventis)

• *Sporanox* (Janssen-Ortho) – itraconazole

Stromectol (Merck) – ivermectin

sulfadiazine – (Eon)

† suramin sodium – *Germanin* (Bayer, Germany)

§ *Tiberal* (Roche, France) – ornidazole

Tindamax (Mission) – tinidazole

tinidazole – *Tindamax* (Mission)

TMP/Sulfa – *Bactrim* (Roche), others

§ triclabendazole – *Egaten* (Novartis)

trimetrexate – *Neutrexin* (US Bioscience)

Continued on next page.

MANUFACTURERS OF DRUGS USED TO TREAT PARASITIC INFECTIONS (continued)

§ *Vansil* (Pfizer) – oxamniquine
• *Vermox* (McNeil) – mebendazole
• *Vibramycin* (Pfizer) – doxycycline
• *Yodoxin* (Glenwood) – iodoquinol

§ *Yomesan* (Bayer, Germany) – niclosamide
• *Zithromax* (Pfizer) – azithromycin

---

* Available in the US only from the manufacturer.
§ Not available in the US; may be available through a compounding pharmacy (see footnote 4).
† Available from the CDC Drug Service, Centers for Disease Control and Prevention, Atlanta, Georgia 30333; 404-639-3670 (evenings, weekends, or holidays: 404-639-2888).
• Also available generically.

DRUGS FOR
Sexually Transmitted Infections

Original publication date – September 2007

Many infections can be transmitted during sexual contact. The text and tables that follow are limited to management of sexually transmitted infections (STIs) other than HIV, viral hepatitis and enteric infections. Guidelines are available from the US Centers for Disease Control and Prevention (CDC) with detailed recommendations for treatment of these diseases.[1]

PARTNER TREATMENT — Complete treatment for STIs should include the sex partners of infected persons. Ideally, partners should themselves be examined and tested for STIs, but that may be difficult to accomplish. An alternate approach is to treat sex partners without direct examination or counseling, either by prescription or by giving the medication for the partner to the index patient, a practice called expedited partner treatment (EPT).[2,3]

CHLAMYDIA — A single 1-g dose of azithromycin (*Zithromax,* and others) or 7 days' treatment with doxycycline (*Vibramycin*, and others) is effective for treatment of uncomplicated urethral or cervical infection caused by *Chlamydia trachomatis*. Ofloxacin (*Floxin*, and others) or levofloxacin *(Levaquin)* for 7 days is an effective but expensive alternative. Erythromycin (*Ery-tab*, and others) frequently causes gastrointestinal (GI) adverse effects.

COST OF SOME DRUGS FOR CHLAMYDIA

Drug	Dosage	Cost[1]
Azithromycin –	1 g PO once	
generic		$26.04
Zithromax (Pfizer)		36.96
Doxycycline –	100 mg PO bid x 7d	
generic		15.26
Vibramycin (Pfizer)		78.12
Levofloxacin –	500 mg PO once/d x 7d	
Levaquin (Ortho-McNeil)		84.91
Ofloxacin –	300 mg PO bid x 7d	
Floxin (Ortho-McNeil)		84.42

1. Cost based on data (June 30, 2007) from retail pharmacies nationwide available from Wolters Kluwer Health.

In Pregnancy – Azithromycin, which is thought to be safe, is now considered the treatment of choice for chlamydial infection during pregnancy.[4,5] Amoxicillin (*Amoxil*, and others) is a safe alternative. Erythromycin is another alternative, but many patients, pregnant or not, may not tolerate its GI effects, and erythromycin estolate is contraindicated in pregnancy. Doxycycline, other tetracyclines and the fluoroquinolones generally should not be used during pregnancy. Treatment failure is more common in pregnancy; repeat testing is recommended. Patients who fail treatment can usually be retreated with the same drug.

In Infancy – Children born to women with cervical *C. trachomatis* infection are at risk for neonatal conjunctivitis and pneumonia. Ophthalmic antibiotics used for gonococcal prophylaxis do not prevent ocular chlamydial infection in the newborn. For treatment of newborns with conjunctivitis or pneumonia caused by *C. trachomatis,* some clinicians have used systemic erythromycin for 14 days, but an association between hypertrophic pyloric stenosis and use of systemic erythromycin has been reported.[6] In one study in 8 infants, a short course of oral azithromycin was effective for treatment of chlamydial conjunctivitis.[7]

Lymphogranuloma Venereum – Infections with the strains of *C. trachomatis* that cause lymphogranuloma venereum, manifested primarily by acute proctitis, have been reported in several urban areas worldwide among men who have sex with men (MSM).[8] A 3-week course of doxycycline is recommended.

Nongonococcal Nonchlamydial Urethritis and Cervicitis — *Mycoplasma genitalium* may cause 10-20% of nongonococcal urethritis (NGU). Other causes include *Ureaplasma urealyticum, Trichomonas vaginalis*, herpes simplex virus or adenovirus, but the etiology of NGU is often unknown.[9] Most cases respond to treatment with azithromycin or doxycycline; azithromycin is more effective for *M. genitalium*. Persistent or recurrent NGU should be treated with azithromycin if doxycycline was used initially.

Cervicitis has been characterized as the female counterpart of NGU in men.[10] Like NGU, cervicitis generally responds to azithromycin or doxycycline. Empiric treatment for *Neisseria gonorrhoeae* should also be given in areas with high prevalence.

GONORRHEA — Resistance of gonococci to fluoroquinolones has markedly increased in recent years, and these drugs are no longer recommended to treat gonorrhea.[11] A single intramuscular (IM) injection of ceftriaxone (*Rocephin*, and others) is the treatment of choice for anogenital and pharyngeal gonorrhea, including infection with penicillin-, fluoroquinolone-, and tetracycline-resistant strains of *N. gonorrhoeae*. Calcium-containing solutions must not be mixed with, given at the same time as, or for up to 48 hours after ceftriaxone; calcium-ceftriaxone precipitates in lungs and kidneys have been fatal in infants. Cefixime

COST OF SOME DRUGS FOR GONORRHEA

Drug	Dosage	Cost[1]
Ceftriaxone –	125 mg IM once	
generic		$10.57[2]
Rocephin (Roche)		17.36[2]
Cefixime[3] –	400 mg PO once	
Suprax (Lupin)		8.83
Cefpodoxime –	400 mg PO once	
Vantin (Pfizer)		13.64

1. Cost based on data (June 30, 2007) from retail pharmacies nationwide available from Wolters Kluwer Health.
2. Cost of a 250-mg vial, the smallest marketed dose.
3. Only the suspension is currently marketed in the US.

(Suprax) is an oral alternative that is effective for infection at all mucosal sites; only the suspension is currently marketed in the US, but the tablet formulation may be reintroduced soon. Cefpodoxime (*Vantin*, and others) is another option for oral therapy, but may be less effective for pharyngeal infection.[12]

Patients with gonorrhea should also be treated for presumptive chlamydial infection, usually with a single 1-g dose of azithromycin or 7 days of doxycycline.[13] Azithromycin 2 g orally is generally effective against both gonorrhea and *C. trachomatis*, but because it is expensive, may be poorly tolerated and may induce macrolide resistance in *N. gonorrhoeae*, it is not recommended for such use, except in pregnant women who are allergic to beta-lactam antibiotics.

Gonococcal ophthalmia, bacteremia, arthritis or meningitis in adults, and all gonococcal infections in children are best treated with appropriate doses of a parenteral third-generation cephalosporin such as ceftriaxone.

In Pregnancy – There are no well-studied, readily available options for treatment of gonorrhea in pregnant women who are allergic to beta-lactam antibiotics. Spectinomycin is no longer available in the US and its reintroduction is uncertain. Azithromycin 2 g appears to be the best option,[5] but the 2-g dose has not been studied in pregnancy and GI intolerance may be a problem. Gentamicin 300 mg IM is a possible alternative. All of these regimens should be followed by a test of cure 2-3 weeks after treatment.

FOLLOW-UP — Early retesting to document cure (3-4 weeks after treatment) is not recommended except for chlamydia or gonorrhea in pregnant women, or when adherence is in doubt. Rescreening or late retesting to detect reinfection or delayed treatment failure should be done 3 months after treatment for all men and women with gonorrhea or chlamydial infection.[14]

EPIDIDYMITIS — Acute epididymitis in men <35 years old is usually caused by *C. trachomatis* or, less frequently, *N. gonorrhoeae*. Older men or those who have had urinary tract instrumentation may have epididymitis due to enteric gram-negative bacilli or *Pseudomonas*. Gram-negative bacilli may also cause urethritis or epididymitis in men who practice insertive anal intercourse. When the organism is not known and gonorrhea is unlikely, epididymitis can be treated empirically with ceftriaxone plus doxycycline.

PELVIC INFLAMMATORY DISEASE — *C. trachomatis* or *N. gonorrhoeae* cause about two thirds of cases of acute pelvic inflammatory disease (PID), but *M. genitalium, M. hominis* and various facultative and anaerobic bacteria may also be involved. Treatment regimens should include antimicrobial agents active against all of these pathogens. Parenteral regimens include cefotetan (*Cefotan*, and others) or cefoxitin (*Mefoxin,* and others) plus doxycycline, or clindamycin *(Cleocin,* and others) plus an aminoglycoside. Parenteral therapy is continued until clinical improvement occurs, and then oral doxycycline is substituted to complete 14 days' total therapy. An oral alternative is doxycycline, with or without metronidazole (*Flagyl*, and others), after an initial IM dose of a cephalosporin such as ceftriaxone. Levofloxacin or ofloxacin should not be used unless infection with fluoroquinolone-resistant *N. gonorrhoeae* has been excluded.

BACTERIAL VAGINOSIS — The role of sexual transmission is unclear in bacterial vaginosis, in which normal H_2O_2-producing *Lactobacillus* sp. are replaced by overgrowth with *Gardnerella vaginalis, Mobiluncus*, various anaerobic bacteria and *M. hominis*.[15] Bacterial vaginosis has also been associated with an increased risk of PID. Oral metronidazole for 7 days or tinidazole for 2 or 5 days[16] is usually effective. Vaginal metronidazole, or oral or vaginal clindamycin, is also effective. With any regimen, recurrence is common; retreatment with the same agent or an alternative is usually effective in the short term, but symptomatic recurrence is common. Maintenance suppressive therapy with metronidazole gel reduces the recurrence rate.[17] No male counterpart has been identified and treatment of patients' male sex partners does not reduce the frequency of recurrence.

In Pregnancy – Since bacterial vaginosis has been associated with premature labor and complications of delivery, symptomatic bacterial vaginosis in pregnancy should be treated.[18] In controlled trials, however, oral metronidazole treatment of asymptomatic bacterial vaginosis in pregnant women has not consistently reduced the frequency of adverse pregnancy outcomes.

VULVOVAGINAL CANDIDIASIS — Vulvovaginal candidiasis, typically caused by *Candida albicans*, is not sexually transmitted but is common in women being evaluated for STIs. Many remedies are available. Uncomplicated candidiasis of mild to moderate severity in immunocompetent women responds well to 1-, 3- and 7-day regimens of intravaginal butoconazole (*Gynazole*), clotrimazole (*Gyne-Lotrimin*, and others), miconazole (*Monistat*, and others), terconazole (*Terazol*, and others) or tioconazole (*Vagistat* and others).[19] A single oral dose of fluconazole (*Diflucan*, and others) 150 mg is as effective as 7 days of intravaginal clotrimazole or miconazole and is preferred by many patients; severe episodes may require additional doses of fluconazole on days 4 and 7.[20]

Complicated vulvovaginal candiasis (recurrent or clinically severe episodes, cases due to azole-resistant *C. glabrata* or other nonalbicans species, or infection in immunodeficient women, those with poorly controlled diabetes, or pregnant women) often requires more aggressive or more prolonged treatment. Further recurrences can be prevented for at least 6 months by prophylaxis with oral fluconazole 150 mg once weekly.

ALTERNATIVE TREATMENTS FOR VAGINAL INFECTIONS — "Broad-spectrum" vaginal preparations and currently available preparations of *Lactobacillus* sp. or dairy products are not reliably effective for treatment or prevention of any vaginal infection. Douching is not effective for prevention or treatment of vaginal infection; it may lead to upper genital tract infection and should be discouraged.

TRICHOMONIASIS — Oral metronidazole has been the treatment of choice for trichomoniasis. Intravaginal treatment with metronidazole gel is not effective. Resistance to metronidazole, especially high-grade resistance, remains rare. Tinidazole *(Tindamax)*, a nitroimidazole similar to metronidazole, is also effective and may be better tolerated; it can be used to treat metronidazole-resistant vaginal infections.[21]

In Pregnancy – Trichomoniasis in pregnancy has been associated with adverse pregnancy outcomes.[22] Metronidazole is now believed to be safe during all stages of pregnancy and should be used to treat symptomatic trichomoniasis in pregnancy.

SYPHILIS — Parenteral penicillin G remains the drug of choice for treating all stages of syphilis. Primary, secondary or latent syphilis known to be of less than one year's duration (early syphilis) should be

COST OF DRUGS FOR TRICHOMONIASIS

Drug	Dosage	Cost[1]
Metronidazole –	2 g PO once	
generic		$2.40
Flagyl (Pfizer)		20.08
Tinidazole –	2 g PO once	
Tindamax		21.40
(Mission Pharmacal)		

1. Cost based on data (June 30, 2007) from retail pharmacies nationwide available from Wolters Kluwer Health.

treated with a single IM injection of benzathine penicillin G, a repository formulation. Doxycycline is also usually effective if compliance is assured. For late syphilis (more than one year's duration) other than neurosyphilis, a longer course of treatment with IM penicillin G benzathine is recommended.

Azithromycin 2 g was as effective as benzathine penicillin against early syphilis in a randomized controlled trial in Tanzania.[23] However, in several locations in North America and Europe, strains of *Treponema pallidum* resistant to azithromycin are common and apparently increasing in prevalence.[24,25] Routine use of azithromycin is not recommended for treatment of syphilis in the US.[26]

Neurosyphilis – Symptomatic neurosyphilis, including ophthalmic infection, requires treatment with high doses of IV aqueous penicillin G or IM procaine penicillin G with probenecid.

Syphilis and HIV – The majority of HIV-infected patients with syphilis respond to standard benzathine penicillin, but some of these patients may need higher doses or longer treatment. Cerebrospinal fluid abnormalities are common in patients with syphilis and HIV, regardless of the stage of syphilis, but whether these patients should receive high-dose IV penicillin is unclear.[27]

IV ceftriaxone for 10 days may be as effective as IV penicillin for treatment of neurosyphilis in HIV-infected patients, but its efficacy for parenchymal or late forms of neurosyphilis has not been studied.[28]

Syphilis in Pregnancy – Syphilis in pregnant women should be treated with penicillin in doses appropriate to the stage of the disease. When pregnant women with syphilis are allergic to penicillin, most experts recommend hospitalization, desensitization and treatment with penicillin. Retreatment in subsequent pregnancies is unnecessary in the absence of clinical or serological evidence of new or persistent infection.

Congenital Syphilis – A positive serological test for syphilis in a newborn without stigmata of syphilis may be due either to passive transfer of maternal antibodies or to prenatal infection. If there is no definite evidence of adequate treatment of the mother with penicillin during the pregnancy, Medical Letter consultants recommend prompt treatment of such infants rather than waiting 3-6 months to see if the antibody titer falls.

CHANCROID — Chancroid, caused by *Haemophilus ducreyi,* is uncommon in the US. A single dose of azithromycin or ceftriaxone is usually effective, but more prolonged therapy may be required in HIV-infected patients.

PEDICULOSIS AND SCABIES — *Phthirus pubis* (pubic lice), which can be found on eyelashes and back, axillary and leg hairs as well as pubic areas, and *Sarcoptes scabiei* (scabies) can both be transmitted by intimate exposure. The drug of choice is topical 1% permethrin (*Nix*, and others) for pubic lice, and 5% permethrin (*Elimite*, and others) for scabies; both of these can be used in pregnancy.

Oral ivermectin *(Stromectol)*, 200 mcg/kg, is also effective as a single dose for treatment of lice or scabies, and can be repeated 10-14 days later for resistant infections with scabies. Crusted scabies, a serious complication usually seen in patients with AIDS or other immunodeficiencies, should be treated with both permethrin and ivermectin.[29] Ivermectin has, however, been placed by the FDA in category C for use during pregnancy and should not be used to treat these disorders in pregnant women.

GENITAL WARTS AND HUMAN PAPILLOMAVIRUS INFECTION — External genital warts are caused by human papillomavirus (HPV), usually type 6 or 11; other types (16, 18 and others) cause dysplasia and neoplasia of the cervix, anus and genital skin. No form of HPV-specific treatment has been shown to eradicate the virus or to modify the risk of cervical dysplasia or cancer, and no single treatment is uniformly effective in removing warts or preventing recurrence. Trichloroacetic acid, podophyllin, and cryotherapy (with liquid nitrogen or a cryoprobe) remain the most widely used treatments for external genital warts, but the response rate is only 60-70%, and at least 20-30% of responders will have a recurrence. Imiquimod 5% cream *(Aldara)*, an immune modulator, and podofilox 0.5% solution or gel *(Condylox)* are no more effective, but they offer the advantage of self-application by patients at home. The HPV vaccine *(Gardasil)*, though highly effective in preventing infection with selected types of HPV,[30,31] does not influence the course of established infection and has no therapeutic role.

No treatment is recommended for subclinical HPV infection in the absence of dysplasia or neoplasia. The transient nature of most HPV infections in young women suggests that these infections and the low-grade cervical dysplasia often associated with them should both be treated conservatively because they often regress spontaneously.[32]

In Pregnancy – Imiquimod, podofilox and podophyllin are not recommended for use during pregnancy. Topical trichloroacetic acid, cryotherapy, electrodesiccation, or electrocauterization are options that can be

COST OF DRUGS FOR GENITAL HERPES[1]

Drug	Dosage	Cost[2]
Acyclovir –	400 mg PO tid x 7-10d	
generic		$40.53
Zovirax (GSK)		88.20
Famciclovir[3] –	250 mg PO tid x 7-10d	
Famvir (Novartis)		111.51
Valacyclovir –	1 g PO bid x 7-10d	
Valtrex (GSK)		155.12

1. Dosage is for initial episodes of genital herpes. For treatment of other stages, see table on page 298.
2. Cost of 7 days' treatment based on the most recent data (June 30, 2007) from retail pharmacies nationwide available from Wolters Kluwer Health.
3. Not FDA-approved for initial treatment of genital herpes.

used in pregnancy. Scissor excision or laser therapy is effective and well-tolerated if the clinician is properly trained.

GENITAL HERPES — Acyclovir *(Zovirax,* and others), famciclovir *(Famvir)* or valacyclovir *(Valtrex)* taken orally for 7-10 days can shorten the duration of pain, systemic symptoms and viral shedding in initial herpes simplex virus (HSV) genital infection. Episodic treatment of symptomatic recurrent lesions with the same drugs can speed healing if treatment is started early.[33-35] Continuous suppressive therapy substantially reduces symptomatic recurrences and subclinical shedding. Suppressive therapy with valacyclovir 500 mg daily has markedly reduced the frequency of HSV transmission to heterosexual partners.[36]

Antiviral-resistant strains of HSV are uncommon; they occur mainly in immunodeficient patients treated with antiviral drugs.[37] Long-term suppressive therapy has prevented emergence of drug-resistant HSV in stem-cell transplant recipients.[38]

DRUGS OF CHOICE FOR SOME SEXUALLY TRANSMITTED INFECTIONS

Type or Stage		Drugs of Choice
CHLAMYDIAL INFECTION AND RELATED CLINICAL SYNDROMES[1]		
Urethritis, cervicitis, conjunctivitis, or proctitis (except lymphogranuloma venereum)		
		Azithromycin[2]
	OR	Doxycycline[2,4-6]
Infection in Pregnancy		
		Azithromycin
	OR	Amoxicillin
Neonatal Ophthalmia or Pneumonia		
		Azithromycin
Lymphogranuloma venereum		
		Doxycycline[4,5]
GONORRHEA[9]		
Urethral, cervical, rectal or pharyngeal		
		Ceftriaxone
	OR	Cefixime[12]
EPIDIDYMITIS		
		Ceftriaxone
		plus
		doxycycline[4,5]

1. Related clinical syndromes include nonchlamydial nongonococcal urethritis (NGU) and cervicitis.
2. For cases of persistent or recurrent nonchlamydial NGU, azithromycin should be used if initial treatment was with doxycycline. Some experts add tinidazole or metronidazole as recommended against trichomoniasis.
3. Should be used only if fluoroquinolone-resistant Neisseria gonorrhoeae has been excluded.
4. Not recommended in pregnancy.
5. Or oral tetracycline 500 mg qid (contraindicated in pregnancy).
6. Less effective than azithromycin against NGU associated with Mycoplasma genitalium.
7. Erythromycin ethylsuccinate 800 mg may be substituted for erythromycin base 500 mg; erythromycin estolate is contraindicated in pregnancy.

Dosage	Some Alternatives
1 g PO once	Ofloxacin[3,4] 300 mg PO bid x 7d
	Levofloxacin[3,4] 500 mg PO once/d x 7d
100 mg PO bid x 7d	Erythromycin[7] 500 mg PO qid x 7d
1 g PO once	Erythromycin[7] 500 mg PO qid x 7d
500 mg PO tid x 7d	
20 mg/kg PO once/d x 3d	Erythromycin 12.5 mg/kg PO qid x 14d[8]
100 mg PO bid x 21d	Erythromycin[7] 500 mg PO qid x 21d
125 mg IM once[10]	Cefpodoxime 400 mg PO once[11]
400 mg PO once	Azithromycin 2 g PO once[13]
	Gentamicin 300 mg IM once[14]
250 mg IM once	Ofloxacin[3,4] 300 mg PO bid x 10d
	Levofloxacin[3,4] 500 mg PO once/d x 10d
100 mg PO bid x 10d	

8. Pyloric stenosis has been associated with use of erythromycin in newborns.
9. All patients should also receive a course of treatment effective for chlamydia.
10. 125 mg is effective, but the smallest marketed dose is 250 mg and some experts use the larger dose.
11. Efficacy uncertain for pharyngeal infection.
12. Only the suspension is currently marketed in the US.
13. Use of azithromycin is recommended only for pregnant women allergic to beta-lactam drugs.
14. Gentamicin 300 mg may be an option for pregnant women with beta-lactam allergy.

Continued on next page.

DRUGS OF CHOICE FOR SOME SEXUALLY TRANSMITTED INFECTIONS (continued)

Type or Stage		Drugs of Choice
PELVIC INFLAMMATORY DISEASE		
Parenteral		Cefotetan or Cefoxitin[16]
		plus doxycycline[4] **followed by** doxycycline[4]
	OR	Clindamycin **plus** gentamicin
		followed by doxycycline[4]
Oral		Ceftriaxone **followed by** doxycycline[4,20]
BACTERIAL VAGINOSIS		
		Metronidazole
	OR	Tinidazole
	OR	Metronidazole gel 0.75%[21]
	OR	Clindamycin 2% cream[21]

15. Parenteral therapy is continued until clinical improvement occurs, and then oral doxycycline is substituted to complete 14 days' total therapy.
16. Cefoxitin has been in short supply.
17. Some clinicians believe the addition of metronidazole is not required.
18. Or clindamycin 450 mg oral qid to complete 14 days.

Dosage	Some Alternatives
2 g IV q12h[15]	Ampicillin/sulbactam 3g IV q6h
2 g IV q6h[15]	**plus** doxycycline[4] 100 mg PO or IV q12h or
	Ofloxacin[3,4] 400 mg IV q12h or
	levofloxacin[3,4] 500 mg IV once/d
	plus metronidazole 500 mg IV q8h[17]
100 mg PO or IV q12h[15]	
	followed by doxycycline[4] 100 mg PO
100 mg PO bid to complete 14d[18]	bid to complete 14d[18]
900 mg IV q8h[15]	
2 mg/kg IV once, then	
1.5 mg/kg IV q8h[15,19]	
100 mg PO bid to complete 14d[18]	
250 mg IM once	Cefoxitin 2g IM once
	plus probenecid 1g PO once
100 mg PO bid x 14d	**followed** by doxycycline[4,20]
	100 mg PO bid x 14d
	Ofloxacin[3,4] 400 mg PO bid x 14d or
	levofloxacin[3,4] 500 mg PO once/d x 14d
	+/- metronidazole[17] 500 mg PO bid x 14d
500 mg PO bid x 7d	Metronidazole ER 750 mg PO once/d x 7d
2 g PO once/d x 2d	Tinidazole 1 g PO once/d x 5d
5 g intravaginally once or twice	Clindamycin 300 mg PO bid x 7d
daily x 5d	Clindamycin ovules[21]
5 g intravaginally at bedtime	100 mg intravaginally at bedtime x 3d
x 3-7d	

19. A single daily dose of 3 mg/kg is likely to be effective, but has not been studied in pelvic inflammatory disease.
20. Some experts would add metronidazole 500 mg bid.
21. In pregnancy, topical preparations have not been effective in preventing premature delivery; oral metronidazole has been effective in some studies.

Continued on next page.

DRUGS OF CHOICE FOR SOME SEXUALLY TRANSMITTED INFECTIONS (continued)

Type or Stage	Drugs of Choice
TRICHOMONIASIS	
	Metronidazole[22]
OR	Tinidazole
SYPHILIS	
Early (Primary, secondary, or latent less than one year)	
	Penicillin G benzathine
Late (more than one year's duration, cardiovascular, gumma, late-latent)	
	Penicillin G benzathine
Neurosyphilis	Penicillin G[24]
Congenital	Penicillin G
OR	Penicillin G procaine
CHANCROID[26]	
	Azithromycin
OR	Ceftriaxone
GENITAL WARTS[27]	
	Trichloroacetic or bichloroacetic acid, or podophyllin[4] or liquid nitrogen
	Imiquimod 5%[4]
	Podofilox 0.5%[4]

22. Limited data support efficacy against trichomoniasis in men.
23. Some experts recommend a repeat dose after 7 days, especially in patients with HIV infection or pregnant women.
24. Patients allergic to penicillin should be desensitized and treated with penicillin.
25. Dose for neonates <7 days old is 50,000 units/kg q12h; dose is q8h for those >7 days old.

Dosage	Some Alternatives
2 g PO once 2 g PO once	Metronidazole 375 or 500 mg PO bid x 7d
2.4 MU IM once[23]	Doxycycline[4] 100 mg PO bid x 14d
2.4 MU IM wkly x 3wks	Doxycycline[4] 100 mg PO bid x 4wks

3 to 4 MU IV q4h or 24 MU
  continuous IV infusion x 10-14d
	Penicillin G procaine 2.4 MU IM once/d
	  plus probenecid 500 mg PO qid,
	  both x 10-14d
	Ceftriaxone 2 g IV once/d x 10-14d

50,000 units/kg IV q8-12h[25]
  for 10-14d
50,000 units/kg IM once/d
  for 10-14d	

1 g PO once 250 mg IM once	Ciprofloxacin[4] 500 mg PO bid x 3d Erythromycin[7] 500 mg PO tid x 7d
1-2x/wk until resolved	Surgical removal Laser surgery
3x/wk x 16wks bid x 3d, 4 days rest, then repeated up to 4x	

26. All regimens, especially single-dose ceftriaxone, are less effective in HIV-infected patients.
27. Recommendations for external genital warts. Liquid nitrogen can also be used for vaginal, urethral, and oral warts. Podofilox or imiquimod can be used for urethral meatus warts. Trichloroacetic or bichloroacetic acid can be used for anal warts.

Continued on next page.

**DRUGS OF CHOICE FOR SOME SEXUALLY TRANSMITTED
INFECTIONS (continued)**

Type or Stage		Drugs of Choice
GENITAL HERPES		
First Episode		Acyclovir
	OR	Famciclovir[28]
	OR	Valacyclovir
Severe (hospitalized patients)		Acyclovir
Suppression[29]		Acyclovir
	OR	Famciclovir
	OR	Valacyclovir
Episodic Treatment[31]		Acyclovir
	OR	Famciclovir
	OR	Valacyclovir

28. Not FDA-approved for treatment of initial episodes of genital herpes.
29. Some Medical Letter consultants discontinue preventive treatment for 1 to 2 months once a year to reassess the frequency of recurrence.
30. Use 500 mg once daily in patients with <10 recurrences per year and 500 mg bid or 1 g daily in patients with ≥10 recurrences per year.

In Pregnancy – Although acyclovir is not approved for treatment of pregnant women, its use during pregnancy has not been associated with an increased risk of congenital abnormalities, and many clinicians prescribe the drug for treatment of first episodes of genital herpes during pregnancy.

PROPHYLAXIS FOLLOWING SEXUAL ASSAULT — Many experts recommend that sexually assaulted adults and adolescents be given treatment to prevent STIs, including therapy for gonorrhea (ceftriaxone or cefixime), chlamydial infection (azithromycin or doxycycline), and bacterial vaginosis and trichomoniasis (metronidazole or tinidazole). Prophylaxis is not recommended for prepubertal children. Treatment should be started within 72 hours.

Dosage	Some Alternatives
400 mg PO tid x 7-10d	Acyclovir 200 mg PO 5x/d x 7-10d
250 mg PO tid x 7-10d	
1g PO bid x 7-10d	
5-10 mg/kg IV q8h x 5-7d	
400 mg PO bid	Acyclovir 200 mg PO 4-5x/d
250 mg PO bid	
500 mg-1g PO once/d[30]	
800 mg PO tid x 2d	
or 400 mg PO tid x 3-5d[32]	
1 g PO bid x 1d[33]	
500 mg PO bid x 3d	

31. Antiviral therapy is variably effective for episodic treatment of recurrences; only effective if started early.
32. No published data are available to support 3 days' use.
33. For recurrent HSV in HIV-positive patients, 500 mg bid for 7d.

1. CDC. Sexually transmitted diseases treatment guidelines, 2006 MMWR Recomm Rep 2006; 55(RR-11):1.
2. MR Golden et al. Effect of expedited treatment of sex partners on recurrent or persistent gonorrhea or chlamydial infection. N Engl J Med 2005; 352:676.
3. P Kissinger et al. Patient-delivered partner treatment for male urethritis: a randomized, controlled trial. Clin Infect Dis 2005; 41:623.
4. L Rahangdale et al. An observational cohort study of Chlamydia trachomatis treatment in pregnancy. Sex Transm Dis 2006; 33:106.
5. HL Johnson et al. Sexually transmitted infections during pregnancy. Curr Infect Dis Rep 2007; 9:125.
6. BE Mahon et al. Maternal and infant use of erythromycin and other macrolide antibiotics as risk factors for infantile hypertrophic pyloric stenosis. J Pediatr 2001; 139:380.
7. MR Hammerschlag et al. Treatment of neonatal chlamydial conjunctivitis with azithromycin. Pediatr Infect Dis J 1998; 17:1049.
8. D Richardson and D Goldmeier. Lymphogranuloma venereum: an emerging cause of proctitis in men who have sex with men. Int J STD AIDS 2007; 18:11.

Drugs for Sexually Transmitted Infections

9. CS Bradshaw et al. Etiologies of nongonococcal urethritis: bacteria, viruses, and the association with orogenital exposure. J Infect Dis 2006; 193:336.

10. P Nyirjesy. Nongonococcal and nonchlamydial cervicitis. Curr Infect Dis Rep 2001; 3:540.

11. Update to CDC's sexually transmitted diseases treatment guidelines, 2006: fluoroquinolones no longer recommended for treatment of gonococcal infections. MMWR Morb Mortal Wkly Rep 2007; 56:332.

12. C Hall et al. Single-dose, oral cefpodoxime proxetil is effective for treatment of uncomplicated urogenital and rectal gonorrhea. 17th Meeting of the International Society for STD Research; July 29-August 1, 2007; Seattle, WA. Abstract P-459.

13. SB Lyss et al. Chlamydia trachomatis among patients infected with and treated for Neisseria gonorrhoeae in sexually transmitted disease clinics in the United States. Ann Intern Med 2003; 139;178.

14. TA Peterman et al. High incidence of new sexually transmitted infections in the year following a sexually transmitted infection: a case for rescreening. Ann Intern Med 2006; 145:564.

15. DN Fredricks et al. Molecular identification of bacteria associated with bacterial vaginosis. N Engl J Med 2005; 353:1899.

16. Tinidazole (Tindamax) – a new oral treatment for bacterial vaginosis. Med Lett Drugs Ther 2007; 49:73.

17. JD Sobel et al. Suppressive antibacterial therapy with 0.75% metronidazole vaginal gel to prevent recurrent bacterial vaginosis. Am J Obstet Gynecol 2006; 194:1283.

18. CC Tebes et al. The effect of treating bacterial vaginosis on preterm labor. Infect Dis Obstet Gynecol 2003; 11:123

19. Drugs for vulvovaginal candidiasis. Med Lett Drugs Ther 2001; 43:3.

20. JD Sobel et al. Treatment of complicated Candida vaginitis: comparison of single and sequential doses of fluconazole. Am J Obstet Gynecol 2001; 185:363.

21. JD Sobel et al. Tinidazole therapy for metronidazole-resistant vaginal trichomoniasis. Clin Infect Dis 2001; 33:1341.

22. D Soper. Trichomoniasis: under control or undercontrolled? Am J Obstet Gynecol 2004; 190:281.

23. G Riedner et al. Single-dose azithromycin versus penicillin G benzathine for the treatment of early syphilis. N Engl J Med 2005; 353:1236.

24. SA Lukehart et al. Macrolide resistance in Treponema pallidum in the United States and Ireland. N Engl J Med 2004; 351:154.

25. SJ Mitchell et al. Azithromycin-resistant syphilis infection: San Francisco, California, 2000-2004. Clin Infect Dis 2006; 42:337.

26. KK Holmes. Azithromycin versus penicillin G benzathine for early syphilis. N Engl J Med 2005; 353:1291.

27. NM Zetola and JD Klausner. Syphilis and HIV infection: an update. Clin Infect Dis 2007; 44:1222.

28. CM Marra et al. A pilot study evaluating ceftriaxone and penicillin G as treatment agents for neurosyphilis in human immunodeficiency virus-infected individuals. Clin Infect Dis 2000; 30:540.

29. P del Giudice. Ivermectin in scabies. Curr Opin Infect Dis 2002; 15:123.

30. A human papillomavirus vaccine. Med Lett Drugs Ther 2006; 48:65.

31. LR Baden et al. Human papillomavirus vaccine—opportunity and challenge. N Engl J Med 2007; 356:1990.

32. AB Moscicki et al. Risks for incident human papillomavirus infection and low-grade squamous intraepithelial lesion development in young females. JAMA 2001; 285:2995.

33. A Wald et al. Two-day regimen of acyclovir for treatment of recurrent genital herpes simplex virus type 2 infection. Clin Infect Dis 2002; 34:944.

34. PA Leone et al. Valacyclovir for episodic treatment of genital herpes: a shorter 3-day treatment course compared with 5-day treatment. Clin Infect Dis 2002; 34:958.

35. FY Aoki et al. Single-day, patient-initiated famciclovir therapy for recurrent genital herpes: a randomized, double-blind, placebo-controlled trial. Clin Infect Dis 2006; 42:8.

36. L Corey et al. Once-daily valacyclovir to reduce the risk of transmission of genital herpes. N Engl J Med 2004; 350:11.

37. M Reyes et al. Acyclovir-resistant genital herpes among persons attending sexually transmitted disease and human immunodeficiency virus clinics. Arch Intern Med 2003; 163:76.

38. V Erard et al. Use of long-term suppressive acyclovir after hematopoietic stem-cell transplantation: impact on herpes simplex virus (HSV) disease and drug-resistant HSV disease. J Infect Dis 2007; 196:266.

ADULT IMMUNIZATION

Original publication date – July 2006

Although immunization programs have produced high vaccination rates in US infants and children, similar successes have not been achieved in adults.[1] Vaccines recommended for routine use in adults[2] are reviewed here. Immunizations for travel were reviewed in a recent issue.[3]

VACCINE PREPARATIONS

Live attenuated vaccines use a weakened form of the pathogen, which replicates after administration to induce an immune response. Their efficacy can be diminished by factors that damage the organism or interfere with replication, such as heat, light or circulating antibody. Compared to inactivated vaccines, live attenuated vaccines tend to have higher rates of adverse effects, particularly fever, but generally produce longer lasting immunity.

Inactivated vaccines are prepared from whole bacteria or virus, or a fractional antigenic component of one. Fractional vaccines are usually either protein- or polysaccharide-based. Protein-based vaccines typically include subunits of microbiologic protein or inactivated bacterial toxins (toxoids). Polysaccharide-based vaccines are generally less immunogenic than protein-based vaccines; they may be conjugated to a toxoid to increase the immune response.

VACCINE PREPARATIONS

Live Attenuated	Measles, Mumps, Rubella, Varicella, Herpes Zoster, Yellow Fever, Intranasal Influenza, Oral Typhoid, Vaccinia
Inactivated	
Whole organism	Polio, Hepatitis A, Rabies
Fractional	
Pure Polysaccharide	Pneumococcal *(Pneumovax),* Meningococcal *(Menomune),* IM Typhoid
Conjugate Polysaccharide	Pneumococcal *(Prevnar),* Meningococcal *(Menactra),* Haemophilus Influenzae type b
Protein	Acellular Pertussis, Tetanus, Diphtheria, Hepatitis B, Influenza, Human Papillomavirus

VACCINES

Five vaccines are currently recommended by the US Advisory Committee on Immunization Practices (ACIP) for routine use in adults: tetanus-diphtheria (Td), pneumococcal, influenza, varicella and measles/mumps/rubella (MMR). For some patients, hepatitis A and B and meningococcal vaccines are also recommended. In addition, vaccines for protection against herpes zoster and human papillomavirus have recently been licensed by the FDA.

TETANUS, DIPHTHERIA AND PERTUSSIS — Tetanus toxoid and diphtheria toxoid were introduced into routine US childhood immunization programs in the late 1940s. Since then, rates of tetanus and diphtheria infection have substantially declined; sporadic cases occur in unvaccinated or incompletely vaccinated patients.[4]

Routine immunization has reduced the incidence of pertussis ("whooping cough") in children, but it is estimated to cause 600,000 cases of respiratory infection each year in adults 19-64 years old in whom vaccine-induced immunity has waned over time.[5] In addition, susceptible adults are an important reservoir for disease in unimmunized or partially immunized infants and children.

Inactivated adsorbed (aluminum-salt-precipitated) tetanus and diphtheria toxoid (Td) has been the standard booster vaccine for adults. A vaccine containing five protein components of acellular pertussis combined with diphtheria and tetanus toxoids (Tdap) was recently approved by the FDA in an adult formulation (*Adacel* – sanofi pasteur) and is now recommended as a one-time booster for adults 19-64 years of age.[6] Pediatric DTaP contains larger amounts of diphtheria and pertussis toxoids than Tdap and is not licensed for use in adults.

Recommendations for Use – The ACIP recommends that persons with an uncertain history of primary vaccination receive 3 doses of a tetanus and diphtheria toxoid vaccine, one of which (preferably the first) should be Tdap. The first 2 doses should be administered at least 4 weeks apart and the third 6-12 months after the second. A booster dose is given every 10 years. Tdap should replace one Td booster in adults and may be given as soon as 2 years after the last Td.

Adverse Effects – Local reactions such as erythema and induration around the injection site are common with the Td vaccine, but usually self-limited. Arthus-type reactions with extensive painful swelling can occur in adults with a history of repeated vaccination. Fever and injection site pain may occur more frequently with Tdap.

INFLUENZA — Influenza vaccine is about 80% (30-40% in the elderly) effective in preventing infection; effectiveness varies annually depending on the match between the vaccine and circulating strains.[7]

All influenza vaccines contain two influenza A strains and one influenza B strain selected annually by the US Public Health Service. Two types of influenza vaccine are available in the US: an inactivated intramuscular vaccine and a live attenuated intranasal vaccine *(FluMist)*.

No commercial vaccine is available for pathogenic strains of avian influenza (H5N1, H7N2, H9N2, H7N3, H7N7). Since standard influenza vaccines usually include N1 and N2, it is biologically plausible that they might offer some protection against avian flu strains with these neuraminidases.

Recommendations for Use – Based on the duration of protective antibodies and the timing of influenza circulation, the optimal time for annual vaccination in the US is in October or November, but the vaccine should be offered until the end of the influenza season in the late spring. In recent years, the vaccine supply has not been sufficient for all adults with indications for vaccination, leading the CDC to recommend that inactivated vaccine available early in the season be targeted to those at high risk of influenza complications, including pregnant women in any trimester, all persons ≥65 years old, and patients of any age with asthma, diabetes or other chronic medical conditions. Household contacts and caregivers of infants <6 months of age, institutionalized patients and healthcare workers should also be vaccinated first. After the high-risk groups, inactivated vaccine should be offered to all adults, particularly those ≥50 years old.

The live attenuated intranasal vaccine is approved only for healthy, nonpregnant patients 5-49 years old. It can be offered each year to all eligible individuals as soon as it is available. It should not be used in patients who are immunosuppressed and is not recommended for those with chronic cardiovascular, pulmonary, renal or metabolic disease.[8]

Adverse Effects – Except for soreness at the injection site, adverse reactions to inactivated influenza vaccine are uncommon. Fever, myalgia and malaise can occur. Whether inactivated influenza vaccine can cause Guillain-Barre syndrome is controversial. The live-attenuated intranasal vaccine is generally well tolerated, but can cause mild rhinorrhea, nasal congestion and sore throat; it has also been reported to cause asthma exacerbations.[9] After receiving the live-virus vaccine, healthcare workers, family members and other close contacts of severely immunosuppressed patients should avoid contact with the immunosuppressed person for 7 days because of the theoretical risk of transmission of vaccine-strain virus. Both types of vaccine are grown in eggs and should not be given to persons with a history of anaphylactic reactions to egg proteins.

PNEUMOCOCCAL — Vaccination against *Streptococcus pneumoniae* can reduce the incidence of invasive pneumococcal disease (pneumonia, bacteremia, meningitis) and decrease morbidity and mortality.[10]

A 23-valent pneumococcal polysaccharide vaccine (PPV23; *Pneumovax* – Merck) has been available for many years for use in adults. PPV23 contains 25 mcg of purified capsular polysaccharide antigen from each of 23 serotypes of *S. pneumoniae*. The serotypes contained in the vaccine account for 85 to 90% of the strains that cause invasive disease.[11] In addition, cross-reactivity occurs with capsular antigens from other strain types that account for an additional 8% of bacteremic disease.

A conjugate vaccine containing 7 serotypes of pneumococcus (*Prevnar* – Wyeth) is FDA-approved for use in infants and toddlers.[12]

Recommendations for Use – A one-time dose of pneumococcal polysaccharide vaccine is recommended by the ACIP for all adults ≥65 years of age. Pneumococcal vaccine is also recommended for persons of any age with chronic illnesses that place them at moderate risk for pneumococcal disease, such as those with diabetes, heart disease, chronic pulmonary disease, chronic liver disease, immunodeficiencies or malignancies and those on immunosuppressive drugs or residing in long-term care facilities.

Persons who receive an initial dose before 65 years of age should be revaccinated once, at least 5 years after initial vaccination. A second

VACCINES FOR ADULTS

Vaccines	Dose
Tetanus, diphtheria (Td)	
Tetanus and Diphtheria Adsorbed for Adult Use (sanofi pasteur)	0.5 mL IM (5 Lf T/2 Lf d)
Tetanus, Diphtheria, Acellular Pertussis (Tdap)	
Adacel (sanofi pasteur)	0.5 mL IM[1]
Influenza[2]	
Inactivated	0.5 mL IM (15 mcg of each antigen)
Fluarix (GSK)	
Fluvirin (Chiron)	
Fluzone (sanofi pasteur)	
Live attenuated	0.25 mL x2 intranasal ($10^{6.5-7.5}$ TCID$_{50}$)
Flumist (MedImmune)	
Pneumococcal	
Pneumovax 23 (Merck)	0.5 mL IM or SC (25 mcg of each antigen)
Measles, Mumps, Rubella (MMR)	
MMR II (Merck)	0.5 mL SC[4]

* **A:** vaccine recommended by the ACIP for ALL adults in the age category who lack evidence of immunity (i.e. lack evidence of immunization or have no prior evidence of infection); **B:** vaccine recommended if another risk factor is present on the basis of medical, occupational, lifestyle, or other indications; **NA:** not available.
1. Each dose of Tdap contains 2.5 mcg of detoxified pertussis toxin, 5 mcg of filamentous hemaglutinin, 3 mcg of peractin, 5 mcg of fimbraie types 2 and 3 in addition to 5 Lf of tetanus toxoid and 2 Lf of diphtheria toxoid.
2. Though annual influenza vaccine is recommended for all adults >50 years, in years of influenza vaccine shortage, the CDC recommends that high risk adults be prioritized first.

Adult Age Range	Recommendation*	Schedule
≥19 yrs	A	1 booster dose q10yrs
19-64 yrs	A	1 booster dose
19-49 yrs	B	1 dose/yr
≥50 yrs[2]	A	1 dose/yr
19-49 yrs	B	1 dose/yr
19-64 yrs	B	1-2 doses[3]
≥65 yrs	A	1 dose
19-49 yrs	A	1-2 doses[5,6]
≥50 yrs	B	1 dose[6,7]

3. One-time revaccination after 5 years for high-risk patients.
4. Each dose contains approximately 1,000 $TCID_{50}$ (50% tissue culture infectious dose) of measles virus; 20,000 $TCID_{50}$ of mumps virus; and 1,000 $TCID_{50}$ of rubella virus.
5. Second dose must be administered at least 28 days after the first. 1-2 doses for measles and mumps and 1 dose for rubella.
6. Recommendations for immunization during a mumps outbreak have been published by the CDC (MMWR Early Release. June 1, 2006. 55:1).
7. One dose for rubella.

Continued on next page.

VACCINES FOR ADULTS (continued)

Vaccines	Dose
Varicella	
Varivax (Merck)	0.5 mL SC (1350 PFU)
Herpes Zoster	
Zostavax (Merck)	0.65 mL SC (19,400 PFU)
Hepatitis B	
Engerix-B (GSK)	1 mL IM (20 mcg)[8]
Recombivax-HB (Merck)	1 mL IM (10 mcg)[8]
Hepatitis A	
Havrix (GSK)	1 mL IM (1440 EL.U.)
Vaqta (Merck)	1 mL IM (50 U)
Hepatitis A/B	
Twinrix (GSK)	1 mL IM (720 EL.U./20 mcg) (1 mL)
Meningococcal[11]	
Menactra (sanofi pasteur)	0.5 mL IM (4 mcg of each antigen)
Menomune (sanofi pasteur)	0.5 mL SC (50 mcg of each antigen)
Human Papillomavirus	
Gardasil (Merck)	0.5 mL IM

8. Dose for hemodialysis is 40 mcg given at 0, 1 and 6 months *(Recombivax)* or 0, 1, 2, and 6 months *(Engerix-B)*.
9. A 4-dose schedule at 0, 1, 2 and 12 months is also FDA-approved.
10. The third dose can be given 2 months after the second dose provided at least 4 months have elapsed since the first dose (CDC. The Pink Book. 9th ed, p. 221).

dose may also be given after 5 years to persons with asplenia or other underlying immunosuppression regardless of age. Additional doses are not generally recommended.

Adverse Effects – Mild to moderate soreness and erythema at the injection site are common. One retrospective study found no increase in adverse effects among persons who received ≥3 doses.[13]

Adult Age Range	Recommendation*	Schedule
19-49 yrs	A	2 doses (0, 4-8 wks)
≥50 yrs	B	2 doses (0, 4-8 wks)
≥60 yrs	NA	1 dose
>19 yrs	B	3 doses (0, 1 and 6 mos)[9,10]
>19 yrs	B	3 doses (0, 1 and 6 mos)[10]
≥19 yrs	B	2 doses (0 and 6-12 mos)
≥19 yrs	B	2 doses (0 and 6-18 mos)
≥18 yrs	B	3 doses (0, 1 and 6 mos)
18-55 yrs	B	1 dose[12]
≥19 yrs	B	1 dose[12]
19-26 yrs	NA	3 doses (0, 2 and 6 mos)

11. Meningococcal conjugate vaccine *(Menactra)* is preferred for adults ≤55 years.
12. Revaccination every 5 years if ongoing risk has been recommended for *Menomune* (no data for *Menactra*, but likely lasts longer than *Menomune*).

MEASLES, MUMPS, RUBELLA (MMR) — Routine vaccination of children with MMR vaccine has decreased rates of measles, mumps and rubella by 99% in the US.[14] Sporadic outbreaks usually originate with a traveler from another country. Congenital rubella syndrome is no longer considered a public health threat, largely due to high rates of immunity in women of childbearing age.

A large mumps outbreak centered in Iowa began in December of 2005 and has spread. About 40% of the cases have been in adults 18-25 years old, many of whom are college students and have been vaccinated. The source of the outbreak is unknown, but the circulating strain (genotype G) is also responsible for an ongoing outbreak in the United Kingdom involving >70,000 people.[15,16]

Each component of MMR is available as a separate monovalent formulation (*Attenuvax* for measles, *Mumpsvax* for mumps, and *Meruvax II* for rubella). The trivalent MMR vaccine is preferred for routine adult vaccination. If a component of the MMR vaccine is specifically contraindicated or if the vaccinee has acceptable evidence of immunity to one or two components of the MMR vaccine, monovalent formulations could be substituted.

Each 0.5-mL subcutaneous dose of MMR vaccine contains live-attenuated measles and mumps virus, both derived from chick embryo cell culture, and rubella virus derived from human diploid cell culture.

Recommendations for Use – In most adults, one dose of MMR is sufficient. A second dose, given at least 28 days after the first, may be required in some situations to ensure protection from the measles or mumps components of the vaccine.

Adults born before 1957 (1970 in Canada) can be considered immune to **measles**. All adults should receive at least 1 dose of vaccine unless they have a physician-documented history of measles or laboratory evidence of immunity. Two doses of vaccine, separated by at least 28 days, are recommended for adults who were previously vaccinated with the killed measles vaccine commonly used in the 1960s, and for students in post-secondary educational institutions, healthcare workers, susceptible travelers to countries where measles is endemic, and susceptible adults with a recent measles exposure.

US adults born before 1957 can also be considered immune to **mumps**. The ACIP now recommends vaccination against mumps for persons born during or after 1957 who do not have a history of physician-diagnosed mumps, laboratory evidence of immunity, or immunity through vaccination, which the ACIP has recently redefined as 1 dose of mumps vaccine for preschool children and adults not at high risk and 2 doses for children in grades K-12 and adults at high risk (healthcare workers, international travelers and post-high-school students).[17]

During a mumps outbreak, a second dose should be considered for children 1-4 years old and for all adults, given at least 28 days after the first dose. The ACIP suggests that healthcare workers who do not have immunity through vaccination or other evidence of immunity receive 2 doses of the vaccine, even if they were born before 1957.[17]

One dose of MMR should be administered to all adult women, especially those of childbearing age regardless of their birth year, whose **rubella** vaccination history is unreliable or who lack evidence of immunity to rubella.

Women who are pregnant and who do not have evidence of immunity should receive MMR vaccine upon completion of pregnancy, ideally before discharge from the healthcare facility.

Adverse Effects – Adverse events associated with MMR vaccination include pain and erythema at the injection site (7-29%), fever and rash (5%, most commonly associated with the measles component), and transient arthralgias (up to 25% of postpubertal women receiving rubella vaccine). Systemic anaphylactic reactions and thrombocytopenia occur very rarely. There is no convincing evidence to support a causal link between MMR vaccination and autism or Guillain-Barre Syndrome.[14,18]

Contraindications – Because the MMR vaccine is a live-attenuated virus vaccine, it is contraindicated in pregnant women and in patients with moderate to severe immunodeficiency. HIV-infected patients who are asymptomatic or who are symptomatic and do not have evidence of severe underlying immunosuppression (CD4 count < 200 cells/mcL, <14% of total) are an exception and should be considered for vaccination if it is indicated.[19] Patients with a history of anaphylaxis to neomycin should not receive the vaccine. Patients with a history of egg allergy without anaphylaxis can be vaccinated.

VARICELLA — Universal childhood vaccination against varicella, introduced in the US in 1995, has resulted in a sharp decline in varicella-related morbidity and mortality in children.[20] Adults with primary varicella infection are at much higher risk than children of developing severe disease.[21]

Each 0.5-mL dose of varicella vaccine containing at least 1350 plaque-forming units of a live attenuated Oka strain of varicella zoster virus (VZV).

Recommendations for Use – All persons born in the US before 1966 are considered immune. Two doses of vaccine separated by 4-8 weeks are recommended for adults without evidence of immunity to varicella: a history of typical varicella, laboratory evidence of immunity, documentation of vaccination, or physician-diagnosed herpes zoster. Adult vaccination programs should target those in close contact with persons at risk for severe disease (healthcare workers or family contacts of immunosuppressed persons), and those at high risk of being exposed to or transmitting the virus, such as teachers, childcare workers, adults living with young children, residents and staff members of institutions, and military personnel.

Adverse Effects – Local injection-site reactions are common in vaccinated adults. Other adverse effects include fever (10%) and injection-site or generalized varicella-like rash (1-5%). Spread of vaccine virus from healthy vaccinees who develop a varicella-like rash to susceptible contacts has been reported. Vaccine recipients should avoid, if possible, contact with susceptible high-risk individuals (immunocompromised persons, pregnant women, neonates of non-immune mothers).

Contraindications – Because it is a live vaccine, *Varivax* is contraindicated in pregnant women and patients with immunosuppression or untreated TB. It should not be given to patients with a history of anaphylaxis to neomycin.

HERPES ZOSTER — The FDA recently approved a high-potency formulation (19,400 plaque-forming units) of varicella vaccine (*Zostavax* – Merck) for prevention of herpes zoster (shingles) in adults ≥60 years old. Approval was based on a study evaluating this vaccine in about 38,000 subjects with a history of varicella. One dose of vaccine decreased the frequency of herpes zoster by about 50% overall. The benefit was highest in patients 60-69 years old and declined with increasing age.[22] Injection-site reactions were the most common adverse effects and occurred in about 30% of patients. Contraindications are the same as those for varicella vaccine.

HEPATITIS B — Transmission of hepatitis B virus occurs through sexual contact, contact with infected blood or other body fluids and through perinatal exposure. Universal vaccination of infants has been standard in the US since 1991, and routine vaccination of adolescents has been recommended since 1996.

Available formulations of hepatitis B vaccine contain hepatitis B surface antigen (HBsAg) protein grown in baker's yeast using recombinant DNA technology, which is then purified and adsorbed to aluminum hydroxide. Each 1.0 mL dose of *Engerix-B* contains 20 mcg of HBsAg, while each 1.0 mL dose of *Recombivax HB* contains 10 mcg of HBsAg. The hepatitis B component in the combined hepatitis A and B vaccine *(Twinrix)* is the same antigenic component as in *Engerix-B*. All available vaccines are equally effective.[23]

ADULT VACCINES ACCORDING TO RISK GROUP

Risk Groups	Td	Influenza
Pregnancy	✓	✓
Malignancy[4] (solid or hematologic); **radiation or chemotherapy[5]; high-dose long-term corticosteroids[3]; congenital immunodeficiency; CSF leaks**	✓	✓
Diabetes; chronic cardiac, pulmonary[6] or liver[7] disease	✓	✓[6]
Asplenia[8,9] (including terminal complement component deficiency)	✓	✓[10]
End-stage renal disease (including hemodialysis); **recipients of clotting factor concentrates**	✓	✓
HIV		
Symptomatic	✓	✓
Asymptomatic	✓	✓
Healthcare workers	✓	✓

✓: Recommended; **RF:** Recommended if another risk factor is present; **C:** Contraindicated
1. Pregnant women who are not immune to rubella and/or varicella should receive one dose of MMR vaccine and/or varicella vaccine after delivery and before discharge from the hospital. Dose 2 of varicella should be given 4-8 weeks after dose 1.
2. Patients with leukemia in remission with no recent history (≥3 months) of chemotherapy are not considered severely immunosuppressed for the purpose of receiving live-virus vaccines.
3. Considered by most clinicians to be equivalent to ≥2 mg/kg/d or ≥20 mg/d of prednisone or its equivalent for ≥14 days. Short-term (<2 weeks treatment), low to moderate doses, long-term alternate day treatment with short-acting preparations, maintenance physiologic doses (replacement therapy), or steroids administered topically, by aerosol or by intrarticular, bursal or tendon injection are not considered contraindications to live-virus vaccines.
4. See also: CDC. Guidelines for preventing opportunistic infections among hematopoietic stem cell transplant recipients. MMWR 2000; 49(RR-10);1.
5. Chemotherapy with alkylating agents or antimetabolites.
6. Chronic pulmonary disease: chronic pneumonitis, chronic obstructive pulmonary disease, chronic bronchitis or asthma; asthma is an indication for annual influenza vaccination but not pneumococcal vaccination.

Recommendations for Use – Hepatitis B immunization is recommended for adults with a medical, occupational or behavorial risk of infection. Medical indications include hemodialysis or treatment with clotting-factor concentrates. Occupational indications include health care or public safety work with potential exposure to blood or body fluids. Behavioral

Pneumo-coccal	MMR	Varicella	Hep B	Hep A	Meningo-coccal
RF	C[1]	C[1]	RF	RF	RF
✓	C[2,3]	C[2,3]	RF	RF	RF
✓[6]	✓	✓	RF	RF	RF
✓	✓	✓	RF	RF	✓
✓	✓	✓	✓[11]	RF	RF
✓	C[12]	C	✓	RF	RF
✓	✓[13]	C	✓	RF	RF
RF	✓	✓	✓	RF	RF

7. Chronic liver disease includes patients with chronic alcoholism.
8. Includes functional or anatomic asplenia, including elective splenectomy. When possible, persons undergoing elective splenectomy should receive the indicated vaccines >2 weeks prior to surgery.
9. *Haemophilus influenzae* type B (Hib) vaccine should also be considered in persons with asplenia.
10. No data exist on the risk for severe or complicated influenza in persons with asplenia. However, influenza is a risk factor for secondary bacterial infections that can be life-threatening in asplenic patients.
11. Hemodialysis patients should receive a 40 mcg/ml or two 20 mcg/ml doses of Hepatitis B vaccine.
12. Should be considered for all symptomatic HIV-infected persons who do not have evidence of severe immunosuppression (CD4 count [%] <200 cells/mcL [<14%]) or of measles immunity.
13. Recommended for asymptomatic HIV-infected persons who do not have evidence of severe immunosuppression (CD4 count [%] <200 cells/mcL [<14%]) for whom measles vaccination would otherwise be indicated.

indications include injection drug use, sex with more than one partner in the previous 6 months, recently acquired sexually transmitted infection, and men who have sex with men. Other populations who should receive hepatitis B vaccination include clients of facilities that treat STIs, HIV or drug abuse, residents and staff members of institutions for the developmentally disabled, inmates of correctional facilities, household contacts and sex partners of those with chronic hepatitis B infection, and travelers who will be in countries with intermediate or high prevalence of hepatitis B infection for more than 6 months, or who may undergo medical or dental procedures in such countries.[3,24]

Primary immunization with hepatitis B vaccine usually consists of 3 doses given at 0, 1, and 6 months. An alternate schedule of 3 doses given at 0, 1 and 2 months, followed by a fourth dose at 12 months, is approved only for *Engerix-B* in the US. An interrupted hepatitis B vaccination series does not have to be restarted. A 3-dose series started with one vaccine may be completed with the other. Immunity is believed to be lifelong for most adults who have completed a primary immunization series.

Adverse Effects – The most common adverse effects of hepatitis B vaccination are pain at the injection site. Fever occurs in <10% of recipients.

HEPATITIS A — Hepatitis A virus (HAV) infection is frequently reported in the US and is endemic in certain communities in the western and southwestern states and in Alaska. In the US, the prevalence of anti-HAV antibodies increases from about 10% in preadolescent children to about 75% in elderly adults.[25] Vaccination is now part of routine pediatric immunization in the US.

Two inactivated hepatitis A whole-virus vaccines *(Vaqta, Havrix)* are available in the US. *Twinrix*, the combination hepatitis A and B vaccine, contains half of the hepatitis A component of *Havrix*. All 3 vaccines are equally effective.

Recommendations for Use – Hepatitis A vaccine is recommended for adults with a medical, occupational or behavioral risk of hepatitis infection. Medical indications include clotting factor disorders or chronic liver disease, including chronic active hepatitis C and/or B virus infection. Occupational indications include work with HAV in a laboratory setting. Behavioral indications include illicit (injection and non-injection) drug users or men who have sex with men. Hepatitis A vaccine is also recommended for susceptible travelers going anywhere other than Canada, Australia, New Zealand, Japan, South Korea or western Europe.

Hepatitis A vaccination in adults usually consists of two doses separated by at least 6 months. After a single dose, *Havrix* provides protection for 12 months, and *Vaqta* for 18 months. Patients who receive *Twinrix* need 3 doses at 0, 1 and 6 months. Patients who have received a first dose of one vaccine will respond to a second dose of the other. Booster doses are not recommended.[26]

Adverse Effects – Local injection site reactions such as pain, swelling or erythema occur in 20-50% of vaccine recipients. Mild systemic complaints such as malaise, low-grade fever or fatigue occur in less than 10%.

MENINGOCOCCAL — About 2000 cases of meningococcal disease occur in the US each year. The case fatality rate is 10% for meningitis and up to 40% for meningococcemia. Rates of meningococcal disease are highest in infancy, but a second peak occurs in adolescence and young adulthood, and about 3% of cases occur in college students, especially freshmen living in dormitories. Five major serogroups of *Neisseria meningitidis* — A, B, C, Y and W-135 — cause most human infection.[27]

Two quadrivalent vaccines are available against *Neisseria meningitidis* serogroups A, C, Y, and W135. *Menomune* contains meningococcal capsular polysaccharides. *Menactra* contains the same capsular polysaccharides conjugated to diptheria toxoid.[28] Neither vaccine provides protection against serogroup B, which does not have an immunogenic polysaccharide capsule.

Each 0.5 mL dose of *Menactra* contains 4 mcg of meningococcal polysaccharide from each of the four serogroups conjugated to 48 mcg of diphtheria toxoid protein. Each dose of *Menomune* contains 50 mcg of meningococcal polysaccharide from each of the four serogroups. In adults, both vaccines are effective and induce serotype-specific antibody responses in over 90% of recipients.[27]

Recommendations for Use – Vaccination is recommended for adults with anatomic or functional asplenia or terminal complement component deficiencies, first-year college students living in dormitories, laboratory personnel routinely exposed to isolates of *N. meningitidis*, military recruits, and persons who travel to or reside in countries in which meningococcal disease is hyperendemic or epidemic, particularly those in the "meningitis belt" of sub-Saharan Africa. The government of Saudi Arabia also requires vaccination for pilgrims during the annual Hajj.

A single dose of vaccine is recommended. The conjugate vaccine is preferred for adults 18-55 years, although the polysaccharide vaccine is an acceptable alternative. For adults vaccinated with the polysaccharide vaccine, revaccination after 5 years is recommended for patients who remain at high risk. The duration of protection with conjugate vaccine is likely to be longer, but data are not yet available.

Adverse Effects – The most common adverse reactions to *Menactra* have been headache, fatigue and malaise, in addition to pain, redness and induration at the site of injection. The rates of these reactions are higher than with *Menomune*, but similar to those with tetanus toxoid. Eight cases of Guillian-Barre syndrome have been reported in adolescents who received *Menactra*, but cause and effect have not been established.[29]

OTHER VACCINES

Haemophilus Influenzae Type b (Hib) – Most adults do not require routine immunization with Hib conjugate vaccine, which is FDA-approved for use only in children. Adults with chronic medical conditions such as sickle cell disease, HIV infection, leukemia or lymphoma, or those with anatomic or functional asplenia are at increased risk for invasive disease due to Hib. Vaccination of these patients could be considered, but its efficacy is unknown.

Human Papillomavirus (HPV) – A new inactivated human papillomavirus (HPV) vaccine (*Gardasil* – Merck) is now available for prevention of HPV infection caused by HPV types 6, 11, 16 and 18 in girls and women 9-26 years old. HPV types 16 and 18 cause 70% of cervical cancers; types 6 and 11 cause 90% of genital warts.[30,31] It is administered in 3 doses at 0, 2 and 6 months. Mild to moderate injection site reactions are common. The duration of immunity is unknown.

1. G Poland et al. Standards for Adult Immunization Practices. Am J Prev Med 2003; 25:144.
2. Centers for Disease Control and Prevention (CDC). Recommended Adult Immunization Schedule — United States, October 2005-September 2006. MMWR Quick Guide 2005; 54:Q1.
3. Advice for Travelers. Treat Guidel Med Lett 2006; 4:25.
4. Centers for Disease Control and Prevention (CDC). National Immunization Program. Epidemiology and Prevention of Vaccine-Preventable Diseases. The Pink Book. 9th Edition. January 2006; pages 57 and 69. Available at www.cdc.gov/nip/publications/pink/default.htm. Accessed June 12, 2006.
5. Provisional recommendations for Tdap in adults. Advisory Committee on Immunization Practices (ACIP) – October 2005. Available at www.cdc.gov/nip. Accessed June 12, 2006.
6. Adacel and Boostrix: Tdap vaccines for adolescents and adults. Med Lett Drugs Ther 2006; 48:5.
7. SA Harper et al. Prevention and control of influenza. Recommendations of the Advisory Committee on Immunization Practices (ACIP). MMWR Recomm Rep 2005; 54(RR-8):1.
8. Influenza vaccine 2005-2006. Med Lett Drugs Ther 2005; 47:85.
9. HS Izurieta et al. Adverse events reported following live, cold-adapted, intranasal influenza vaccine. JAMA 2005; 294:2720.
10. DN Fisman et al. Prior pneumococcal vaccination is associated with reduced death, complications, and length of stay among hospitalized adults with community-acquired pneumonia. Clin Infect Dis 2006; 42:1093.
11. Prevention of pneumococcal disease: recommendations of the Advisory Committee on Immunization Practices (ACIP). MMWR Recomm Rep 1997; 46(RR-8):1.
12. Pneumococcal vaccine (Prevnar) for otitis media. Med Lett Drugs Ther 2003; 45:27.
13. FJ Walker et al. Reactions after 3 or more doses of pneumococcal polysaccharide vaccine in adults in Alaska. Clin Infect Dis 2005; 40:1730.
14. JC Watson et al. Measles, Mumps, and Rubella — Vaccine use and strategies for elimination of measles, rubella, and congenital rubella syndrome and control of mumps: recommendations of the Advisory Committee on Immunization Practices (ACIP). MMWR Recomm Rep 1998; 47(RR-8);1.
15. Centers for Disease Control and Prevention (CDC). Update: Multistate outbreak of mumps – United States, January 1-May 2, 2006. MMWR Morb Mortal Wkly Rep May 26, 2006, 55:559.

16. RK Gupta et al. Mumps and the UK epidemic 2005. BMJ 2005; 330:1132.

17. Centers for Disease Control and Prevention (CDC). Notice to readers: Updated recommendations of the Advisory Committee on Immunization Practices (ACIP) for the control and elimination of mumps. MMWR Early release. June 1, 2006; 55:1.

18. KM Madsen and M Vestergaard. MMR vaccination and autism: what is the evidence for a causal association? Drug Saf 2004; 27:831.

19. WL Atkinson et al. General recommendations on immunization. Recommendations of the Advisory Committee on Immunization Practices (ACIP) and the American Academy of Family Physicians (AAFP). MMWR Recomm Rep 2002; 51(RR-2):1.

20. HQ Nguyen et al. Decline in mortality due to varicella after implementation of varicella vaccination in the United States. N Engl J Med 2005; 352:450.

21. AA Gershon and S Hambleton. Varicella vaccine for susceptible adults: do it today. Clin Infect Dis 2004; 39:1640.

22 MN Oxman et al. A Vaccine to Prevent Herpes Zoster and Postherpetic Neuralgia in Older Adults. N Engl J Med 2005; 352:2271.

23. Twinrix: a combination hepatitis A and B vaccine. Med Lett Drugs Ther 2001; 43:67.

24. Provisional recommendations for hepatitis B vaccination of adults. Advisory Committee on Immunization Practices (ACIP) – October 2005. Available at www.cdc.gov/nip. Accessed June 12, 2006.

25. Advisory Committee on Immunization Practices (ACIP). Prevention of hepatitis A through active or passive immunization: recommendations of the Advisory Committee on Immunization Practices (ACIP). MMWR Recomm Rep 2006; 55(RR-7):1.

26. P Van Damme et al. Hepatitis A booster vaccinations: is there a need? Lancet 2003; 362:1065.

27. OO Bilukha et al. Prevention and control of meningococcal disease. Recommendations of the Advisory Committee on Immunization Practices (ACIP). MMWR Recomm Rep 2005; 54(RR-7):1.

28. Menactra: a meningococcal conjugate vaccine. Med Lett Drugs Ther 2005; 47:29.

29. Center for Disease Control and Prevention (CDC). Update: Guillain-Barre syndrome among recipients of Menactra meningococcal conjugate vaccine—United States, October 2005-February 2006. MMWR Morb Mortal Wkly Rep 2006; 55:364.

30. LL Villa et al. Prophylactic quadrivalent human papillomavirus (types 6, 11, 16, and 18) L1 virus-like particle vaccine in young women: a randomised double-blind placebo-controlled multicentre phase II efficacy trial. Lancet Oncol 2005; 6:271.

31. FE Skjeldestad for the Future II Steering Committee. Prophylactic quadrivalent human papillomavirus (HPV) (types 6, 11, 16, 18) L1 virus-like particle (VLP) vaccine (Gardasil) reduces cervical intraepithelial neoplasia (CIN) 2/3 risk. 43rd annual meeting of IDSA, October 6-9, 2005, San Francisco. Abstract LB-8a. Available at www.idsociety.org. Accessed June 12, 2006.

Herpes Zoster Vaccine *(Zostavax)*
Originally published in The Medical Letter – September 2006; 48:73

A live attenuated varicella-zoster vaccine (*Zostavax* – Merck) has been approved by the FDA for prevention of herpes zoster (HZ; zoster; shingles) in persons ≥60 years old. Each dose of *Zostavax* contains about 14 times as much varicella-zoster virus (VZV) as *Varivax*, which has been used in the US since 1995 to vaccinate against varicella (chicken pox).

HERPES ZOSTER — Following primary infection (varicella), VZV persists in a latent form in sensory ganglia. VZV-specific cell-mediated immunity (VZV-CMI), which develops in response to varicella infection, prevents the latent virus from reactivating and multiplying to cause herpes zoster. When VZV-CMI falls below a critical threshold, as it does in older persons and immunosuppressed patients, latent VZV can reactivate, multiply and spread within the ganglion, causing neuronal necrosis, intense inflammation and often severe neuralgia. Postherpetic neuralgia (PHN), a debilitating neuropathic pain syndrome that can persist for months or even years, occurs in about one-third of patients with HZ who are ≥60 years of age.

Currently more than 90% of adults in the US have had varicella and are at risk for HZ.[1] More than one million new cases of HZ are estimated to occur in the US each year, more than half in people ≥60 years old.[2] Second episodes of HZ are uncommon in immunocompetent persons because the marked increase in VZV-CMI induced by HZ usually protects the patient against another episode of the disease.

THE VACCINE — Several clinical studies have demonstrated that immunization with VZV vaccines boosts waning VZV-CMI in older adults.[3-5] The Shingles Prevention Study, a VA cooperative study, randomized 38,546 adults ≥60 years old with a history of varicella to *Zostavax* or placebo to determine whether boosting VZV-CMI protects against herpes zoster and postherpetic neuralgia. The mean duration of surveillance was about 3 years.

The vaccine reduced the severity and duration of pain and discomfort ("the burden of illness") caused by HZ, which was the primary endpoint of the study, by 61%.[2] HZ occurred in 315 vaccine recipients and in 642 who received placebo. Vaccine-virus DNA was not detected in any of the HZ cases. PHN developed in 27 vaccine recipients and in 80 placebo recipients. The reductions in HZ and PHN with the vaccine were both statistically significant. The vaccine was effective in preventing HZ (51% overall, 64% in patients 60-69 years old and 38% in those ≥70). Its efficacy overall in preventing PHN was 67%, and was virtually the same in patients 60-69 and ≥70 years old.

ADVERSE EFFECTS — Reactions to the vaccine at the injection site (erythema, pain, tenderness, swelling and pruritus) were generally mild. Varicella-like rash at the injection site occurred in 20 subjects who received the vaccine and in 7 who received placebo. Transmission of the vaccine virus from vaccine recipients to other susceptible persons has not been reported with *Zostavax*, but has occurred very rarely in contacts of *Varivax* recipients who developed a varicella-like rash after vaccination.

RECOMMENDATIONS AND COST — *Zostavax* is given as a single subcutaneous dose (0.65 mL), which costs about $150. It is indicated for immunocompetent persons ≥60 years old. Adults who have not had varicella (who are VZV-seronegative) should be immunized against varicella with two doses of *Varivax*.

Zostavax is contraindicated in persons who are immunosuppressed as a result of disease (e.g., AIDS, lymphoproliferative malignancies) or treatment (cytotoxic chemotherapy, systemic corticosteroids) and in those with a history of an anaphylactic reaction to gelatin, neomycin or other components of the vaccine.

CONCLUSION — *Zostavax* appears to be safe and effective in patients ≥60 years old for protecting against herpes zoster and postherpetic neuralgia, especially in reducing the severity and duration of the disease. The duration of protection and the need for booster vaccination remain to be determined.

1. JW Gnann, Jr and RJ Whitley. Clinical practice. Herpes zoster. N Engl J Med 2002; 347:340.
2. MN Oxman et al. A vaccine to prevent herpes zoster and post-herpetic neuralgia in older adults. N Eng J Med 2005; 352:2271.
3. MN Oxman. Immunization to reduce the frequency and severity of herpes zoster and its complications. Neurology 1995; 45 (12 suppl 8):S41.
4. MJ Levin et al. Use of a live attenuated varicella vaccine to boost varicella-specific immune responses in seropositive people 55 years of age and older: duration of booster effect. J Infect Dis 1998; 178 suppl 1:S109.
5. E Trannoy et al. Vaccination of immunocompetent elderly subjects with a live attenuated Oka strain of varicella zoster virus: a randomized, controlled, dose-response trial. Vaccine 2000; 18:1700.

A Human Papillomavirus Vaccine
Originally published in The Medical Letter – August 2006; 48:65

A recombinant quadrivalent human-papillomavirus-like particle vaccine, *Gardasil* (Merck), has been approved by the FDA for use in girls and women 9-26 years old to prevent diseases associated with infection with human papillomavirus (HPV) types 6, 11, 16, and 18, including genital warts, precancerous cervical, vaginal or vulvar lesions, and cervical cancer.

BACKGROUND — HPV is sexually transmitted; it is acquired by young women soon after initiation of sexual activity, with a cumulative incidence of 40% within 16 months.[1] Although most HPV infections are cleared without clinical sequelae, persistent infection can cause abnormalities in the cervical epithelium that may progress to cancer.

More than 30 types of HPV can infect the genital tract. Types 16 and 18 are responsible for more than 70% of cervical cancers and high-grade cervical intraepithelial neoplasia (CIN), a precursor of cervical cancer. Types 6 and 11 cause about 90% of genital warts.

CLINICAL STUDIES — HPV 16 is common in young women and is difficult to clear. A randomized, placebo-controlled trial evaluated a prototype HPV 16 vaccine in 1533 women 16-23 years old with no evidence of HPV infection at enrollment. At follow-up a median of 17 months after the third vaccine dose, 41 cases of persistent HPV 16 infection and 9 cases of CIN grade 1/2 were found in the placebo group, compared to no cases of either one among those who were vaccinated.[2] A further follow-up at 48 months found no cases of HPV 16-related CIN grade 2/3 among women who were vaccinated, compared to 12 in the placebo group.[3]

A randomized, double-blind, 3-year trial compared a quadrivalent HPV vaccine (equivalent to *Gardasil*) with placebo in women 16-23 years old; women with previous HPV infection were not excluded. The primary endpoint, persistent infection with HPV 6, 11, 16 or 18, or cervical or external genital HPV-associated disease, occurred in 4 of 235 women who received the vaccine and in 36 of 233 who received placebo, a 90% reduction.[4]

A randomized, placebo-controlled trial of the new quadrivalent human papillomavirus vaccine in more than 12,000 women evaluated its efficacy in preventing HPV 16/18-related CIN 2/3 and cervical cancer. At 2 years, there was no HPV 16/18-related CIN 2/3 among the 5301 women who were vaccinated and 21 cases among the 5258 who received placebo.[5] There were 59 cases of genital warts among the women who received placebo, and one among those who were vaccinated.

No clinical data are available in girls younger than 16. The FDA apparently inferred efficacy in this age group from immunogenicity studies in girls 9-15 years old.

ADVERSE EFFECTS — Adverse reactions at the injection site included pain, swelling, erythema and pruritus; discontinuation of the vaccine series was uncommon. Fever occurred 1-15 days post-vaccination in 10.3% of women who received the vaccine and in 8.6% who received placebo.

RECOMMENDATIONS — Although HPV vaccine would ideally be administered before the onset of sexual activity, girls and women who are already sexually active should also be vaccinated. The US Advisory Committee on Immunization Practices (ACIP) recommends vaccination in all girls and women 11-26 years old. Girls 11 and 12 years old can begin the vaccine series during their routine young adolescent visit where they are already scheduled to receive 2 other vaccinations (Tdap and meningococcal vaccine). The ACIP has suggested that vaccination could be started as early as age 9 at the discretion of the healthcare provider.[6] HPV vaccine should not be given to women who are pregnant.

DOSAGE, ADMINISTRATION AND COST — *Gardasil* is administered in 3 separate 0.5-mL intramuscular injections at 0, 2 and 6 months. It should be injected into the deltoid or anterolateral thigh. Each dose costs about $120; the cost of a full course will be about $360.

CONCLUSION — The new quadrivalent HPV vaccine *(Gardasil)* is nearly 100 percent effective in girls and women in preventing persistent infection with HPV types 6, 11, 16 and 18 and associated precancerous cervical and external genital lesions. Whether immunity will persist long enough, without a booster, to provide lifelong protection against development of cervical cancer, and whether males should also be vaccinated, remain to be determined.

1. RL Winer et al. Genital human papillomavirus infection: incidence and risk factors in a cohort of female university students. Am J Epidemiol 2003; 157:218.
2. LA Koutsky et al. A controlled trial of a human papillomavirus type 16 vaccine. N Engl J Med 2002; 347:1645.
3. C Mao et al. Efficacy of human papillomavirus-16 vaccine to prevent cervical intraepithelial neoplasia: a randomized controlled trial. Obstet Gynecol 2006; 107:18.
4. LL Villa et al. Prophylactic quadrivalent human papillomavirus (types 6, 11, 16, and 18) L1 virus-like particle vaccine in young women: a randomised double-blind placebo-controlled multicentre phase II efficacy trial. Lancet Oncol 2005; 6:271.
5. FE Skjeldestad for the Merck phase 3 HPV vaccine steering committee (FUTURE II). Prophylactic quadrivalent human papillomavirus (HPV) (types 6, 11, 16, 18) L1 virus-like particle (VLP) vaccine (Gardasil) reduces cervical intraepithelial neoplasia (CIN 2/3) risk. Presented at: Infectious Disease Society of America Late Breaker Session 66, LB-8A; October 7, 2005; San Francisco, CA.
6. CDC's advisory committee recommends human papillomavirus vaccination. June 29, 2006. Availabe at: www.cdc.gov/od/oc/media/pressrel/r060629.htm (accessed on August 7, 2006).

Mumps Outbreak Recommendations
Originally published in The Medical Letter – June 2006; 48:45

A large mumps outbreak that began in Iowa in December 2005 has spread.[1] About 40% of the cases have been in people 18-25 years old, many of whom are college students and had been vaccinated against the disease.

THE DISEASE — Mumps is transmitted by droplet or fomite exposure with an average incubation period of 16-18 days. The illness has a prodrome of headache, malaise, anorexia and fever, followed within 1 day by unilateral or bilateral salivary gland swelling, particularly of the parotid. About 20% of cases are asymptomatic. Oophoritis (5% of postpubertal women), orchitis (25% of postpubertal men), a usually benign meningitis ($\leq$10%), and transient high-frequency deafness (4% of adults) can occur.[2]

THE VACCINE — The attenuated live-virus mumps vaccine was first approved in the US in 1967 for use in adolescents.[3] In 1977 it was incorporated into the routine vaccination recommendations for young children. A single dose of measles, mumps and rubella (MMR) vaccine is about 80% effective in preventing mumps; two doses increase protection to 90%. Antibodies may not reach protective levels until 2-4 weeks after vaccination.

ROUTINE CHILDHOOD IMMUNIZATION — The US Advisory Committee on Immunization Practices (ACIP) recommends one dose of MMR at 12-15 months of age and a second dose at 4-6 years. Since 2000, most states have required 2 doses of MMR before school entry. Many colleges now also require a second dose before matriculation.

SOURCE OF OUTBREAK — The source of the current outbreak is unknown, but the circulating strain (genotype G) is responsible for an ongoing outbreak in the United Kingdom that has involved >70,000 people, many of them young adults. Mumps vaccine was not introduced in the UK until 1988, and there was a worldwide shortage of mumps vaccine and MMR in the early 1990s.[4]

US AGE DISTRIBUTION — In the recent outbreak in the US, the cases in young people who had received 1 or 2 doses of the vaccine are thought to be due to the close living conditions in college dormitories and the documented 10-20% failure rate of mumps vaccine. The relatively low incidence in older people might be due to superior immunity from natural infection.

RECOMMENDATIONS — In addition to routine immunization, the CDC now recommends MMR vaccine for persons born after 1957 who do not have a history of physician-diagnosed mumps infection, laboratory evidence of immunity, or immunity through vaccination, which the ACIP has recently redefined as 1 dose of mumps vaccine for preschool children and adults not at high risk and 2 doses for children in grades K-12 and adults at high risk (healthcare workers, international travelers and post-high-school students).

During an outbreak, a second dose should be considered for all adults and children 1-4 years old, given at least 28 days after the first dose. The CDC suggests that unvaccinated healthcare workers born before 1957 who do not have other evidence of immunity should also receive 2 doses of the vaccine. Both mumps and MMR vaccine are contraindicated during pregnancy and in patients with moderate to severe immunodeficiency.

1. CDC. Update: multistate outbreak of mumps – United States, January 1-May 2, 2006. MMWR Morb Mortal Wkly Rep 2006; 55:559.
2. N Litman and SG Baum in GL Mandell et al eds. Mumps virus. *Principles and Practice of Infectious Diseases*, 6th ed. Philadelphia, PA: Elsevier Churchill Livingstone; 2005, page 2003.
3. Mumps virus vaccine. Med Lett Drugs Ther 1968; 10:14.
4. CDC. Mumps epidemic – United Kingdom 2004-2005. MMWR Morb Mortal Wkly Rep 2006; 55:173.

A Second Dose of Varicella Vaccine
Originally published in The Medical Letter – September 2006; 48:80

The US Advisory Committee on Immunization Practices (ACIP) has recommended the addition of a routine second dose of varicella vaccine for children <13 years old. Varicella vaccine has been used in the US since 1995, but varicella outbreaks have continued to occur among school children vaccinated with a single dose. In one such outbreak, the attack rate was 100% in unvaccinated children and 18% in those previously vaccinated.[1] In vaccinated children, the typical maculopapular-vesicular rash of varicella may be only maculopapular with few or no vesicles, but these children could still transmit virus to susceptible contacts.

EVIDENCE OF VARICELLA IMMUNITY

Prior vaccination:
  1 dose for pre-school children ≥12 months old
  2 doses for school-aged children, adolescents and adults

Laboratory evidence of varicella infection

History of varicella or herpes zoster infection

Born in US before 1980*

*But this evidence alone is insufficient for healthcare workers and pregnant women.

RECOMMENDATIONS — The first dose of varicella vaccine given at 12-15 months of age should now be followed by a second dose at age 4-6 years.[2] Two doses of varicella vaccine have been shown to be well tolerated, significantly more immunogenic than a single dose, and more than 3 times as effective in preventing disease.[3]

The ACIP now recommends that children, adolescents and adults who have previously received only a single dose of the vaccine receive a "catch-up" dose, at least 3 months after the first in children <13 years, and that all unvaccinated people ≥13 years old without a history of varicella or evidence of immunity be vaccinated with 2 doses of vaccine given 4-8 weeks apart.

Varicella vaccine is not recommended for pregnant women (who, if not immune, should be vaccinated after delivery) or immunocompromised patients, except for children with mild to moderate HIV infection.

THE VACCINE — Live attenuated varicella vaccine can be given alone (*Varivax* – Merck) or as part of a combined measles-mumps-rubella-varicella vaccine (*ProQuad* – Merck), which is as immunogenic as giving separate injections of MMR and varicella vaccine.[4] The two-dose varicella vaccination schedule now coincides with the MMR series.

CONCLUSION — Vaccination against varicella now requires giving 2 doses of varicella vaccine.

1. AS Lopez et al. One dose of varicella vaccine does not prevent school outbreaks: is it time for a second dose? Pediatrics 2006; 117:e1070.
2. ACIP provisional recommendations for prevention of varicella, available at (www.cdc.gov/nip/vaccine/varicella/varicella_acip_recs_prov_ june_2006.pdf).
3. B Kuter et al. Ten year follow-up of healthy children who received one or two injections of varicella vaccine. Pediatr Infect Dis J 2004; 23:132.
4. M Knuf et al. Immunogenicity and safety of two doses of tetravalent measles-mumps-rubella-varicella vaccine in healthy children. Pediatr Infect Dis J 2006; 25:12.

Tdap, DTaP Mix-Ups
Originally published in The Medical Letter – January 2007; 49:8

Medical Letter consultants have brought to our attention some confusion that has accompanied the release of *Adacel*, a combination of tetanus toxoid, diphtheria toxoid and acellular pertussis antigens (Tdap) recently approved for use as a booster in adolescents and adults 11-64 years old (Med Lett Drugs Ther 2006; 48:5). Another Tdap vaccine, *Boostrix*, is approved for use in adolescents 10-18 years old. Some adults have inadvertently been immunized with *Daptacel* or *Infanrix* (DTaP), which are intended for active immunization of infants and children 6 weeks to 6 years old. Such mix-ups were reported by the Institute for Safe Medication Practices (www.ismp.org) in the August 24 and December 2006 issues of its newsletter.

TDAP VS. DTAP

| | SANOFI/PASTEUR | | GLAXOSMITHKLINE | |
| | *Adacel* (Tdap) 11-64 yrs | *Daptacel* (DTaP) 6 wks-6 yrs | *Boostrix* (Tdap) 10-18 yrs | *Infanrix* (DTaP) 6 wks-6 yrs |
COMPONENT				
Tetanus toxoid	5.0 Lf	5.0 Lf	5.0 Lf	10.0 Lf
Diphtheria toxoid	2.0 Lf	15.0 Lf	2.5 Lf	25.0 Lf
Detoxified pertussis toxin	2.5 mcg	10.0 mcg	8.0 mcg	25.0 mcg
Other pertussis antigens				
Filamentous hemagglutinin	5 mcg	5 mcg	8 mcg	25 mcg
Pertactin	3 mcg	3 mcg	2.5 mcg	8 mcg
Fimbriae types 2 and 3	5 mcg	5 mcg	none	none

Lf: Limit of flocculation unit

Tdap, DTaP Mix-Ups

The problem with giving these pediatric vaccines to adults is that they contain *more* diphtheria and pertussis antigens than the adult vaccine, and adults may have untoward reactions to these higher antigen levels. One consultant who inadvertently gave the pediatric vaccine to 80 adults reports that a few developed fever to 102°F, and several developed severe erythema and swelling at the injection site. In the absence of a comparative trial, whether these reactions were due to the higher antigen load can only be a matter of speculation.

The reasons for the mix-ups, according to the Institute, include the similarities in the brand names and packaging of *Adacel* and *Daptacel* in addition to the similar component antigens in the 2 products (the components of *Adacel* are listed in a different order and are labeled as "reduced" diphtheria toxoid and acellular pertussis). The manufacturer of *Adacel* and *Daptacel* intends to make changes in the packaging and labeling to clarify the differences between the products. The inadvertent administration of *Infanrix* to adults was caused by an electronic order entry program's failure to differentiate between the adult and pediatric vaccines.

VariZIG for Prophylaxis After Exposure to Varicella
Originally published in The Medical Letter – August 2006; 48:69

The US manufacturer of varicella zoster immune globulin (VZIG; Massachusetts Public Health Biologic Laboratories, Boston, MA) recently discontinued its production. A Canadian formulation, *VariZIG* (Varicella Zoster Immune Globulin [Human] – Cangene Corporation, Winnipeg) is now available in the US under an investigational new drug application expanded access protocol.[1]

VIRUS TRANSMISSION — Patients with varicella are most contagious from 1-2 days before to shortly after the onset of rash, and virus can be transmitted until the lesions are crusted. Varicella can also be contracted from patients with recent-onset (about 7 days) herpes zoster lesions.

RECOMMENDATIONS — The US Advisory Committee on Immunization Practices (ACIP) recommends that healthy nonimmune adults and children exposed to varicella-zoster virus (VZV) receive prophylaxis with live-attenuated varicella vaccine *(Varivax)*, preferably within 96 hours of exposure.[2] Exposed patients for whom varicella vaccine is contraindicated and who are at high risk for complications of varicella infection (see table) should receive *VariZIG*. *VariZIG* is approved in Canada only for use in pregnant women.

If *VariZIG* cannot be obtained for these patients within 96 hours of exposure, the ACIP recommends considering use of intravenous immune globulin (IVIG) at a dose of 400 mg/kg once (also within 96 hours of exposure). Individual lots of IVIG are not routinely tested for varicella antibody, and IVIG is not FDA-approved for this indication.

CLINICAL STUDIES — A randomized 6-week study compared *VariZIG* (either IM or IV) to VZIG (IM) for prevention of varicella within 14 days of exposure in 57 pregnant women seronegative for VZV. The rate of symptomatic varicella infection with *VariZIG* (29%) was

PATIENTS ELIGIBLE FOR *VARIZIG**

Neonates whose mothers had signs or symptoms of varicella between 5 days before and 2 days after delivery
Premature infants >28 weeks gestation who are exposed to VZV in the neonatal period and whose mothers do not have evidence of immunity
Premature infants <28 weeks gestation or who weigh <1000 g at birth who are exposed in the neonatal period, regardless of mother's immune status
Immunocompromised patients of any age
Nonimmune pregnant women

*According to the US Advisory Committee on Immunization Practices

lower than the rate with VZIG (42%), but the difference was not statistically significant. Among patients who developed varicella, those treated within 1-4 days of exposure had milder symptoms.[3]

SAFETY AND ADVERSE EFFECTS — *VariZIG*, like VZIG, is prepared from pooled human plasma, which is screened for disease-causing viruses such as HIV or the hepatitis viruses. Virus filtration and inactivation methods are highly effective for reducing the risk of transmission of known viral agents, but the possibility remains that this product could still transmit known or unknown infectious agents.

In clinical trials, adverse effects included pain at the injection site (17%), headache (7%) and rash (5%). Myalgias, nausea, rigors, flushing, and fatigue were less common. Rare hypersensivity reactions can occur in patients with hypersensitivity to immune globulins or IgA deficiency.

There are no other known risks to pregnant women from *VariZIG*. Administration of VZIG and Rho(D) immune globulin during pregnancy has not been associated with reproductive adverse effects.

DOSAGE, ADMINISTRATION AND COST — *VariZIG* is supplied as a lyophilized powder for reconstitution in 125-unit vials. The recommended dose is 125 units/ 10 kg body weight given IM, with a maximum dose of 625 units (5 vials). The ACIP recommends that infants weighing less than 10 kg receive 125 units. *VariZIG* should be given as soon as possible after exposure; treatment more than 96 hours (4 days) after exposure is of uncertain value. In Canada, a 125-unit vial costs CAN$158.00, according to Canadian Blood Services (distributor for Cangene).

OBTAINING *VariZIG* — Since *VariZIG* (unlike VZIG) is an investigational product and is available in the US under an expanded access protocol, central institutional review board (IRB) approval has been obtained. Many institutions may require additional approval by their internal IRB. FFF Enterprises (24-hour telephone: 800-843-7477, Temecula, California) is the sole authorized US distributor of *VariZIG*. After a review of eligibility, it can be delivered, according to the distributor, within 24 hours of a request. Informed consent and a total of 4 visits are required. Whether to permit a healthcare provider to obtain an inventory of *VariZIG* for future use is under review by the FDA.

OTHER CONSIDERATIONS — *VariZIG* may prolong the incubation period of varicella (usually 14-16 days) by more than a week. Vaccination with live vaccines, such as measles, mumps and rubella (MMR), should be delayed for at least 3 months after *VariZIG* or IVIG administration. The ACIP recommends that varicella vaccination be offered after 5 months.

CONCLUSION — Varicella zoster immune globulin *(VariZIG)* is recommended for prophylaxis of persons at high risk of severe varicella who are exposed to varicella or herpes zoster and have contraindications to use of varicella vaccine. For healthy adults and others with no contraindications, varicella vaccine, which provides long-lasting protection, is preferred.

VariZIG for Prophylaxis After Exposure to Varicella

1. Centers for Disease Control and Prevention (CDC). A new product (VariZIG) for postexposure prophylaxis of varicella available under an investigational new drug application expanded access protocol. MMWR Morb Mortal Wkly Rep 2006; 55:209.
2. Centers for Disease Control and Prevention (CDC). Prevention of varicella. Update recommendations of the Advisory Committee on Immunization Practices (ACIP). MMWR Recomm Rep 1999; 48 (RR-6):1.
3. G Koren et al. Serum concentrations, efficacy, and safety of a new, intravenously administered varicella zoster immune globulin in pregnant women. J Clin Pharmacol 2002; 42:267.

ADVICE FOR
Travelers

Original publication date – May 2006

Patients planning to travel to other countries often ask physicians for information about immunizations and prevention of diarrhea and malaria. More detailed advice for travelers is available from the Centers for Disease Control and Prevention at 877-FYI-TRIP (877-394-8747) or www.cdc.gov/travel.

IMMUNIZATIONS

Common travel immunizations are listed in the table on page 344. In addition to receiving travel-specific vaccines, all travelers (including children) should be up to date on routine immunizations. Guidelines for routine adult immunization will be published in a future issue of *Treatment Guidelines*. Immunocompromised or pregnant patients generally should not receive live virus vaccines, such as those for measles and yellow fever, although in some situations the benefit might outweigh the risk.

CHOLERA — The risk of cholera in tourists is very low. The parenteral vaccine licensed in the US is no longer available. An oral vaccine called *Dukoral* is available in some European countries (Chiron) and in Canada (Sanofi Pasteur). It is not currently recommended for routine use in travelers. Vaccination might be considered for travelers who plan to work in refugee camps or as health care providers in endemic areas.

HEPATITIS A — Hepatitis A vaccine, which is now part of routine childhood immunization in the US, is recommended for all unvaccinated travelers going anywhere other than Canada, Australia, New Zealand, South Korea, Japan or western Europe. The majority of hepatitis A cases imported into the US by travelers are related to travel in Mexico and Central America.[1]

Vaccination of adults and children usually consists of two IM doses separated by 6-18 months. Additional booster doses are not needed.[2] Two hepatitis A vaccines are available in the US. Patients who received a first dose of one vaccine will respond to a second dose of the other. Second doses given up to 8 years after the first dose have produced protective antibody levels.[3,4]

Antibodies reach protective levels 2-4 weeks after the first dose. Even when exposure to the disease occurs sooner than 4 weeks after vaccination, the traveler is usually protected because of the relatively long incubation period of hepatitis A (average 28 days).[5] Children under 1 year of age and other travelers who cannot receive the vaccine should be given immune globulin (IG) (0.02 mL/kg IM if traveling for <3 months, 0.06 mL/kg IM if traveling for >3 months).

HEPATITIS B — Vaccination against hepatitis B is recommended for unvaccinated travelers going to intermediately or highly endemic areas if they plan to stay for a long time, return frequently, or live among the local population. It is also recommended for short-stay travelers planning to receive medical or dental care, or to undergo cosmetic needle punctures for tattoos or body piercing. Anyone who might have unprotected sexual contact with new partners should be immunized against hepatitis B.

Primary immunization consists of 3 doses given IM at 0, 1 and 6 months. An accelerated schedule of 3 doses given at 0, 1 and 2 months, followed by a fourth dose at 12 months, is approved for *Engerix-B* in the US. An accelerated schedule of 0, 7 and 21 days with a fourth dose at 12 months

LOW-RISK REGIONS FOR HEPATITIS A & B*

Hepatitis A	Hepatitis B
United States	United States[1]
Canada	Canada[1]
Western Europe (all countries)	Mexico
South Korea	Costa Rica
Japan	Chile
Australia	Argentina
New Zealand	Paraguay
	Uruguay
	Western Europe[2]
	Hungary
	Australia
	New Zealand

* All other areas are intermediate to high risk; vaccine is indicated.
1. Risk is high in Alaska natives and indigenous populations of northern Canada.
2. Risk is intermediate in Greece, Italy, Portugal, Malta and Spain.

can also be used if necessary, but is not FDA-approved. A 2-dose schedule of adult *Recombivax* at 0 and 4-6 months is approved in the US for adolescents 11-15 years old.[6]

An interrupted hepatitis B vaccination series does not need to be restarted. A 3-dose series started with one vaccine may be completed with the other. Post-vaccination serologic testing is recommended for health care workers.

HEPATITIS A/B — A combination vaccine *(Twinrix)* containing the same antigenic components as *Engerix-B* and pediatric *Havrix* is available for patients ≥18 years old. It is given in 3 doses at 0, 1 and 6 months; at least 2 doses should be given before travel. An accelerated schedule of 0, 1 and 3 weeks with a fourth dose at 12 months can be used if necessary, but is not FDA-approved.[7]

The combination vaccine can be used to complete an immunization series started with monovalent hepatitis A and B vaccines. *Twinrix Junior* is available outside the US for children 1-15 years old.

INFLUENZA — Influenza may be a risk in the tropics year-round and in temperate areas of the Southern Hemisphere from April to October. Outbreaks have occurred on cruise ships and on organized group tours in any latitude or season.[8]

Influenza vaccine against strains in the Northern Hemisphere is sometimes available in the US until the end of June. High-risk patients (>50 years or 6-23 months old, pregnant women, or anyone ≥6 months old with chronic disease) from the Northern Hemisphere who travel to the Southern Hemisphere during that region's influenza season should consider being immunized on arrival because the vaccine active against strains in the Southern Hemisphere is rarely available in the Northern. There is no commercial influenza vaccine available for pathogenic strains of avian influenza (H5N1, H7N2, H9N2, H7N3, H7N7). Since standard commercially available influenza vaccines include N1 and N2, it is biologically plausible that they might offer some protection against avian flu strains with these neuraminidases.

JAPANESE ENCEPHALITIS — Japanese encephalitis is an uncommon but potentially fatal mosquito-borne viral disease that occurs in rural Asia, especially near pig farms and rice paddies. It is usually seasonal (May-October), but may occur year-round in equatorial regions. The attack rate in travelers has been very low.[9] A vaccine is available in the US *(JE-Vax)* and should be considered for travelers >1 year old who expect a long stay (usually considered ≥4 weeks) in rural areas or heavy exposure to mosquitoes (such as adventure travelers).

Three doses are given over 2 to (preferably) 4 weeks. Local injection-site reactions, mild systemic adverse effects such as fever, headache and myalgias, and allergic reactions including urticaria and angioedema, can occur in up to 20% of patients. Whenever possible, the last dose should be given at least 10 days before departure due to the unpredictable allergic adverse effects. The duration of immunity is unknown; a booster can be given after 24 months.

MEASLES — Adults born after 1956 (1970 in Canada) who have not received 2 doses of live measles vaccine (not the killed vaccine that was commonly used in the 1960s) after their first birthday and do not have a physician-documented history of infection or laboratory evidence of immunity should receive a single dose of measles or measles-mumps-rubella (MMR) vaccine before traveling. Both are attenuated live-virus vaccines.

Children ≥12 months old should receive 2 doses of MMR vaccine at least 28 days apart before traveling outside the US. Children 6-11 months old should receive 1 dose before traveling, but will still need two subsequent doses for routine immunization, one at 12-15 months and one at 4-6 years.

MENINGOCOCCAL — Meningococcal vaccine is recommended for adults and children at least 2 years old who are traveling to areas where epidemics are occurring, or to the "meningitis belt" (semi-arid areas of sub-Saharan Africa extending from Senegal and Guinea eastward to Ethiopia) from December to June. Saudi Arabia requires a certificate of immunization for pilgrims during the Hajj. Immunization should also be considered for travelers to other areas who will have prolonged contact with the local population, such as those living in a dormitory or refugee camp, or working in a health care setting.[10,11]

Two quadrivalent vaccines are available against *Neisseria meningitidis* serogroups A, C, Y, and W135. *Menomune* contains meningococcal capsular polysaccharides. *Menactra* contains capsular polysaccharides conjugated to diphtheria toxoid.[12]

SOME IMMUNIZATIONS FOR TRAVEL

Vaccines	Adult Dose (Volume)	Pediatric Age
HEPATITIS A		
Havrix (GSK)	1440 EU IM (1 mL)	1-18 yrs
Vaqta (Merck)	50 U IM (1 mL)	1-18 yrs
HEPATITIS B		
Engerix-B (GSK)	20 mcg IM (1 mL)	Birth-19 yrs
Recombivax-HB (Merck)	10 mcg IM (1 mL)	Birth-19 yrs
HEPATITIS A/B		
Twinrix (GSK)	720 EU/20 mcg IM (1 mL)	Not approved for <18 yrs
JAPANESE ENCEPHALITIS		
JE-Vax (Sanofi Pasteur)	1 mL SC	1-3 yrs >3 yrs
MENINGOCOCCAL		
Menomune (Sanofi Pasteur)	50 mcg of each antigen SC (0.5 mL)	≥2 yrs
Menactra (Sanofi Pasteur)	4 mcg of each antigen IM (0.5 mL) (18-55 yrs)	11-17 yrs
RABIES		
Imovax (Sanofi Pasteur)	≥2.5 IU of rabies antigen IM (1 mL)	Birth
RabAvert (Chiron)	≥2.5 IU of rabies antigen IM (1 mL)	Birth

Pediatric Dose (Volume)	Standard Primary Schedule	Duration of Protection
720 EU IM (0.5 mL) 25 U IM (0.5 mL)	0 and 6-12 mos 0 and 6-18 mos	Probably lifelong after completion of primary series[1]
10 mcg IM (0.5 mL) 5 mcg IM (0.5 mL)	0, 1 and 6 mos 0, 1 and 6 mos	Probably lifelong after completion of primary series
—	0, 1 and 6 mos	Probably lifelong after completion of primary series
0.5 mL SC 1 mL SC	0, 7 and 14 or (preferably) 30 days	Not established; a single booster is usually given after 24 months if ongoing risk
50 mcg of each antigen SC (0.5 mL)	Single dose	Repeat every 5 yrs if ongoing risk
4 mcg of each antigen IM (0.5 mL)	Single dose	No data. Likely longer than *Menomune*
≥2.5 IU of rabies antigen IM (1 mL)	0, 7 and 21 or 28 days[2]	Routine boosters not necessary; for those engaging in frequent high-risk activities (cavers, veterinarians, laboratory workers), serologic testing is recommended every 2 yrs with booster doses if low levels[3]
≥2.5 IU of rabies antigen IM (1 mL)	0, 7 and 21 or 28 days[2]	

Continued on next page.

SOME IMMUNIZATIONS FOR TRAVEL (continued)

Vaccines	Adult Dose (Volume)	Pediatric Age
TYPHOID		
Typhim Vi (Sanofi Pasteur)	25 mcg IM (0.5 mL)	≥2 yrs
Vivotif Berna (Berna Products)	1 cap PO (contains 2-6x10⁹ viable CFU of *S. typhi* Ty21a)	≥6 yrs
YELLOW FEVER		
YF-Vax (Sanofi Pasteur)	4.74 log₁₀ plaque forming units of 17D204 attenuated YF virus SC (0.5 mL)	≥9 mos

1. Protection likely lasts at least 12 months after a single dose.
2. Regimen for pre-exposure prophylaxis. If a previously vaccinated traveler is exposed to a potentially rabid animal, post-exposure prophylaxis with 2 additional vaccine doses separated by 3 days should be initiated as soon as possible.

The most common adverse reactions to *Menactra* have been headache, fatigue and malaise, in addition to pain, redness and induration at the site of injection. The rates of these reactions are higher than with *Menomune*, but similar to those with tetanus toxoid. Eight cases of Guillian-Barre syndrome have been reported in adolescents who received *Menactra*, but cause and effect have not been established.[13]

POLIO — Adults who have not previously been immunized against polio should receive a primary series of inactivated polio vaccine (IPV) if traveling to areas where polio is endemic (Nigeria, India, Pakistan, Afghanistan) or to areas with documented outbreaks. Previously unimmunized children should also receive a primary series of IPV. If protection is needed within 4 weeks, a single dose of IPV is recommended, but

Pediatric Dose (Volume)	Standard Primary Schedule	Duration of Protection
25 mcg IM (0.5 mL)	Single dose	Repeat every 2 yrs if ongoing risk
1 cap PO (contains 2-6x10^9 viable CFU of *S. typhi* Ty21a)	1 cap every other day x 4 doses	Repeat every 5 yrs if ongoing risk
4.74 $\log_{10}$ plaque forming units of 17D204 attenuated YF virus SC (0.5 mL)	Single dose	Booster dose every 10 yrs if ongoing risk

3. Antibody levels below complete virus neutralization at a 1:5 serum dilution by the rapid fluorescent focus inhibition test.

provides only partial protection. Adult travelers to risk areas who have previously completed a primary series and have never had a booster should receive a booster dose of IPV.

RABIES — Rabies is highly endemic in Africa, Asia (particularly India) and parts of Latin America, but the risk to travelers is low. Pre-exposure immunization against rabies is recommended for travelers with an occupational risk of exposure, for those planning extended stays in endemic areas where immediate access to medical care might be limited, especially children, and for outdoor-adventure travelers.[14,15] The 2 vaccines available in the US *(Imovax, RabAvert)* are both given in the deltoid (not gluteal) muscle at 0, 7 and 21 or 28 days.

After a bite or skin-penetrating scratch from a potentially rabid animal, patients who received pre-exposure prophylaxis should promptly receive 2 additional doses of vaccine at days 0 and 3. The CDC has published a list of cell culture rabies vaccines available outside the US.[16] Without pre-exposure immunization, treatment requires rabies immune globulin (RIG) and 5 doses (over 28 days) of an approved vaccine. Most rabies vaccines available globally are safe and effective. RIG is a blood product and its purity and potency may be less reliable in developing countries.

TETANUS, DIPHTHERIA AND PERTUSSIS (DTaP) — Children should receive 3 or (preferably) 4 doses of DTaP prior to travel. An accelerated schedule can be used beginning at age 6 weeks, with the second and third doses given 4 weeks after the previous dose.

A single dose of one of two new combination vaccines, *Adacel* and *Boostrix*, that include tetanus toxoid, diphtheria toxoid and acellular pertussis antigens (Tdap), is now recommended as a replacement for a routine tetanus-diphtheria (Td) booster in adolescents 11-18 years old (*Adacel* or *Boostrix*) and in adults 19-64 years old *(Adacel)*, but is not specifically indicated for travelers.[17]

TICK-BORNE ENCEPHALITIS (TBE) — TBE occurs in Scandinavia, western and central Europe and countries of the former USSR, mainly in rural forested areas.[18] Risk is greatest from March to November. Humans acquire the disease through the bite of a tick or, rarely, from eating unpasteurized dairy (mostly goat) products. Immunization is recommended only for travelers who will spend extensive time outdoors in rural areas. The vaccine, which is not approved in the US, is usually given in 3 doses over 9-12 months, but can be given over as few as 2 or 3 weeks, and is available in Europe (*Encepur* – Chiron; *FSME-Immun Inject* – Baxter AG). It can be obtained in Canada through the Emergency Drug Release Program by contacting the Special Access Programme, Health Protection Branch (613-941-2108).

TYPHOID — Typhoid vaccine is recommended for travelers to the Indian Subcontinent and other developing countries in Central and South America, the Caribbean, Africa and Asia, especially if they will be visiting friends or relatives or traveling outside routine tourist destinations.[19,20] A purified capsular polysaccharide parenteral vaccine *(Typhim Vi)* for adults and children ≥2 years old is given as a single IM dose at least 2 weeks before departure. Re-vaccination is recommended every 2 years (3 years in Canada).

A live-attenuated oral vaccine *(Vivotif Berna)* is available for adults and children ≥6 years old. It is taken every other day as a single capsule (at least 1 hour before eating) for a total of 4 capsules, beginning no later than 2 weeks before departure; it protects for about 5 years. The capsules must be refrigerated. Antibiotics should be avoided from the day before the first capsule until 7 days after the last.

YELLOW FEVER — Yellow fever vaccine *(YF-Vax)*, a single-dose attenuated live virus vaccine prepared in eggs, should be given at least 10 days before travel to endemic areas, which include much of tropical South America and sub-Saharan Africa between 15°N and 15°S.[21] Some countries in Africa require an International Certificate of Vaccination (or physician's waiver letter) against yellow fever from all entering travelers; other countries in Africa, South America and Asia require evidence of vaccination from travelers coming from or traveling through endemic or infected areas. The vaccine is available in the US only from providers certified by state health departments.[22] Boosters are given every 10 years, but immunity probably lasts much longer. If other live vaccines (measles, MMR) are not administered simultaneously with yellow fever vaccine, administration should be separated by one month to avoid a diminished immune response to the vaccines.

Yellow fever vaccine is contraindicated in travelers who are immunocompromised or have egg allergy. Yellow fever vaccine-associated viscerotropic disease, a severe systemic illness that can cause fatal organ failure, has been reported rarely. It has occurred only in first-time recipients, especially those with thymus disorders. Vaccine-associated encephalitis has also occurred, primarily in infants; for this reason the vaccine should be avoided if possible in infants <9 months old and it is contraindicated in infants <6 months old. Travelers >60 years of age have a greater risk of systemic adverse effects.

TRAVELERS' DIARRHEA

The most common cause of travelers' diarrhea, usually a self-limited illness lasting several days, is infection with noninvasive enterotoxigenic (ETEC) or enteroaggregative (EAEC) strains of *Escherichia coli*. *Campylobacter*, *Shigella*, *Salmonella*, *Aeromonas*, viruses and parasites are less common. Children tend to have more severe illness and are particularly susceptible to dehydration. Travelers to areas where hygiene is poor should avoid raw vegetables, fruit they have not peeled themselves, unpasteurized dairy products, cooked food not served steaming hot, and tap water, including ice.

Treatment – For mild diarrhea, loperamide (*Imodium*, and others), an over-the-counter synthetic opioid (4-mg loading dose, then 2 mg orally after each loose stool to a maximum of 16 mg/d for adults), often relieves symptoms in <24 hours. It should not be used if fever or bloody diarrhea are present, and some patients complain of constipation after use. Loperamide is approved for use in children >2 years old.

If diarrhea is moderate to severe, persistent (>3 days) or associated with fever or bloody stools, self-treatment for 1-3 days with ciprofloxacin, levofloxacin, norfloxacin or ofloxacin is usually recommended.[23] Azithromycin is an alternative[24] and is the drug of choice for travelers to areas with a high prevalence of fluoroquinolone-resistant *Campylobacter*, such as Thailand and India.[25] It can also be used in pregnant women and children (10 mg/kg/d x 3d), and patients who do not respond to a fluoroquinolone in 48 hours.

SOME DRUGS FOR TREATMENT OF TRAVELERS' DIARRHEA

Drug	Dosage	Cost[1]
Azithromycin –	1000 mg once	$34.64
Zithromax (Pfizer)	or 500 mg once/d x 3d	51.96
Ciprofloxacin –	500 mg bid x 1-3d	
average generic		30.48
Cipro (Bayer)		35.28
sustained release		
Cipro XR	1000 mg once/d x1-3d	32.16
Levofloxacin –	500 mg once/d x 1-3d	34.65
Levaquin (Ortho-McNeil)		
Norfloxacin – Noroxin (Merck)	400 mg bid x 1-3d	22.56
Ofloxacin – Floxin (Ortho-McNeil)	300 mg bid x 1-3d	37.26
Rifaximin – Xifaxan (Salix)	200 mg tid x 3d	33.39

1. Cost for 3 days (except *Zithromax* 1000 mg), based on the most recent data (February 28, 2006) from retail pharmacies nationwide available from Wolters Kluwer Health.

A non-absorbed oral antibiotic derived from rifampin, rifaximin[26] is approved for treatment of travelers' diarrhea caused by noninvasive strains of *E. coli* in travelers ≥12 years of age. In clinical trials it has been similar in efficacy to ciprofloxacin, with fewer adverse effects.[27] It should not be used in infections associated with fever or blood in the stool or those caused by *Campylobacter jejuni*.

Packets of oral rehydration salts (*Ceralyte*, *ORS*, and others) mixed in potable water can help maintain electrolyte balance, particularly in children and the elderly. They are available from suppliers of travel-related products and some pharmacies in the US, and from pharmacies overseas.

Prophylaxis – Medical Letter consultants generally do not prescribe antibiotic prophylaxis for travelers' diarrhea, but rather instruct the patient to begin self-treatment when symptoms are distressing or persistent. Some travelers, however, such as immunocompromised patients, might benefit from prophylaxis. In such patients, ciprofloxacin 500 mg, levofloxacin 500 mg, ofloxacin 300 mg or norfloxacin 400 mg can be given once-daily during travel and for 2 days after return and are generally well tolerated.

In one 2-week study among travelers to Mexico, rifaximin (200 mg 1-3x/d) was effective in preventing travelers' diarrhea.[28] Bismuth subsalicylate (*Pepto-Bismol*, and others) can prevent diarrhea in travelers who take 2 tablets 4 times a day for the duration of travel, but it is less effective than antibiotics.

MALARIA

No drug is 100% effective for prevention of malaria; travelers should be told to take other protective measures against mosquito bites in addition to medication.[29] Countries with a risk of malaria are listed in the table. Some countries with endemic malaria transmission may not have malaria in the most frequently visited major cities and rural tourist resorts. Insect bite prevention is an important adjunct to malaria prophylaxis. Travelers to malarious areas should be reminded to seek medical attention if they have fever either during their trip or up to a year (especially during the first 2 months) after they return.

CHLOROQUINE-SENSITIVE MALARIA — Chloroquine is the drug of choice for prevention of malaria in the few areas that still have chloroquine-sensitive malaria (see Table: Countries with a risk of malaria, footnotes 4, 5, and 6).

CHLOROQUINE-RESISTANT MALARIA — Three drugs of choice with similar efficacy, listed with their dosages in the table on page 354, are available in the US for prevention of chloroquine-resistant malaria.

COUNTRIES WITH A RISK OF MALARIA[1]

AFRICA

Angola	Democratic	Kenya	São Tomé
Benin	Republic of the	Liberia	and Príncipe
Botswana	Congo	Madagascar	Senegal
Burkina Faso	Djibouti	Malawi	Sierra Leone
Burundi	Equatorial	Mali	Somalia
Cameroon	Guinea	Mauritania	South Africa[3]
Cape Verde[2]	Eritrea[3]	Mauritius[3]	Sudan
Central African	Ethiopia[3]	Mayotte	Swaziland
Republic	Gabon	Mozambique	Tanzania
Chad	Gambia, The	Namibia	Togo
Comoros	Ghana	Niger	Uganda
Congo	Guinea	Nigeria	Zambia
Côte d'Ivoire	Guinea-Bissau	Rwanda	Zimbabwe[3]

AMERICAS

Argentina[3,4]	Dominican	Guyana	Paraguay[3,4]
Belize[3,4]	Republic[3,4]	Haiti[4]	Peru[3]
Bolivia[3]	Ecuador[3]	Honduras[3,4]	Suriname[3]
Brazil	El Salvador[3,4]	Mexico[3,4]	Venezuela[3]
Colombia[3]	French Guiana	Nicaragua[3,4]	
Costa Rica[3,4]	Guatemala[3,4]	Panama[3,5]	

ASIA

Afghanistan	Georgia[3,4]	Malaysia[3]	Thailand[3]
Armenia[3,4]	India	Myanmar[3]	Turkey[3,4]
Azerbaijan[3,4]	Indonesia[3]	Nepal[3]	Turkmenistan[3,4]
Bangladesh[3]	Iran[3]	Pakistan	Uzbekistan[4]
Bhutan[3]	Iraq[3,4]	Philippines[3]	Vietnam[3]
Cambodia[3]	Korea, North[3,4]	Saudi Arabia[3]	Yemen[3]
China, People's	Korea, South[3,4]	Sri Lanka	
Republic[3,6]	Kyrgystan[3]	Syria[3,4]	
East Timor	Laos[3]	Tajikistan	

OCEANIA

Papua New	Solomon Islands	Vanuatu
Guinea		

1. Only includes countries for which prophylaxis is recommended. Regional variation in risk may exist within a country. More detailed information is available at www.cdc.gov/malaria and by phone for medical personnel from the Malaria Branch of the CDC at 770-488-7788.
2. Island of Saõ Tiago only (limited risk).
3. No malaria in major urban areas.
4. Chloroquine is the drug of choice for prophylaxis.
5. Chloroquine is recommended west of the Canal Zone.
6. Chloroquine is recommended except in Hainan and Yunnan provinces.

DRUGS OF CHOICE FOR PREVENTION OF MALARIA

Drug	Adult dosage
CHLOROQUINE-RESISTANT AREAS[†]: **Drug of Choice[1]:**	
Atovaquone/proguanil[2] – *Malarone, Malarone Pediatric*	1 adult tablet once/d[3]
OR Mefloquine[4] – *Lariam,* and others	1 tablet once/wk[5]
OR Doxycycline – *Vibramycin,* and others	100 mg once/d
Alternative[8]: Primaquine phosphate[9,10]	30 mg base daily[11]
CHLOROQUINE-SENSITIVE AREAS[†]: **Drug of Choice[1]:**	
Chloroquine phosphate[12] *Aralen,* and others	300 mg base[13] once/wk

† Chloroquine-resistant *Plasmodium falciparum* occurs in all malarious areas except Central America (excluding Panama east of the Canal Zone), Mexico, Haiti, the Dominican Republic, Paraguay, northern Argentina, North and South Korea, Georgia, Armenia, most of rural China and some countries in the Middle East (chloroquine resistance has been reported in Yemen, Oman, Saudi Arabia and Iran).

1. For prevention of relapse after departure ("presumptive anti-relapse therapy"; "terminal prophylaxis") from areas where *P. vivax* and *P. ovale* are endemic, some experts prescribe in addition primaquine phosphate 30 mg base/d or, for children, 0.5 mg base/kg/d for 14 days after departure from the malarious area. Others prefer to rely on surveillance to detect cases when they occur, particularly when exposure was limited or doubtful. See also footnote 10.

2. There have been several isolated reports of *P. falciparum* resistance in Africa (E Schwartz et al, Clin Infect Dis 2003; 37:450; A Farnert et al, BMJ 2003; 326:628).

3. Available as a fixed-dose combination: adult tablets (*Malarone;* 250 mg atovaquone/100 mg proguanil) and pediatric tablets (*Malarone Pediatric;* 62.5 mg atovaquone/25 mg proguanil). To enhance absorption, it should be taken with food or a milky drink.

4. Resistance to mefloquine is a significant problem in the malarious areas of Thailand and in the areas of Myanmar and Cambodia that border on Thailand.

Pediatric dosage	Duration
11-20 kg: 1 peds tab/d[3] 21-30 kg: 2 peds tabs/d[3] 31-40 kg: 3 peds tabs/d[3] ≥41 kg: 1 adult tab/d[3]	Start: 1-2d before travel Stop: 1 wk after leaving malarious zone
≤9 kg: 4.6 mg/kg base (5 mg/kg salt) once/wk[5,6] 10-19 kg: ¼ tablet once/wk[5,6] 20-30 kg: ½ tablet once/wk[5,6] 31-45 kg: ¾ tablet once/wk[5,6] >46 kg: 1 tablet once/wk[5,6]	Start: 1-2 wks before travel Stop: 4 wks after leaving malarious zone
2 mg/kg/d[7] (up to 100 mg/d)	Start: 1-2d before travel Stop: 4 wks after leaving malarious zone
0.5 mg/kg base/d[11]	Start: 1d before travel Stop: 7d after leaving malarious zone
5 mg/kg base (8.3 mg/kg salt) once/wk[13] (up to 300 mg base/wk)	Start: 1-2 wks before travel Stop: 4 wks after leaving malarious zone

5. In the US, a 250-mg tablet of mefloquine contains 228 mg mefloquine base. Outside the US, each 275-mg tablet contains 250 mg base.
6. For pediatric doses <1/2 tablet, it may be advisable to have a pharmacist crush the tablet, estimate doses by weighing, and package them in gelatin casules.
7. Not recommended for children <8 years old.
8. The combination of weekly chloroquine (300 mg base) and daily proquanil (200 mg) is recommended by the World Health Organization (www.WHO.int) for use in selected areas. The combination is no longer recommended by the CDC. Proguanil (*Paludrine* – Wyeth Ayerst, Canada; AstraZeneca, United Kingdom) is not available alone in the US but is widely available in Canada and Europe. Prophylaxis is recommended during exposure and for 4 weeks afterwards.
9. Not approved for this indication by the FDA, but recommended for use by the CDC.
10. Patients should be screened for G-6-PD deficiency before treatment.
11. In the US, a 26.3 mg tablet of primaquine phosphate contains 15 mg primaquine base. Nausea and abdominal pain can be diminished by taking with food.
12. Atovaquone/proquanil, mefloquine, doxycycline or primaquine may be used in patients who are unable to take chloroquine.
13. In the US, a 500-mg tablet of chloroquine phosphate contains 300 mg chloroquine base.

A fixed-dose combination of **atovaquone and proguanil**, *Malarone,* taken once daily, is generally the best tolerated drug,[30] but it can cause headache, GI disturbances and mouth ulcers. Single case reports of Stevens-Johnson syndrome and hepatitis have been published.[31,32] Atovaquone/proguanil should not be given to patients with severe renal impairment (CrCl <30 mL/min).

Mefloquine (*Lariam*, and others) has the advantage of once-a-week dosing, but is contraindicated in patients with a history of any psychiatric disorder, and also in those with a history of seizures or cardiac conduction abnormalities. Dizziness, headache, insomnia and disturbing dreams are the most common CNS adverse effects. The drug's adverse effects in children are similar to those in adults.[33] If a patient develops psychological or behavioral abnormalities such as depression, restlessness or confusion while taking mefloquine, another drug should be substituted. Mefloquine should not be given together with quinine, quinidine or halofantrine due to potential prolongation of the QT interval; caution is required when using these drugs to treat patients who have taken mefloquine prophylaxis.

Doxycycline (*Vibramycin*, and others), which frequently causes GI disturbances and can cause photosensitivity and vaginitis, offers an inexpensive once-daily alternative. Doxycycline should not be taken concurrently with antacids, oral iron or bismuth salts.

A fourth drug, **primaquine phosphate**, is available for patients unable to take other antimalarial drugs. Several studies have shown that daily primaquine can provide effective prophylaxis against chloroquine-resistant *Plasmodium falciparum* and *P. vivax*.[34] Primaquine can cause hemolytic anemia in patients with glucose-6-phosphate dehydrogenase (G-6-PD) deficiency, which is most common in African, Asian, and Mediterranean peoples. Travelers should be screened for G-6-PD deficiency before treatment with the drug. Primaquine should be taken with food to reduce GI effects.

MEFLOQUINE-RESISTANT MALARIA — Doxycycline or ato-vaquone/proguanil are recommended for prophylaxis against meflo-quine-resistant malaria, which occurs in the malarious areas of Thailand and in the areas of Myanmar and Cambodia that border on Thailand.

PREGNANCY — Malaria in pregnancy is particularly serious for both mother and fetus; prophylaxis is indicated if travel cannot be avoided. The safety of atovaquone/proguanil in pregnancy is unknown; outcomes were normal in 24 women treated with the combination in the second and third trimester.[35] Proguanil has been used in pregnancy without evidence of toxicity. Mefloquine is not approved for use during pregnancy. It has, however, been reported to be safe for prophylactic use during the second or third trimester of pregnancy and possibly during early pregnancy as well.[36,37] Chloroquine has been used extensively and safely for prophylaxis during pregnancy. Doxycycline and primaquine are contraindicated in pregnancy.

INSECT BITE PROTECTION

To minimize insect bites, travelers should wear light-colored, long-sleeved shirts, pants, socks and covered shoes. They should sleep in air conditioned or screened areas and use insecticide-impregnated bed nets. Mosquitoes that transmit malaria are most active between dusk and dawn; those that transmit dengue fever bite during the day, particularly during early morning and late afternoon.

DEET — The most effective topical insect repellent is N, N-diethyl-m-toluamide (DEET).[38,39] Applied on exposed skin, DEET repels mosquitoes, as well as ticks, chiggers, fleas, gnats and some flies. DEET is available in formulations of 5-40% and 100%. Medical Letter consultants prefer concentrations of 30-35%; higher concentrations protect longer but do not improve efficacy. A long-acting DEET formulation originally developed for the US Armed Forces (US Army Extended

Duration Topical Insect and Arthropod Repellent – EDTIAR) containing 25-33% DEET *(Ultrathon)* can protect for 6-12 hours. A microencapsulated sustained-release formulation containing 20% DEET *(Sawyer Controlled Release)* is also available and can provide longer protection than similar concentrations of other DEET formulations.

According to the CDC, DEET in concentrations of up to 50% is probably safe in children and infants >2 months old; the American Academy of Pediatrics recommends use of concentrations containing no more than 30%. DEET should not be used in infants <2 months old. One study found that applying DEET regularly during the second and third trimesters of pregnancy did not result in any adverse effects on the fetus.[40] DEET has been shown to decrease the effectiveness of sunscreens when it is applied after the sunscreen. Applying a sunscreen before or after a DEET-containing insect repellent did not reduce the effectiveness of the insect repellent.[41]

PICARIDIN — Picaridin has been available in Europe and Australia for many years. No data are available concerning the 7% and 15% formulations *(Cutter Advanced)* currently sold in the US.[42] They might be as effective against mosquitoes as low concentrations of DEET, providing protection for 1-4 hours. Higher concentrations sold in Europe have been shown to protect against mosquitoes for up to 8 hours.[43-45]

PERMETHRIN — An insecticide available in liquid and spray form, permethrin *(Duranon, Permanone,* and others) can be used on clothing, mosquito nets, tents and sleeping bags for protection against mosquitoes and ticks. After application to clothing, it remains active for several weeks through multiple launderings. Using permethrin-impregnated mosquito nets while sleeping is helpful when rooms are not screened or air-conditioned. If bednets or tents are immersed in the liquid, the effect can last for about 6 months. In combination with use of DEET on exposed skin, permethrin on clothing provides increased protection.

SOME OTHER INFECTIONS

DENGUE — Dengue fever is a viral disease transmitted by mosquito bites that occurs worldwide in tropical and subtropical areas, including cities.[46] Epidemics have occurred in recent years in the Indian Subcontinent, Southeast Asia, sub-Saharan Africa, the South Pacific and Australia, Central and South America and the Caribbean. It has also been reported in travelers from the US vacationing at popular tourist destinations in Hawaii, Puerto Rico, the US Virgin Islands and Mexico.[47] Prevention of mosquito bites during the day, particularly in early morning and late afternoon, is the primary way to protect against dengue fever; no vaccine is currently available.

LEPTOSPIROSIS — Leptospirosis, a bacterial disease that occurs in many domestic and wild animals, is endemic worldwide, but the highest incidence is in tropical and subtropical areas. Transmission to humans usually occurs through contact with water or damp soil contaminated by the urine of infected animals.[48] Travelers at increased risk, such as adventure travelers and those who engage in recreational water activities, should consider chemoprophylaxis with doxycycline 200 mg orally once a week, beginning 1-2 days before and continuing throughout the period of exposure. No human vaccine is available in the US.

RESPIRATORY INFECTIONS — After febrile and GI illness, respiratory infection is the most common infectious disease affecting travelers.[49] In the winter of 2003 a new coronavirus caused severe acute respiratory syndrome (SARS) and disrupted travel to much of Southeast Asia and Canada. Although cases of SARS have not been seen since April 2004, the CDC recommends that travelers to China avoid visiting live animal markets.

Currently, outbreaks of avian influenza in poultry merit monitoring. To date avian influenza has been spread to humans primarily from direct contact with sick birds or their feces. The CDC recommends that travelers to countries with documented outbreaks of avian influenza avoid live poultry markets, farms, and contact with sick or dead poultry and surfaces that appear to be contaminated with poultry feces, and only eat poultry products that are well cooked.[50] Travelers should wash their hands frequently with soap and water or use an alcohol-based hand rub. The CDC does not recommend traveling with a supply of antiviral drugs.

NON-INFECTIOUS RISKS OF TRAVEL

Many non-infectious risks are associated with travel. Injuries, particularly **traffic accidents** and **drowning**, which account for the majority of travel-related deaths, and **sunburn** occur in many travelers.

HIGH ALTITUDE ILLNESS — Rapid exposure to altitudes >8,000 feet (2500 meters) can cause acute mountain sickness (headache, fatigue, nausea, anorexia, insomnia, dizziness); pulmonary and cerebral edema are uncommon.[51] Sleeping altitude appears to be especially important in determining whether symptoms develop. The most effective preventive measure is pre-acclimatization by a 2- to 4-day stay at intermediate altitude (6000-8000 feet) and gradual ascent to higher elevations.

Acetazolamide, a carbonic anhydrase inhibitor, taken in a dosage of 125-250 mg b.i.d. (or 500 mg daily with the slow-release formulation *Diamox Sequels*) beginning 1-2 days before ascent and continuing at high altitude for 48 hours or longer, decreases the incidence and severity of acute mountain sickness.[52] The recommended dose for children is 5 mg/kg/d in 2 or 3 divided doses. Although acetazolamide, a sulfone, has little cross-reactivity with sulfa drugs, hypersensitivity reactions to acetazolamide are more likely to occur in those who have had severe (life-threatening) allergic reactions to sulfa drugs.[53]

Symptoms can be treated after they occur by descent to a lower altitude or by giving supplemental oxygen, especially during sleep. When descent is impossible, dexamethasone (*Decadron*, and others) 4 mg q6h, acetazolamide 250-500 mg q12h, or the two together, may help.

VENOUS THROMBOEMBOLISM — Prolonged immobilization, particularly during air travel, increases the risk of lower extremity deep vein thrombosis (DVT). Travelers with risk factors for thrombosis (past history of thrombosis, obesity, malignancy, increased platelets) are at even higher risk. Nevertheless, flight-related symptomatic pulmonary embolism is rare.[54]

To minimize the risk, travelers should be advised to walk around or, if necessary, exercise while sitting by flexing/extending ankles and knees, to drink extra fluids and to avoid alcohol and caffeine. Compression stockings can decrease the risk of asymptomatic DVT.[55] Giving a single dose of a low-molecular-weight heparin as prophylaxis to travelers at high risk reduced the incidence of DVT in a clinical trial.[56]

JET LAG — Disturbance of body and environmental rhythms resulting from a rapid change in time zones gives rise to jet lag, which is characterized by insomnia, decreased quality of sleep, loss of concentration, and irritability. It is usually more severe after eastward travel.

A variety of interventions have been tried, but none is proven to be effective. Shifting daily activities to correspond to the time zone of the destination country before arrival along with taking short naps, remaining well hydrated, avoiding alcohol and pursuing activities in sunlight on arrival, may help. The dietary supplement melatonin (2-3 mg started on the first night of travel and continued for 1-5 days after arrival) has been reported to facilitate the shift of the sleep-wake cycle and decrease symptoms in some patients. Slow-release forms of melatonin were not effective.[57,58] As a dietary supplement in the US, however, its purity and potency are suspect. In one study, zolpidem *(Ambien)* started the first night after travel and taken for 3 nights was helpful.[59]

MOTION SICKNESS — Therapeutic options for motion sickness remain limited.[60] The prescription cholinergic blocker scopolamine in a patch or oral formulation can decrease symptoms. *Transderm Scop* is applied to the skin behind the ear 6-8 hours before exposure and changed every 3 days. The oral 8-hour tablet *(Scopace)* is taken 1 hour before exposure. Oral promethazine *(Phenergan*, and others) is a highly sedating alternative. Over-the-counter drugs such as dimenhydrinate *(Dramamine*, and others) or meclizine *(Bonine*, and others) are less effective, but may be helpful for milder symptoms.

1. R Steffen. Changing travel-related global epidemiology of hepatitis A. Am J Med 2005; 118 suppl 10A:46S.
2. P Van Damme et al. Hepatitis A booster vaccination: is there a need? Lancet 2003; 362:1065.
3. S Iwarson et al. Excellent booster response 4 to 8 years after a single primary dose of an inactivated hepatitis A vaccine. J Travel Med 2004; 11:120.
4. S Iwarson. Are we giving too many doses of hepatitis A and B vaccines? Vaccine 2002; 20:2017.
5. BA Connor. Hepatitis A vaccine in the last-minute traveler. Am J Med 2005; 118 Suppl 10A:58S.
6. JS Keystone. Travel-related hepatitis B: risk factors and prevention using an accelerated vaccination schedule. Am J Med 2005; 118 suppl 10A:63S.
7. JN Zuckerman et al. Hepatitis A and B booster recommendations: implications for travelers. Clin Infect Dis 2005; 41:1020.
8. DO Freedman and K Leder. Influenza: changing approaches to prevention and treatment in travelers. J Travel Med 2005; 12:36.
9. Centers for Disease Control and Prevention (CDC). Japanese encephalitis in a U.S. traveler returning from Thailand, 2004. MMWR Morb Mortal Wkly Rep 2005; 54:123.
10. A Wilder-Smith. Meningococcal disease in international travel: vaccine strategies. J Travel Med 2005; 12 Suppl 1:S22.
11. OO Bilukha and N Rosenstein; National Center for Infectious Diseases, Centers for Disease Control and Prevention (CDC). Prevention and control of meningococcal disease. Recommendations of the Advisory Committee on Immunization Practices (ACIP). MMWR Recomm Rep 2005; 54 (RR-7):1.
12. Menactra: a meningococcal conjugate vaccine. Med Lett Drugs Ther 2005; 47:29.
13. Center for Disease Control and Prevention (CDC). Update: Guillain-Barre syndrome among recipients of Menactra meningococcal conjugate vaccine — United States, October 2005-February 2006. MMWR Morb Mortal Wkly Rep 2006; 55:364.
14. CE Rupprecht and RV Gibbons. Clinical practice. Prophylaxis against rabies. N Engl J Med 2004; 351:2626.
15. FX Meslin. Rabies as a traveler's risk, especially in high-endemicity areas. J Travel Med 2005; 12 Suppl 1:S30.

16. Human rabies prevention—United States, 1999 Recommendations of the Advisory Committee on Immunization Practices (ACIP). MMWR Recomm Rep 1999; 48 (RR-1):1.

17. Adacel and Boostrix: Tdap vaccines for adolescents and adults. Med Lett Drugs Ther 2006; 48:5.

18. P Rendi-Wagner. Risk and prevention of tick-borne encephalitis in travelers. J Travel Med 2004; 11:307.

19. B Basnyat et al. Enteric (typhoid) fever in travelers. Clin Infect Dis 2005; 41:1467.

20. C Luxemburger and AK Dutta. Overlapping epidemiologies of hepatitis A and typhoid fever: the needs of the traveler. J Travel Med 2005; 12 Suppl 1:S12.

21. TP Monath and MS Cetron. Prevention of yellow fever in persons traveling to the tropics. Clin Infect Dis 2002; 34:1369.

22. Directory available at: www2.ncid.cdc.gov/travel/yellowfever

23. HL Dupont. Travellers' diarrhoea: contemporary approaches to therapy and prevention. Drugs 2006; 66:303.

24. JA Adachi et al. Azithromycin found to be comparable to levofloxacin for the treatment of US travelers with acute diarrhea acquired in Mexico. Clin Infect Dis 2003; 37:1165.

25. D Jain et al. Campylobacter species and drug resistance in a north Indian rural community. Trans R Soc Trop Med Hyg 2005; 99:207.

26. Rifaximin (Xifaxan) for travelers' diarrhea. Med Lett Drugs Ther 2004; 46:74.

27. AL Pakyz. Rifaximin: a new treatment for travelers' diarrhea. Ann Pharmacother 2005; 39:284.

28. HL Dupont et al. A randomized, double-blind, placebo-controlled trial of rifaximin to prevent travelers' diarrhea. Ann Intern Med 2005; 142:805.

29. LH Chen and JS Keystone. New strategies for the prevention of malaria in travelers. Infect Dis Clin North Am 2005; 19:185.

30. P Schlagenhauf et al. Tolerability of malaria chemoprophylaxis in non-immune travellers to sub-Saharan Africa: multicentre, randomised, double blind, four arm study. BMJ 2003; 327:1078.

31. M Emberger et al. Stevens-Johnson syndrome associated with Malarone antimalarial prophylaxis. Clin Infect Dis 2003; 37:e5.

32. M Grieshaber et al. Acute hepatitis and atovaquone/proguanil. J Travel Med 2005; 12:289.

33. TA Albright et al. Side effects of and compliance with malaria prophylaxis in children. J Travel Med 2002; 9:289.

34. JK Baird et al. Primaquine for prevention of malaria in travelers. Clin Infect Dis 2003; 37:1659.

35. R McGready et al. The pharmacokinetics of atovaquone and proguanil in pregnant women with acute falciparum malaria. Eur J Clin Pharmacol 2003; 59:545.

36. CDC. Health Information for International Travel 2005-2006, p 205.

37. BL Smoak et al. The effects of inadvertent exposure of mefloquine chemoprophylaxis on pregnancy outcomes and infants of US Army servicewomen. J Infect Dis 1997; 176:831.

38. Insect repellents. Med Lett Drugs Ther 2003; 45:41.

39. MS Fradin and JF Day. Comparative efficacy of insect repellents against mosquito bites. N Engl J Med 2002; 347:13.

40. R McGready et al. Safety of the insect repellent N,N-diethyl-M-toluamide (DEET) in pregnancy. Am J Trop Med Hyg 2001; 65:285.
41. ME Murphy et al. The effect of sunscreen on the efficacy of insect repellent: a clinical trial. J Am Acad Dermatol 2000; 43:219.
42. Picardin—a new insect repellent. Med Lett Drugs Ther 2005; 47:46.
43. A Badolo et al. Evaluation of the sensitivity of Aedes aegypti and Anopheles gambiae complex mosquitoes to two insect repellents: DEET and KBR 3023. Trop Med Int Health 2004; 9:330.
44. SP Frances et al. Laboratory and field evaluation of commercial repellent formulations against mosquitoes (diptera: culcidae) in Queensland, Australia. Aust J Entomol 2005; 44:431.
45. C Constantini et al. Field evaluation of the efficacy and persistence of insect repellents DEET, IR3535, and KBR 3023 against Anopheles gambiae complex and other Afrotropical vector mosquitoes. Trans R Soc Trop Med Hyg 2004; 98:644.
46. A Wilder-Smith and E Schwartz. Dengue in travelers. N Engl J Med 2005; 353:924.
47. Center for Disease Control and Prevention (CDC). Travel-associated dengue infections—United States, 2001-2004. MMWR Morb Mortal Wkly Rep 2005; 54: 556.
48. AJ McBride et al. Leptospirosis. Curr Opin Infect Dis 2005; 18:376.
49. DO Freedman et al. Spectrum of disease and relation to place of exposure among ill returned travelers. N Engl J Med 2006; 354:119.
50. http://www.cdc.gov/travel/other/avian_influenza_se_asia_2005.htm.
51. SA Gallagher and PM Hackett. High-altitude illness. Emerg Med Clin North Am 2004; 22:329.
52. B Basnyat et al. Acetazolamide 125 mg BD is not significantly different from 375 mg BD in the prevention of acute mountain sickness: The Prophylactic Acetazolamide Dosage Comparison for Efficacy (PACE) Trial. High Alt Med Biol 2006; 7:17.
53. BL Strom et al. Absence of cross-reactivity between sulfonamide antibiotics and sulfonamide nonantibiotics. N Engl J Med 2003; 349:1628.
54. MT Ansari et al. Traveler's thrombosis: a systematic review. J Travel Med 2005; 12:142.
55. E Ferrari and G Morgan. Travel as a risk factor for venous thromboembolic disease. Eur J Med Res 2004; 9:146.
56. MR Cesarone et al. Venous thrombosis from air travel: the LON-FLIT3 study–prevention with aspirin vs low-molecular-weight heparin (LMWH) in high-risk subjects: a randomized trial. Angiology 2002; 53:1.
57. A Herxheimer and KJ Petrie. Melatonin for the prevention and treatment of jet lag. Cochrane Database Syst Rev 2002; 2:CD001520.
58. N Buscemi et al. Efficacy and safety of exogenous melatonin for secondary sleep disorders and sleep disorders accompanying sleep restriction: meta-analysis. BMJ 2006; 332:385.
59. AD Jamieson et al. Zolpidem reduces the sleep disturbance of jet lag. Sleep Med 2001; 2:423.
60. JF Golding and MA Gresty. Motion sickness. Curr Opin Neurol 2005; 18:29.

PRINCIPAL ADVERSE EFFECTS OF ANTIMICROBIAL DRUGS

Adverse effects of antimicrobial drugs vary with dosage, duration of administration, concomitant therapy, renal and hepatic function, immune competence, and the age of the patient. The principal adverse effects of antimicrobial agents are listed in the following table. The designation of adverse effects as "frequent," "occasional" or "rare" is based on published reports and on the experience of Medical Letter consultants. Information about adverse interactions between drugs, including probable mechanisms and recommendations for clinical management, are available in The Medical Letter Adverse Drug Interactions Program.

ABACAVIR (*Ziagen*)
Frequent: hypersensitivity reaction with fever, GI or respiratory symptoms and rash
Occasional: arthralgias; anemia; lactic acidosis
Rare: anaphylaxis; pancreatitis; hyperglycemia

ABACAVIR-LAMIVUDINE (*Epzicom*) — See individual drugs

ACYCLOVIR (*Zovirax*, others)
Frequent: local irritation at infusion site
Occasional: local reactions with topical use; rash, nausea, diarrhea, headache, vertigo and arthralgias with oral use; decreased renal function sometimes progressing to renal failure; metabolic encephalopathy; bone marrow depression; abnormal hepatic function in immunocompromised patients
Rare: lethargy or agitation; tremor, disorientation; hallucinations; transient hemiparesthesia

ADEFOVIR (*Hepsera*)
Frequent: asthenia; headache; abdominal pain
Occasional: exacerbation of hepatitis B with drug discontinuation
Rare: increased serum creatinine; renal tubular dysfunction with high doses (>60 mg/d)

ALBENDAZOLE (*Albenza*)
Occasional: abdominal pain; increased aminotransferases; reversible alopecia
Rare: leukopenia; rash; renal toxicity

AMANTADINE (*Symmetrel*, others)
Frequent: livedo reticularis and ankle edema; insomnia; dizziness; lethargy
Occasional: depression; psychosis; confusion; slurred speech; visual disturbance; sudden loss of vision; increased seizures in epilepsy; congestive heart failure; orthostatic hypotension; urinary retention; GI disturbance; rash
Rare: seizures; leukopenia; neutropenia; eczematoid dermatitis; photosensitivity; oculogyric episodes;

AMIKACIN (*Amikin*)
Occasional: vestibular damage; renal damage; fever; rash
Rare: auditory damage; CNS reactions; blurred vision; neuromuscular blockade and apnea, may be reversible with calcium salts; paresthesias; hypotension; nausea; vomiting

AMINOSALICYLIC ACID (*Paser*)
Frequent: GI disturbance
Occasional: allergic reactions; liver damage; renal irritation; hematologic abnormalities; thyroid enlargement; malabsorption syndrome

Principal Adverse Effects of Antimicrobial Drugs

Rare: acidosis; hypokalemia; encephalopathy; vasculitis; hypoglycemia in diabetics

AMOXICILLIN — See Penicillins

AMOXICILLIN/CLAVULANIC ACID — See Penicillins

AMPHOTERICIN B DEOXYCHOLATE (*Fungizone*, others)
Frequent: renal damage; hypokalemia; thrombophlebitis at site of peripheral vein infusion; anorexia; nausea; weight loss; bone marrow suppression with reversible decline in hematocrit; headache; chills, fever, vomiting during infusion, possibly with delirium, hypotension or hypertension, wheezing, and hypoxemia, especially in cardiac or pulmonary disease
Occasional: hypomagnesemia; normocytic, normochromic anemia
Rare: hemorrhagic gastroenteritis; rash; blurred vision peripheral neuropathy; seizures; anaphylaxis; arrhythmias; acute liver failure; reversible nephrogenic diabetes insipidus; hearing loss; acute pulmonary edema; spinal cord damage with intrathecal use

AMPHOTERICIN B LIPID FORMULATIONS (*Ambisone, Abelcet, Amphotec*) — See page 156.

AMPICILLIN — See Penicillins

AMPICILLIN/SULBACTAM — See Penicillins

AMPRENAVIR (*Agenerase*)
Frequent: GI disturbance; oral and perioral paresthesias; rash; hypersensitivity with fever
Occasional: hyperglycemia; increased aminotransferases; hyperlipidemia; abnormal fat distribution
Rare: severe rash including Stevens-Johnson syndrome; hemolytic anemia

ANIDULAFUNGIN (*Eraxis*)
Occasional: Infusion-related rash; urticaria; flushing; pruritus; dyspnea and hypotension; fever; nausea; vomiting; hypokalemia
Rare: hepatitis

ARTEMETHER (*Artenam*)
Occasional: neurological toxicity; (possible increase in length of coma in cerebral malaria, seizures); QTc prolongation

ARTESUNATE
Occasional: neurological toxicity; ataxia; slurred speech; possible increase in length of coma in cerebral malaria; seizures; QTc prolongation

ATAZANAVIR (*Reyataz*)
Frequent: hyperbilirubinemia; nausea; rash
Occasional: increased cholesterol and triglycerides; depression; headache; dizziness; fatigue; fever
Rare: insomnia; peripheral neuropathy; PR prolongation; heart block; angioedema; alopecia; Stevens-Johnson syndrome; gout; myasthenia; hepatitis; pancreatitis; diabetes

ATOVAQUONE (*Mepron, Malarone* [with *proguanil*])
Frequent: rash; nausea
Occasional: diarrhea; increased aminotransferases; cholestasis

AZITHROMYCIN (*Zithromax*)
Occasional: nausea; diarrhea; abdominal pain; headache; dizziness; vaginitis
Rare: angioedema; cholestatic jaundice; photosensitivity; reversible dose-related hearing loss; QTc prolongation

AZT — See Zidovudine

AZTREONAM (*Azactam*)
Occasional: local reaction at injection site; rash; diarrhea; nausea; vomiting; increased aminotransferases
Rare: thrombocytopenia

BACITRACIN — many manufacturers
Frequent: nephrotoxicity; GI disturbance
Occasional: rash; hematologic abnormalities
Rare: anaphylaxis

BENZNIDAZOLE (Rochagan)
Frequent: rash; dose-dependent polyneuropathy; GI disturbance; psychic disturbances

BITHIONOL (Bitin)
Frequent: photosensitivity reactions; vomiting; diarrhea; abdominal pain; urticaria
Rare: leukopenia; hepatitis

CAPREOMYCIN (Capastat)
Occasional: renal damage; eighth nerve damage; hypokalemia and other electrolyte abnormalities; pain, induration, excessive bleeding, and sterile abscess at injection site
Rare: allergic reactions; leukocytosis, leukopenia; neuromuscular blockade and apnea with large IV doses, reversed by neostigmine

CARBENICILLIN — See Penicillins

CASPOFUNGIN (Cancidas)
Occasional: fever; rash; increased aminotransferases; GI disturbance; facial flushing
Rare: anaphylaxis

CEPHALOSPORINS
(cefaclor - Ceclor; cefadroxil - Duricef, others; cefazolin - Ancef, others; cefdinir - Omnicef; cefditoren pivoxil - Spectracef; cefepime - Maxipime; cefixime - Suprax; cefoperazone - Cefobid; cefotaxime - Claforan; cefotetan; cefoxitin - Mefoxin; cefpodoxime - Vantin; cefprozil - Cefzil; ceftazidime - Fortaz, Tazidime, Tazicef, Ceptaz; ceftibuten - Cedax; ceftizoxime - Cefizox; ceftriaxone - Rocephin; cefuroxime - Kefurox, Zinacef; cefuroxime axetil - Ceftin; cephalexin - Keflex, others; cephapirin -

Cefadyl, others; cephradine - Velosef, others; loracarbef - Lorabid
Frequent: thrombophlebitis with IV use; serum-sickness-like reaction with prolonged parenteral administration; moderate to severe diarrhea, especially with cefoperazone and cefixime
Occasional: allergic reactions, rarely anaphylactic; pain at injection site; GI disturbance; hypoprothrombinemia,hemorrhage with cefamandole, cefoperazone or cefotetan; rash and arthritis ("serum-sickness") with cefaclor or cefprozil, especially in children; cholelithiasis with ceftriaxone; vaginal candidiasis (especially with cefdinir); carnitine deficiency with prolonged use of cefditoren
Rare: hemolytic anemia; blood dyscrasias; hepatic dysfunction; renal damage; acute interstitial nephritis; CDAD; seizures; toxic epidermal necrolysis

CHLORAMPHENICOL (Chloromycetin, others)
Occasional: hematologic abnormalities; gray syndrome (cardiovascular collapse); GI disturbance
Rare: fatal aplastic anemia, even with eye drops or ointment; allergic and febrile reactions; peripheral neuropathy; optic neuritis and other CNS injury; pseudomembranous colitis

CHLOROQUINE HCL and **CHLOROQUINE PHOSPHATE** (Aralen, others)
Occasional: pruritus; vomiting; headache; confusion; depigmentation of hair; partial alopecia; skin eruptions; corneal opacity; weight loss; extraocular muscle palsies; exacerbation of psoriasis, eczema, and other exfoliative dermatoses; myalgias; photophobia; QTC prolongation
Rare: irreversible retinal injury (especially when total dosage exceeds 100 grams); discoloration of nails and mucus membranes; nerve-type deafness; peripheral neuropathy and myopathy; heart block; torsades de pointes; hematologic abnor-

malities; hematemesis; seizures; neuropsychiatric changes

CIDOFOVIR *(Vistide)*
Frequent: nephrotoxicity; ocular hypotony; neutropenia
Occasional: metabolic acidosis; uveitis; Fanconi syndrome

CIPROFLOXACIN *(Cipro, others)* — See Fluoroquinolones

CLARITHROMYCIN *(Biaxin, others)*
Occasional: nausea; diarrhea; abdominal pain; abnormal taste; headache; dizziness; QTc prolongation
Rare: reversible dose-related hearing loss; pseudomembranous colitis; pancreatitis; torsades de pointes

CLINDAMYCIN *(Cleocin, others)*
Frequent: diarrhea; allergic reactions
Occasional: CDAD, sometimes severe, can occur even with topical use
Rare: hematologic abnormalities; esophageal ulceration; hepatotoxicity

CLOFAZIMINE *(Lamprene)*
Frequent: ichthyosis; pigmentation of skin, cornea and retina; urine discoloration; dryness and irritation of eyes; GI disturbance
Occasional: headache; retinal degeneration
Rare: splenic infarction, bowel obstruction, and GI bleeding with high doses

CLOXACILLIN — See Penicillins

COLISTIMETHATE — See Polymyxins

CROTAMITON *(Eurax)*
Occasional: rash

CYCLOSERINE *(Seromycin, others)*
Frequent: anxiety; depression; confusion; disorientation; paranoia; hallucinations; somnolence; headache
Occasional: peripheral neuropathy; liver damage; malabsorption syndrome; folate deficiency
Rare: suicide; seizures; coma

DAPSONE
Frequent: rash; headache; GI irritation; anorexia; infectious mononucleosis-like syndrome
Occasional: cyanosis due to methemoglobinemia and sulfhemoglobinemia; other hematologic abnormalities, including hemolytic anemia; nephrotic syndrome; liver damage; peripheral neuropathy; hypersensitivity reactions; increased risk of lepra reactions; insomnia; irritability; uncoordinated speech; agitation; acute psychosis
Rare: renal papillary necrosis; severe hypoalbuminemia; epidermal necrolysis; optic atrophy; agranulocytosis; neonatal hyperbilirubinemia after use in pregnancy

DAPTOMYCIN *(Cubicin)*
Occasional: GI disturbances; rash; injection site reaction; fever; headache; insomnia; dizziness
Rare: increased CPK and rhabdomyolysis; eosinophilia

DARUNAVIR *(Prezista)*
Frequent: diarrhea; nausea
Occasional: headache; increased aminotransferases; increased cholesterol and triglycerides; rash
Rare: Stevens-Johnson syndrome

DELAVIRDINE *(Rescriptor)* — Similar to nevirapine, but rash may be less severe and hepatotoxicity is less common

DEMECLOCYCLINE — See Tetracyclines

DICLOXACILLIN — See Penicillins

DIDANOSINE (ddI; *Videx*)
Frequent: peripheral neuropathy; diarrhea; nausea; vomiting; abdominal pain
Occasional: pancreatitis; hyperuricemia; increased aminotransferases; constipation;

loss of taste; hypokalemia; headache;
fever; rash; lactic acidosis; retinal
depigmentation
Rare: hepatic failure; retinal atrophy in
children

DIETHYLCARBAMAZINE CITRATE
(Hetrazan)
Frequent: severe allergic or febrile reac-
tions in patients with microfilaria in the
blood or the skin; GI disturbance
Rare: encephalopathy

DILOXANIDE FUROATE *(Furamide)*
Frequent: flatulence
Occasional: nausea; vomiting; diarrhea
Rare: diplopia; dizziness; urticaria;
pruritus

DORIPENEM *(Doribax)—* Similar to
imipenem, but may be less likely to cause
seizures

DOXYCYCLINE — See Tetracyclines

EFAVIRENZ *(Sustiva)*
Frequent: dizziness; headache; inability
to concentrate; insomnia and somnolence;
rash
Occasional: vivid dreams; nightmares;
hallucinations; hypersensitivity reaction
with fever, GI or respiratory symptoms
and rash; Stevens-Johnson syndrome in
children; increased cholesterol and
triglycerides
Rare: pancreatitis; peripheral neuropathy;
psychiatric symptoms; photosensitivity
reactions; gynecomastia

EFAVIRENZ-EMTRICITABINE-
TENOFOVIR *(Atripla)* — See individual
drugs.

EFLORNITHINE
(Difluoromethylornithine, DFMO, *Ornidyl)*
Frequent: anemia; leukopenia
Occasional: diarrhea; thrombocytopenia;
seizures
Rare: hearing loss

EMTRICITABINE (FTC, *Emtriva)*
Frequent: headache; dizziness; insomnia;
weakness; rash; GI disburbance; increased
CPK
Occasional: dream disturbances; increased
triglycerides; hyperpigmentation of palms
and soles; lactic acidosis; hepatomegaly
with fatty liver; exacerbation of hepatitis B
with drug discontinuation

EMTRICITABINE-TENOFOVIR
(Truvada) — See individual drugs.

ENFUVIRTIDE *(Fuzeon)*
Frequent: injection site reactions; insomnia; depression; increased triglycerides;
neuropathy
Occasional: rash; eosinophilia
Rare: hypersensitivity reactions; increased
bacterial pneumonias

ENTECAVIR *(Baraclude)*
Occasional: headache; fatigue; nausea;
dizziness; exacerbation of hepatitis B with
drug discontinuation

ERTAPENEM *(Invanz)*
Occasional: phlebitis; nausea; vomiting;
diarrhea
Rare: seizures

ERYTHROMYCIN (*Ery-Tab*, others)
Frequent: GI disturbance
Occasional: stomatitis; cholestatic hepatitis especially with erythromycin estolate
in adults; QTc prolongation
Rare: allergic reactions, including severe
respiratory distress; pseudomembranous
colitis; hemolytic anemia; hepatitic pancreatitis; transient hearing loss with high
doses, prolonged use, or in patients with
renal insufficiency; ventricular arrhythmias and torsades de pointes; aggravation of myasthenia gravis; hypothermia; hypertrophic pyloric stenosis following treatment of infants

ETHAMBUTOL *(Myambutol)*
Occasional: optic neuritis; allergic reac-

Principal Adverse Effects of Antimicrobial Drugs

tions; GI disturbance; mental confusion; precipitation of acute gout
Rare: peripheral neuritis; possible renal damage; thrombocytopenia; toxic epidermal necrolysis; lichenoid skin eruption

ETHIONAMIDE (*Trecator-SC*)
Frequent: GI disturbance
Occasional: liver damage; CNS disturbance, including peripheral neuropathy; allergic reactions; gynecomastia; depression; myalgias; hypotension
Rare: hypothyroidism; optic neuritis; arthritis; impotence

FAMCICLOVIR (*Famvir*)
Occasional: headache; nausea; diarrhea

FLUCONAZOLE (*Diflucan*)
Occasional: nausea; vomiting; diarrhea; abdominal pain; increased aminotransferases; headache; rash;
Rare: severe hepatic toxicity; exfoliative dermatitis; anaphylaxis; Stevens-Johnson syndrome; toxic epidermal necrolysis; hair loss

FLUCYTOSINE (*Ancobon*)
Frequent: blood dyscrasias, including pancytopenia and fatal agranulocytosis; GI disturbance, including severe diarrhea and ulcerative colitis; hepatic dysfunction; rash
Occasional: confusion; hallucinations
Rare: anaphylaxis

FLUOROQUINOLONES
(ciprofloxacin – *Cipro*, others; gemifloxacin *(Factive)* ; levofloxacin – *Levaquin*; lomefloxacin – *Maxaquin*; moxifloxacin – *Avelox*; norfloxacin – *Noroxin*; ofloxacin – *Floxin*)
Occasional: nausea; vomiting; diarrhea; abdominal pain; dizziness; headache; tremors; restlessness; confusion; rash; Candida infections of the pharynx and vagina; eosinophilia; neutropenia; leukopenia; increased hepatic enzymes; hyper- and hypoglycemia; increased serum creatinine concentration; insomnia; photosensitivity reactions, especially with

lomefloxacin; QTc prolongation
Rare: hallucinations; delirium; psychosis; vertigo; seizures; paresthesias; blurred vision and photophobia; severe hepatitis; hyper- and hypoglycemia; pseudomembranous colitis; interstitial nephritis; vasculitis; possible exacerbation of myasthenia gravis; serum-sickness-like reaction; anaphylaxis; toxic epidermal necrolysis; anemia; tendinitis or tendon rupture; ventricular tachycardia and torsades de pointes; rhabdomyolysis with ofloxacin

FOSAMPRENAVIR (*Lexiva*)
Frequent: headache; fatigue; rash; GI disturbance
Occasional: depression; increased triglycerides; increased lipase and aminotransferases; perioral numbness or tingling
Rare: neutropenia; Stevens-Johnson syndrome

FOSCARNET (*Foscavir*)
Frequent: renal dysfunction; anemia; nausea; disturbances of Ca, P, Mg, and K metabolism
Occasional: headache; vomiting; fatigue; genital ulceration; seizures; neuropathy
Rare: Nephrogenic diabetes insipidus; cardiac arrhythmias; hypertension

FOSFOMYCIN (*Monurol*)
Frequent: diarrhea
Occasional: vaginitis

FURAZOLIDONE (*Furoxone*)
Frequent: nausea; vomiting
Occasional: allergic reactions, including pulmonary infiltrates; hypotension; urticaria; fever; vesicular rash; hypoglycemia; headache
Rare: hemolytic anemia in G-6-PD deficiency and neonates; disulfiram-like reaction with alcohol; MAO-inhibitor interactions; polyneuritis

GANCICLOVIR (*Cytovene*)
Frequent: neutropenia; thrombocytopenia
Occasional: anemia; fever; rash; abnormal

liver function; neurological toxicity; phlebitis
Rare: hypertension; cardiac arrhythmias; nausea; vomiting; abdominal pain; diarrhea; eosinophilia; hypoglycemia; alopecia; pruritus; urticaria; renal toxicity; psychiatric disturbances; seizures

GEMIFLOXACIN — See Fluoroquinolones

GENTAMICIN
Occasional: vestibular damage; renal damage; rash
Rare: auditory damage; neuromuscular blockade and apnea, reversible with calcium or neostigmine; neurotoxicity; polyneuropathy; anaphylaxis

GRISEOFULVIN *(Fulvicin-U/F, others)*
Occasional: GI disturbance; allergic and photosensitivity reactions
Rare: proteinuria; hematologic abnormalities; confusion; paresthesias; exacerbation of lupus; fixed-drug eruption; reversible liver damage; lymphadenopathy; exacerbation of leprosy

HALOFANTRINE *(Halfan)*
Occasional: diarrhea; abdominal pain; pruritus; QTc and PR prolongation
Rare: cardiac arrhythmias and torsades de pointes

IMIPENEM-CILASTATIN *(Primaxin)*
Occasional: phlebitis; pain at injection-site; fever; urticaria; rash; pruritus; diarrhea; nausea, vomiting and transient hypotension during intravenous infusion
Rare: seizures

IMIQUIMOD *(Aldara)*
Frequent: local erythema; erosion; excoriation; itching; burning and pain

INDINAVIR *(Crixivan)*
Frequent: hyperbilirubinemia; dysuria; kidney stones; flank pain; hematuria; crystalluria

Occasional: pyuria; interstitial nephritis; hemolytic anemia; increased aminotransferases; GI disturbance; reflux esophagitis; glucose intolerance; hyperlipidemia; abnormal fat distribution; increased bleeding in hemophiliacs; paronychia; alopecia; dry skin and mucous membranes
Rare: rash; hyperprolactinemia; cholelithiasis

INTERFERON ALFA *(Alferon N, Infergen, Intron A, Roferon-A, Rebetron with ribavirin; Pegylated interferon alfa 2b-Peg-Intron)*
Frequent: Transient flu-like syndrome; fatigue; anorexia; nausea; diarrhea; increased aminotransferases; rash; dry skin or pruritus; bone marrow suppression; depression; anxiety; insomnia
Occasional: Paresthesias; alopecia; diaphoresis; reactivation of herpes labialis; hypo- and hyperthyroidism; tinnitus; activation of autoimmune diseases, including diabetes
Rare: Visual disturbance and retinopathy; hypertension; cardiac arrhythmias; renal failure; nephrotic syndrome; hearing loss; capillary leak syndrome with monoclonal gammopathy

IODOQUINOL *(Yodoxin, others)*
Occasional: rash; acne; slight enlargement of the thyroid gland; nausea; diarrhea; cramps; anal pruritus
Rare: optic neuritis, atrophy and loss of vision; peripheral neuropathy after prolonged use in high dosage (months); hypersensitivity reactions in patients with iodine sensitivity

ISONIAZID *(Nydrazid, others)*
Occasional: peripheral neuropathy; liver damage, may be chronic, progressive or fatal, risk increases with age; glossitis and GI disturbance; allergic reactions; fever
Rare: hematologic abnormalities; red cell aplasia; depression; agitation; auditory and visual hallucinations; paranoia; optic neuritis; hyperglycemia; folate and vitamin B_6

deficiency; pellagra-like rash; keratitis; lupus erythematosus-like syndrome; Stevens-Johnson syndrome

ITRACONAZOLE (*Sporanox*)
Occasional: nausea; epigastric pain; hepatic toxicity; headache; dizziness; edema; hypokalemia; rash
Rare: congestive heart failure

IVERMECTIN (*Stromectol*)
Occasional: Mazzotti-type reaction seen in onchocerciasis, including fever, pruritus, tender lymph nodes, headache, and joint and bone pain
Rare: hypotension; hepatitis

KANAMYCIN (*Kantrex*, others)
Occasional: eighth-nerve damage affecting mainly hearing that may be irreversible and may not be detected until after therapy has been stopped (more likely with renal impairment); renal damage
Rare: rash; fever; peripheral neuritis; parenteral or intraperitoneal administration may produce neuromuscular blockade and apnea, not reversed by neostigmine or calcium gluconate

KETOCONAZOLE (*Nizoral*, others)
Frequent: nausea; vomiting
Occasional: decreased testosterone synthesis; gynecomastia; oligospermia and impotence in men; rash; pruritus; dizziness; abdominal pain; hepatitis; constipation; diarrhea; fever and chills; photophobia; headache
Rare: hepatotoxicity and jaundice; increased aminotransferases or fatal hepatic necrosis; severe epigastric burning and pain; may interfere with adrenal function; anaphylaxis

LAMIVUDINE (3TC; *Epivir*)
Rare: headache; dizziness; nasal symptoms; rash; nausea; pancreatitis in children; neuropathy; lactic acidosis

LEVOFLOXACIN— See Fluoroquinolones

LINCOMYCIN (*Lincocin*, others)
Frequent: diarrhea
Occasional: CDAD; hypersensitivity reactions
Rare: hematologic abnormalities; hypotension with rapid IV injection; amphylaxis

LINEZOLID (*Zyvox*)
Frequent: GI disturbance; bone marrow suppression particularly thrombocytopenia, risk greater with treatment >10 days; increased aminotransferases
Rare: peripheral nerve and optic neuropathy; bradycardia

LOPINAVIR/RITONAVIR (*Kaletra*)
Similar to ritonavir, but adverse effects are less common; nephrotoxicity has not been reported
Rare: pancreatitis, may be fatal; bradyarrhythmia

LORACARBEF — See Cephalosporins

MALATHION (*Ovide*)
Occasional: local irritation

MARAVIROC (*Selzentry*)
Occasional: cough; pyrexia; upper respiratory tract infection; rash; musculoskeletal symptoms; abdominal pain; postural dizziness
Rare: hepatotoxicity; cardiovascular events

MEBENDAZOLE (*Vermox*)
Occasional: diarrhea; abdominal pain
Rare: leukopenia; agranulocytosis; hypospermia

MEFLOQUINE (*Lariam*)
Frequent: nausea, other GI disturbances; vertigo; lightheadedness; nightmares; visual disturbances; headache; insomnia
Occasional: confusion
Rare: psychosis; hypotension; convulsions; coma; paresthesias; pneumonitis

MEGLUMINE ANTIMONIATE
(*Glucantime*) — Similar to sodium stibogluconate

MELARSOPROL (Mel B)
  Frequent: myocardial damage; albuminuria; hypertension; colic; Herxheimer-type reaction; encephalopathy; vomiting; peripheral neuropathy
  Rare: shock

MEROPENEM (Merrem)— Similar to imipenem, but may be less likely to cause seizures

METHENAMINE MANDELATE
(*Mandelamine*, others) and
METHENAMINE HIPPURATE (*Hiprex, Urex*)
  Occasional: GI disturbance; dysuria; hypersensitivity reactions

METHICILLIN— See Penicillins

METRONIDAZOLE (*Flagyl*, others)
  Frequent: nausea; headache; anorexia; metallic taste
  Occasional: vomiting; diarrhea; dry mouth; stomatitis; insomnia; weakness; vertigo; tinnitus; paresthesias; rash; dark urine; urethral burning; disulfiram-like reaction with alcohol; candidiasis
  Rare: leukopenia; pancreatitis; seizures; peripheral neuropathy; encephalopathy; cerebellar syndrome with ataxia, dysarthria and MRI abnormalities

MICAFUNGIN (*Mycamine*)
  Occasional: fever; headache; GI disturbance; leukopenia; phlebitis at injection site; increased aminotransferases
  Rare: rash; pruritus; facial swelling; anaphylaxis; hemolysis

MICONAZOLE (*Monistat*)
  Occasional: intense, persistent pruritus; rash; local burning and irritation; abdominal cramps
  Rare: hypersensitivity reactions

MINOCYCLINE— See Tetracyclines

MOXIFLOXACIN— See Fluoroquinolones

NAFCILLIN— See Penicillins

NALIDIXIC ACID (*NegGram*, others)
  Frequent: GI disturbance; rash; visual disturbance
  Occasional: CNS disturbance; acute intracranial hypertension in young children and rarely in adults; photosensitivity reactions, sometimes persistent; seizures; hyperglycemia
  Rare: cholestatic jaundice; blood dyscrasias; fatal immune hemolytic anemia; arthralgia or arthritis; lupus-like syndrome; confusion; depression; excitement; visual hallucinations

NELFINAVIR (*Viracept*)
  Frequent: mild to moderate diarrhea
  Occasional: increased aminotransferases; rash; nausea; glucose intolerance; increased bleeding in hemophiliacs; hyperlipidemia; abnormal fat distribution

NEOMYCIN
  Occasional: eighth-nerve and renal damage, same as with kanamycin but hearing loss may be more frequent and severe and may occur with oral, intraarticular, irrigant, or topical use; GI disturbance; malabsorption with oral use; contact dermatitis with topical use
  Rare: neuromuscular blockade and apnea that may be reversed by intravenous neostigmine or calcium gluconate

NEVIRAPINE (*Viramune*)
  Frequent: rash, can progress to Stevens-Johnson syndrome
  Occasional: fever; nausea; headache; hepatotoxicity, which can be fatal; vivid dreams

NICLOSAMIDE (*Niclocide*)
  Occasional: nausea; abdominal pain

Principal Adverse Effects of Antimicrobial Drugs

NIFURTIMOX *(Lampit)*
Frequent: anorexia; vomiting; weight loss; loss of memory; sleep disorders; tremor; paresthesias; weakness; polyneuritis
Rare: convulsions; fever; pulmonary infiltrates and pleural effusion

NITAZOXANIDE *(Alinia)*
Occasional: GI disturbance; headache
Rare: yellow discoloration of sclera; hypersensitivity reactions; increased creatinine; dizziness; flatulence; malaise; salivary gland enlargement

NITROFURANTOIN *(Macrodantin*, others)
Frequent: GI disturbance; allergic reactions, including pulmonary infiltrates
Occasional: lupus-like syndrome; hematologic abnormalities; hemolytic anemia; peripheral neuropathy, sometimes severe; interstitial pneumonitis and pulmonary fibrosis
Rare: cholestatic jaundice; chronic active hepatitis, sometimes fatal; focal nodular hyperplasia of liver; pancreatitis; lactic acidosis; parotitis; trigeminal neuralgia; crystalluria; increased intracranial pressure; severe hemolytic anemia in G-6-PD deficiency

NORFLOXACIN— See Fluoroquinolones

NYSTATIN *(Mycostatin*, others)
Occasional: hypersensitivity reactions; fixed
drug eruption; GI disturbance

OFLOXACIN— See Fluoroquinolones

ORNIDAZOLE *(Tiberal)*
Occasional: dizziness; headache; GI disturbance
Rare: reversible peripheral neuropathy

OSELTAMIVIR PHOSPHATE *(TamiFlu)*
Occasional: nausea; vomiting; headache
Rare: neuropsychiatric events, including suicide, in children and adolescents

OXACILLIN— See Penicillins

OXAMNIQUINE *(Vansil)*
Occasional: fever; headache; dizziness; somnolence and insomnia; rash; nausea; diarrhea; increased aminotransferases; ECG changes; EEG changes; orange-red discoloration of urine
Rare: seizures; neuropsychiatric disturbances

OXYTETRACYCLINE — See Tetracyclines

PARA-AMINOSALICYLIC ACID — See Aminosalicylic acid

PAROMOMYCIN (aminosidine; *Humatin*)
Frequent: GI disturbance with oral use
Rare: eighth-nerve damage (mainly auditory) and renal damage when aminosidine is given IV; vertigo; pancreatitis

PENICILLINS
(amoxicillin – *Amoxil*, others; amoxicillin/clavulanic acid – *Augmentin*; ampicillin – *Principen*, others; ampicillin/sulbactam – *Unasyn*; carbenicillin indanyl – *Geocillin*; cloxacillin; dicloxacillin – *Dycill*, others; methicillin; mezlocillin – *Mezlin*; nafcillin – *Nafcil*, others; oxacillin; penicillin G; penicillin V; piperacillin – *Pipracil*; piperacillin/ tazobactam – *Zosyn*; ticarcillin – *Ticar*; ticarcillin/ clavulanic acid – *Timentin*)
Frequent: allergic reactions, rarely anaphylaxis, erythema multiforme or Stevens Johnson syndrome; rash (more common with ampicillin and amoxicillin than with other penicillins); diarrhea (most common with ampicillin and amoxicillin/clavulanic acid); nausea and vomiting with amoxicillin/clavulanic acid
Occasional: hemolytic anemia; neutropenia; platelet dysfunction with high doses of piperacillin, ticarcillin, nafcillin, or methicillin; cholestatic hepatitis with amoxicillin/clavulanic acid; CDAD (more

common with ampicillin)

Rare: hepatic damage with semisynthetic penicillins; granulocytopenia or agranulocytosis with semisynthetic penicillins; renal damage with semisynthetic penicillins and penicillin G; muscle irritability and seizures, usually after high doses in patients with impaired renal function; hyperkalemia and arrhythmias with IV potassium penicillin G given rapidly; bleeding diathesis; Henoch-Schönlein purpura with ampicillin; thrombocytopenia with methicillin and mezlocillin; terror, hallucinations, disorientation, agitation, bizarre behavior and neurological reactions with high doses of procaine penicillin G, oxacillin, or ticarcillin; hypokalemic alkalosis and/or sodium overload with high doses of ticarcillin or nafcillin; hemorrhagic cystitis with methicillin; GI bleeding with dicloxacillin; tissue damage with extravasation of nafcillin

PENTAMIDINE ISETHIONATE (*Pentam 300, NebuPent*, others)

Frequent: hypotension; hypoglycemia often followed by diabetes mellitus; vomiting; hematologic abnormalities; renal damage; pain at injection site; GI disturbance

Occasional: may aggravate diabetes; shock; hypocalcemia; liver damage; cardiotoxicity; delirium; rash; QTc prolongation

Rare: Herxheimer-type reaction; anaphylaxis; acute pancreatitis; hyperkalemia; torsades de pointes

PERMETHRIN (*Nix*, others)

Occasional: burning; stinging; numbness; increased pruritus; pain; edema; erythema; rash

PIPERACILLIN — See Penicillins

PIPERACILLIN/TAZOBACTAM — See Penicillins

POLYMYXINS

(colistimethate – *Coly-Mycin*, polymyxin B – generic)

Occasional: renal damage; peripheral neuropathy; thrombophlebitis at IV injection site with polymyxin B

Rare: allergic reactions; neuromuscular blockade and apnea with parenteral administration, not reversed by neostigmine but may be by IV calcium chloride

POSACONAZOLE (*Noxafil*)

Frequent: nausea; vomiting; diarrhea; abdominal pain; headache

Occasional: rash; dry skin; taste disturbance; dizziness; paresthesias; flushing; QTc prolongation

Rare: angioedema; anaphylaxis; toxic epidermal necrolysis; hemolytic uremic syndrome/thrombotic thrombocytopenic purpura; arrhythmias

PRAZIQUANTEL (*Biltricide*)

Frequent: abdominal pain; diarrhea; malaise; headache; dizziness

Occasional: sedation; fever; sweating; nausea; eosinophilia

Rare: pruritus; rash; edema; hiccups

PRIMAQUINE PHOSPHATE

Frequent: hemolytic anemia in G-6-PD deficiency

Occasional: neutropenia; GI disturbance; methemoglobinemia

Rare: CNS symptoms; hypertension; arrhythmias

PROGUANIL (*Paludrine; Malarone* [with atovaquone])

Occasional: oral ulceration; hair loss; scaling of palms and soles; urticaria

Rare: hematuria (with large doses); vomiting; abdominal pain; diarrhea (with large doses); thrombocytopenia

PYRANTEL PAMOATE (*Antiminth*, others)

Occasional: GI disturbance; headache; dizziness; rash; fever

Principal Adverse Effects of Antimicrobial Drugs

PYRAZINAMIDE
  Frequent: arthralgia; hyperuricemia
  Occasional: liver damage; GI disturbance; acute gouty arthritis; rash
  Rare: photosensitivity reactions; acute hypertension

PYRETHRINS with PIPERONYL BUTOXIDE (*RID*, others)
  Occasional: hypersensitivity reactions

PYRIMETHAMINE (*Daraprim*)
  Occasional: hematologic abnormalities; folic acid deficiency
  Rare: rash; vomiting; seizures; shock; possibly pulmonary eosinophilia; fatal cutaneous reactions with pyrimethamine-sulfadoxine (*Fansidar*)

QUINACRINE
  Frequent: disulfiram-like reaction with alcohol; nausea; vomiting; colors skin and urine yellow
  Occasional: headache; dizziness
  Rare: rash; fever; psychosis; extensive exfoliative dermatitis in patients with psoriasis

QUININE SULFATE — See Quinine dihydrochloride

QUININE DIHYDROCHLORIDE
  Frequent: cinchonism (tinnitus, headache, nausea, abdominal pain, visual disturbance)
  Occasional: deafness; hemolytic anemia and other hematologic abnormalities; photosensitivity reactions; hypoglycemia; arrhythmias; hypotension; fever
  Rare: blindness; sudden death if injected too rapidly; hypersensitivity reaction with TTP-HUS

QUINUPRISTIN/DALFOPRISTIN (*Synercid*)
  Frequent: local irritation and thrombophlebitis with peripheral IV administration; arthralgias; myalgias; increase in conjugated bilirubin

Occasional: nausea; rash; increased aminotransferases

RALTEGRAVIR (*Isentress*)
  Occasional: diarrhea; nausea; headache
  Rare: increases in serum creatine kinase; myopathy; rhabdomyolysis

RIBAVIRIN (*Copegus, Rebetol, Virazole, Rebetron* [with interferon alfa])
  Occasional: anemia; headache; depression; fatigue; abdominal cramps; nausea; elevation of bilirubin; teratogenic and embryolethal in animals and mutagenic in mammalian cells; rash; conjunctivitis; bronchospasm with aerosol use; hyperuricemia

RIFABUTIN (*Mycobutin*) — Similar to rifampin; also iritis, uveitis, leukopenia, arthralgia

RIFAMPIN (*Rifadin, Rimactane*)
  Frequent: colors urine, tears, saliva, CSF, contact lenses, and lens implants red-orange
  Occasional: liver damage; GI disturbance; hypersensitivity reactions
  Rare: flu-like syndrome, sometimes with thrombocytopenia, hemolytic anemia, shock, and renal failure, particularly with intermittent therapy; acute organic brain syndrome; acute adrenal crisis in patients with adrenal insufficiency; renal damage; severe proximal myopathy

RIFAMPIN-ISONIAZID (*Rifamate*) — See individual drugs

RIFAMPIN-ISONIAZID-PYRAZINAMIDE (*Rifater*) — See individual drugs

RIFAPENTINE (*Priftin*) — Similar to rifampin; higher rate of hyperuricemia

RIFAXIMIN (*Xifaxan*)
  Occasional: headache
  Rare: abnormal dreams; allergic dermatitis; hypersensitivity reactions; photosensitivity; motion sickness

Principal Adverse Effects of Antimicrobial Drugs

RIMANTADINE *(Flumadine)* — Similar to amantadine, but lower risk of CNS effects

RITONAVIR *(Norvir)*
  Frequent: nausea; diarrhea; vomiting; asthenia; elevated serum triglycerides, cholesterol
  Occasional: abdominal pain; anorexia; altered taste; dyspepsia; increased aminotransferases; cholestasis; glucose intolerance; abnormal fat distribution; circumoral and peripheral paresthesias; rash; increased bleeding in hemophiliacs
  Rare: nephrotoxicity; hyperprolactinemia

SAQUINAVIR *(Invirase; Fortovase)*
  Occasional: diarrhea; abdominal discomfort; nausea; glucose intolerance; hyperlipidemia; abnormal fat distribution; increased aminotransferases; increased bleeding in hemophiliacs
  Rare: rash; hyperprolactinemia

SODIUM STIBOGLUCONATE
(Pentostam)
  Frequent: muscle and joint pain; fatigue; nausea; increased aminotransferases; pancreatitis; T-wave flattening or inversion;
  Occasional: weakness; vomiting; abdominal pain; liver damage; bradycardia; leukopenia; thrombocytopenia; rash
  Rare: diarrhea; pruritus; myocardial damage; hemolytic anemia; renal damage; shock; sudden death

SPECTINOMYCIN *(Trobicin)*
  Occasional: soreness at injection site; urticaria; dizziness; insomnia; nausea; chills; fever; decreased urine output; hypersensitivity reactions

SPIRAMYCIN *(Rovamycine)*
  Occasional: GI disturbance
  Rare: hypersensitivity reactions

STAVUDINE (D4T; *Zerit)*
  Frequent: peripheral neuropathy
  Occasional: increased aminotransferases; lactic acidosis; loss of subcutaneous fat
  Rare: rash; pancreatitis

STREPTOMYCIN
  Frequent: eighth-nerve damage (mainly vestibular), sometimes permanent; paresthesias; rash; fever; eosinophilia
  Occasional: pruritus; anaphylaxis; renal damage
  Rare: hematologic abnormalities; neuromuscular blockade and apnea with parenteral administration, usually reversed by neostigmine; optic neuritis; hepatic necrosis; myocarditis; hemolytic anemia; renal failure; toxic erythema; Stevens-Johnson syndrome

SULFONAMIDES
  Frequent: hypersensitivity reactions (rash, photosensitivity, fever)
  Occasional: kernicterus in newborn; renal damage; liver damage; Stevens-Johnson syndrome (particularly with long-acting sulfonamides); hemolytic anemia; other hematologic abnormalities; vasculitis
  Rare: transient acute myopia; CDAD; reversible infertility in men with sulfasalazine; CNS toxicity with trimethoprim/sulfamethoxazole in patients with AIDS

SURAMIN SODIUM
  Frequent: vomiting; pruritus; urticaria; paresthesias; hyperesthesia of hands and feet; peripheral neuropathy; photophobia
  Occasional: kidney damage; hematologic abnormalities; shock; optic atrophy

TELITHROMYCIN *(Ketek)*
  Frequent: GI disturbance; headache; dizziness
  Occasional: visual disturbances including blurred vision, diplopia; difficulty focusing; rash
  Rare: serious hepatotoxicity; anaphylaxis; edema; muscle cramps; QTc prolongation; exacerbation of myasthenia gravis

TENOFOVIR *(Viread)*
  Occasional: diarrhea; nausea; vomiting; flatulence

Principal Adverse Effects of Antimicrobial Drugs

TERBINAFINE *(Lamisil)*
   Frequent: headache; GI disturbance
   Occasional: taste disturbance; increased aminotransferases; rash; pruritus; urticaria; toxic epidermal necrolysis; erythema multiforme
   Rare: hepatitis; anaphylaxis; pancytopenia; agranulocytosis; severe neutropenia; changes in ocular lens and retina; parotid swelling; congestive heart failure

TETRACYCLINES
(demeclocycline – *Declomycin*; doxycycline – *Vibramycin*, others; minocycline – *Minocin*, others; oxytetracycline – *Terramycin*, others; tetracycline hydrochloride – *Sumycin*, others)
   Frequent: GI disturbance; bone lesions and staining and deformity of teeth in children up to 8 years old, and in the newborn when given to pregnant women after the fourth month of pregnancy
   Occasional: malabsorption; enterocolitis; photosensitivity reactions (most frequent with demeclocycline); vestibular toxicity with minocycline; increased azotemia with renal insufficiency (except doxycycline, but exacerbation of renal failure with doxycycline has been reported); renal insufficiency with demeclocycline in cirrhotic patients; hepatitis; parenteral doses may cause serious liver damage, especially in pregnant women and patients with renal disease receiving ≥1 gram/day; esophageal ulcerations; cutaneous and mucosal hyperpigmentation; tooth discoloration in adults with minocycline
   Rare: hypersensitivity reactions, including serum sickness and anaphylaxis; CDAD; hemolytic anemia and other hematologic abnormalities; drug-induced lupus with minocycline; autoimmune hepatitis; increased intracranial pressure; fixed-drug eruptions; diabetes insipidus with demeclocycline; transient acute myopia; blurred vision, diplopia, papilledema; photoonycholysis and onycholysis; acute interstitial nephritis with

minocycline; aggravation of myasthenic symptoms with IV injection, reversed with calcium; possibly transient neuropathy

THIABENDAZOLE *(Mintezol)*
   Frequent: nausea; vomiting; vertigo; headache; drowsiness; pruritus
   Occasional: leukopenia; crystalluria; hallucinations and other psychiatric reactions; visual and olfactory disturbance; rash; erythema multiforme
   Rare: shock; tinnitus; intrahepatic cholestasis; seizures; angioneurotic edema; Stevens-Johnson syndrome

TICARCILLIN — See Penicillins

TICARCILLIN/CLAVULANIC ACID — See Penicillins

TIGECYCLINE *(Tygacil)* — See also Tetracyclines
   Frequent: nausea; vomiting; diarrhea; abdominal pain; permanent discoloration of teeth when given during tooth development (last half of pregnancy, infancy, and childhood to age 8 yrs)
   Occasional: photosensitivity; pseudotumor cerebri; pancreatitis; injection site reactions
   Rare: CDAD

TINIDAZOLE *(Tindamax)*
   Occasional: metallic taste; GI symptoms; rash
   Rare: weakness

TIPRANAVIR *(Aptivus)*/ **RITONAVIR** — See also Ritonavir
   Frequent: diarrhea; nausea; elevated serum triglycerides, cholesterol; increased aminotransferases
   Occasional: fatigue; vomiting; abdominal pain; dyspepsia; anorexia; hyperglycemia; rash; abnormal fat distribution; increased bleeding in hemophiliacs
   Rare: hepatitis and hepatic failure; nephrotoxicity

Principal Adverse Effects of Antimicrobial Drugs

TOBRAMYCIN (*Nebcin*, others) —
Similar to gentamicin
  Rare: delirium

TRIFLURIDINE (*Viroptic*)
  Occasional: burning or stinging; palpebral edema
  Rare: epithelial keratopathy; hypersensitivity reactions

TRIMETHOPRIM (*Proloprim*, others)
  Frequent: nausea, vomiting with high doses
  Occasional: megaloblastic anemia; thrombocytopenia; neutropenia; rash; fixed drug eruption
  Rare: pancytopenia; hyperkalemia

**TRIMETHOPRIM/SULFAMETHOXA-
ZOLE** (*Bactrim, Septra*, others)
  Frequent: rash; fever; nausea and vomiting
  Occasional: hemolysis in G-6-PD deficiency; acute megaloblastic anemia; granulocytopenia; thrombocytopenia; CDAD; kernicterus in newborn; hyperkalemia
  Rare: agranulocytosis; aplastic anemia; hepatotoxicity; pancreatitis; Stevens-Johnson syndrome; aseptic meningitis; fever; confusion; depression; hallucinations; intrahepatic cholestasis; methemoglobinemia; ataxia; CNS toxicity in patients with AIDS; deterioration in renal disease; renal tubular acidosis; hyperkalemia

VALACYCLOVIR (*Valtrex*) — Generally same as acyclovir
  Rare: thrombotic thrombocytopenic purpura/hemolytic uremic syndrome in severely immunocompromised patients treated with high doses

VALGANCICLOVIR (*Valcyte*) —
Generally same as ganciclovir

VANCOMYCIN (*Vancocin*, others)
  Frequent: thrombophlebitis; fever, chills
  Occasional: eighth-nerve damage (mainly hearing) especially with large or continued doses (> than 10 days), in presence of renal damage, and in the elderly; neutropenia; renal damage; hypersensitivity reactions; rash; "redman" syndrome
  Rare: peripheral neuropathy; hypotension with rapid IV administration; exfoliative dermatitis; thrombocytopenia

VORICONAZOLE (*Vfend*)
  Frequent: transient visual disturbances
  Occasional: rash; increased aminotransferases
  Rare: photosensitivity with prolonged use

ZALCITABINE (ddC; *Hivid*)
  Frequent: peripheral neuropathy
  Occasional: stomatitis; esophageal ulceration; nausea; abdominal pain; diarrhea; headache; fever; fatigue; rash
  Rare: pancreatitis; hypersensitivity reactions

ZANAMIVIR (*Relenza*)
  Occasional: nasal and throat discomfort; headache; cough; broncospasm in patients with asthma

ZIDOVUDINE (*Retrovir*)
  Frequent: anemia; granulocytopenia; nail pigment changes; nausea; fatigue
  Occasional: headache; insomnia; confusion; diarrhea; rash; fever; myalgias; myopathy; light-headedness; lactic acidosis
  Rare: seizures; Wernicke's encephalopathy; cholestatic hepatitis; transient ataxia and nystagmus with acute large overdosage

ZIDOVUDINE—LAMIVUDINE
(*Combivir*) — See individual drugs

**ZIDOVUDINE—LAMIVUDINE—
ABACAVIR** (*Trizivir*) — See individual drugs

SAFETY OF ANTIMICROBIAL DRUGS IN PREGNANCY

Drug	Toxicity in Pregnancy	Recommendation	FDA†
Abacavir (Ziagen)	Teratogenic in animals	Caution*	C
Acyclovir (Zovirax)	None known	Caution	B
Adefovir (Hepsera)	Embryotoxic in rats	Caution*	C
Albendazole (Albenza)	Teratogenic and embryotoxic in animals	Contraindicated	C
Amantadine (Symmetrel)	Teratogenic and embryotoxic in rats	Caution*; contraindicated in 1st trimester	C
Amikacin (Amikin)	Possible 8th-nerve toxicity in fetus	Caution*	D
Amoxicillin (Amoxil)	None known	Probably safe	B
Amoxicillin/ clavulanic acid (Augmentin)	None known	Probably safe	B
Ampicillin (Principen)	None known	Probably safe	B
Ampicillin/ sulbactam (Unasyn)	None known	Probably safe	B
Amphotericin B deoxycholate (Fungizone)	None known	Caution	B
Amphotericin B cholesteryl sulfate (Amphotec)	Unknown	Caution	B
Amphotericin B lipid complex (Abelcet)	Unknown	Caution	B

* Use only for strong clinical indication in the absence of suitable alternative.
N/A = FDA pregnancy category not available

Continued on next page.

Safety of Antimicrobial Drugs in Pregnancy

Drug	Toxicity in Pregnancy	Recommendation	FDA†
Liposomal Amphotericin B (*AmBisome*)	Higher rate of spontaneous abortion in rabbits	Caution*	B
Amprenavir (*Agenerase*)	Teratogenic in animals	Caution*; oral solution is contraindicated	C
Anidulafungin (*Eraxis*)	Skeletal abnormalities in rats; reduced fetal weight in rabbits	Caution*	C
Artemether/ lumefantrine (*Coartem, Riamet*)	Unknown	Contraindicated during 1st trimester; caution 2nd and 3rd trimesters*	N/A
Artesunate	Embryocidal and teratogenic in rats	Contraindicated during 1st trimester; caution 2nd and 3rd trimesters*	N/A
Atazanavir (*Reyataz*)	None known	Caution	B
Atovaquone (*Mepron*)	Maternal and fetal toxicity in animals	Caution*	C
Atovaquone/ proguanil (*Malarone*)	Maternal and fetal toxicity in animals	Caution*	C
Azithromycin (*Zithromax*)	None known	Probably safe	B
Aztreonam (*Azactam*)	None known	Probably safe	B
Benznidazole (*Rochagan*)	Unknown	Contraindicated	N/A
Capreomycin (*Capastat*)	Teratogenic in animals	Caution*	C
Carbenicillin indanyl (*Geocillin*)	None known	Probably safe	B
Caspofungin (*Cancidas*)	Embryotoxic in animals	Caution*	C

Continued on next page.

Drug	Toxicity in Pregnancy	Recommendation	FDA†
Cephalosporins[1]	None known	Probably safe	B
Chloramphenicol	Unknown – gray syndrome in newborn	Caution,* especially at term	C
Chloroquine (*Aralen*)	None known with doses recommended for malaria prophylaxis; embryotoxic and teratogenic in rats	Caution*	C
Cidofovir (*Vistide*)	Embryotoxic and teratogenic in rats and rabbits	Caution*	C
Ciprofloxacin (*Cipro*)	Arthropathy in immature animals; available data suggest teratogenic risk unlikely	Probably safe	C
Clarithromycin (*Biaxin*)	Teratogenic in animals	Contraindicated	C
Clindamycin (*Cleocin*)	None known	Caution	B
Cloxacillin	None known	Probably safe	B
Crotamiton (*Eurax*)	Unknown	Caution*	C
Cycloserine (*Seromycin*)	Unknown	Caution*	C
Dapsone	None known; carcinogenic in rats and mice; hemolytic reactions in neonates	Caution,* especially at term	C
Daptomycin (*Cubicin*)	None known	Caution	B
Darunavir (*Prezista*)	None known	Caution	B
Delavirdine (*Rescriptor*)	Teratogenic in rats	Caution*	C

* Use only for strong clinical indication in the absence of suitable alternative.
N/A = FDA pregnancy category not available
1. Cefaclor, cefadroxil (*Duricef*), cefazolin (*Ancef, others*), cefepime (*Maxipime*), cefdinir (*Omnicef*), cefditoren (*Spectracef*), cefixime (*Suprax*), cefoperazone (*Cefobid*), cefotaxime (*Claforan*), cefotetan (*Cefotan*), cefoxitin (*Mefoxin*), cefpodoxime (*Vantin*), cefprozil (*Cefzil*), ceftazadime (*Fortaz*), ceftibuten (*Cedax*), ceftizoxime (*Cefizox*), ceftriaxone (*Rocephin*), cefuroxime (*Zinacef*), cefuroxime axetil (*Ceftin*), cephalexin (*Keflex*), cephradine (*Velosef*), loracarbef (*Lorabid*). Experience with newer agents is limited.

Continued on next page.

Safety of Antimicrobial Drugs in Pregnancy

Drug	Toxicity in Pregnancy	Recommendation	FDA†
Demeclocycline (*Declomycin*)	Tooth discoloration and dysplasia, inhibition of bone growth in fetus; hepatic toxicity and azotemia with IV use in pregnant patients with decreased renal function or with overdosage	Contraindicated	D
Dicloxacillin (*Dycill*)	None known	Probably safe	B
Didanosine (ddI; *Videx*)	None known	Caution	B
Diloxanide (*Furamide*)	Safety not established	Caution*	N/A
Dirithromycin (*Dynabac*)	Retarded fetal development in rodents with high doses	Caution	B
Doripenem (*Doribax*)	Unknown	Caution	B
Doxycycline (*Vibramycin*)	Tooth discoloration and dysplasia, inhibition of bone growth in fetus; hepatic toxicity and azotemia with IV use in pregnant patients with decreased renal function or with overdosage	Contraindicated	D
Efavirenz (*Sustiva*)	Neural tube defects	Caution,* contraindicated in 1st trimester	D
Eflornithine (*Ornidyl*)	Embryocidal in animals	Contraindicated	C
Emtricitabine (*Emtriva*)	None known	Caution	B
Enfuvirtide (*Fuzeon*)	None known	Caution	B
Enoxacin (*Penetrex*)	Arthropathy in immature animals	Caution*	C
Entecavir (*Baraclude*)	Skeletal abnormalities in rats at very large doses	Caution	C

Continued on next page.

Safety of Antimicrobial Drugs in Pregnancy

Drug	Toxicity in Pregnancy	Recommendation	FDA†
Ertapenem (*Invanz*)	Decreased total weight in animals	Caution	B
Erythromycin estolate	Risk of cholestatic hepatitis appears to be increased in pregnant women	Contraindicated	B
Erythromycin (*Ery-Tab*)	None known; neonatal use has been associated with pyloric stenosis	Probably safe	B
Ethambutol (*Myambutol*)	Teratogenic in animals	Caution*	C
Ethionamide (*Trecator-SC*)	Teratogenic in animals	Caution*	C
Famciclovir (*Famvir*)	Carcinogenic in animals	Caution	B
Fluconazole (*Diflucan*)	Teratogenic	Contraindicated for high-dose; caution* for single dose	C
Flucytosine (*Ancobon*)	Teratogenic in rats	Contraindicated	C
Fosamprenavir (*Lexiva*)	Increased rate of abortion and skeletal abnormalities in rabbits	Caution*	C
Foscarnet (*Foscavir*)	Animal toxicity	Caution*	C
Fosfomycin (*Monurol*)	Fetal toxicity in rabbits with maternally toxic doses	Caution	B
Ganciclovir (*Cytovene*; *Vitrasert*)	Teratogenic and embryotoxic in animals	Caution*	C
Gemifloxacin (*Factive*)	Arthropathy in immature animals	Caution*	C
Gentamicin	Possible 8th-nerve toxicity in fetus	Caution*	C
Griseofulvin (*Fulvicin U/F*)	Embryotoxic and teratogenic in animals; carcinogenic in rodents	Contraindicated	C

* Use only for strong clinical indication in the absence of suitable alternative.
N/A = FDA pregnancy category not available

Continued on next page.

Safety of Antimicrobial Drugs in Pregnancy

Drug	Toxicity in Pregnancy	Recommendation	FDA†
Hydroxychloro-quine (*Plaquenil*)	None known with doses recommended for malaria prophylaxis	Caution*	C
Imipenem-cilastatin (*Primaxin*)	Toxic in some pregnant animals	Caution*	C
Indinavir (*Crixivan*)	None known	Caution*	C
Interferon alfa (*Intron A*)	Large doses cause abortions in animals	Caution*	C
Pegylated interferon (*PEG-Intron, Pegasys*)	As above	As above	C
Iodoquinol (*Yodoxin*)	Unknown	Caution*	C
Isoniazid (*Nydrazid, others*)	Embryocidal in some animals	Probably safe	C
Itraconazole (*Sporanox*)	Teratogenic and embryotoxic in rats	Caution*	C
Ivermectin (*Stromectol*)	Teratogenic in animals	Contraindicated	C
Kanamycin (*Kantrex*)	Possible 8th-nerve toxicity in fetus	Caution*	D
Ketoconazole (*Nizoral*)	Teratogenic and embryotoxic in rats	Contraindicated; topical probably safe	C
Lamivudine (3TC; *Epivir*)	Unknown	Caution*	C
Levofloxacin (*Levaquin*)	Arthropathy in immature animals	Caution*	C
Lindane	Absorbed from the skin; potential CNS toxicity in fetus	Contraindicated	C
Linezolid (*Zyvox*)	Decreased fetal survival in rats	Caution*	C
Lomefloxacin (*Maxaquin*)	Arthropathy in immature animals	Caution*	C

Continued on next page.

Drug	Toxicity in Pregnancy	Recommendation	FDA†
Lopinavir/ ritonavir (*Kaletra*)	Animal toxicity	Caution*	C
Loracarbef (*Lorabid*)	None known	Probably safe	B
Malathion, topical (*Ovide*)	None known	Probably safe	B
Maraviroc (*Selzentry*)	Unknown	Caution	B
Mebendazole	Teratogenic and embryo-toxic in rats	Caution*	C
Mefloquine (*Lariam*)[2]	Teratogenic in animals	Caution*	C
Meglumine (*Glucantime*)	Not known	Caution*	N/A
Meropenem (*Merrem*)	Unknown	Caution	B
Methenamine mandelate (*Mandelamine*)	Unknown	Probably safe	C
Metronidazole (*Flagyl*)	None known – carcinogenic in rats and mice	Caution	B
Micafungin (*Mycamine*)	Teratogenic and embryocidal in rabbits	Caution*	C
Miconazole (*Monistat i.v.*)	None known	Caution*; topical probably safe	C
Miltefosine (*Impavido*)	Teratogenic in rats and induces abortions in animals	Contraindicated; effective contraception must be used for 2 months after the last dose	N/A

* Use only for strong clinical indication in the absence of suitable alternative.
N/A = FDA pregnancy category not available
2. Mefloquine should not be used for treatment of malaria during pregnancy unless there is no other treatment option because of increased risk of stillbirth (F Nosten et al, Clin Infect Dis 1999; 28:808). Mefloquine has not been approved for use during pregnancy. However, it has been reported to be safe for prophylactic use during the second or third trimester of pregnancy and possibly during early pregnancy as well (CDC Health Information for International Travel, 2003-2004, page 111; BL Smoak et al, J Infect Dis 1997; 176:831).

Continued on next page.

Safety of Antimicrobial Drugs in Pregnancy

Drug	Toxicity in Pregnancy	Recommendation	FDA†
Minocycline (*Minocin*)	Tooth discoloration and dysplasia, inhibition of bone growth in fetus; hepatic toxicity and azotemia with IV use in pregnant patients with decreased renal function or with overdosage	Contraindicated	D
Moxifloxacin (*Avelox*)	Arthropathy in immature animals	Caution*	C
Nafcillin (*Nafcil*)	None known	Probably safe	B
Nalidixic acid (*NegGram*)	Arthropathy in immature animals; increased intracranial pressure in newborn, teratogenic and embryocidal in rats	Contraindicated	C
Nelfinavir (*Viracept*)	None known	Caution	B
Nevirapine (*Viramune*)	Decrease in fetal weight in rats	Caution*, 3	C
Nitazoxanide (*Alinia*)	None known	Probably safe	B
Nitrofurantoin (*Macrodantin*)	Hemolytic anemia in newborn	Caution*; contraindicated at term	B
Norfloxacin (*Noroxin*)	Arthropathy in immature animals	Probably safe	C
Nystatin (*Mycostatin*)	None known	Probably safe	C
Ofloxacin (*Floxin*)	Arthropathy in immature animals	Probably safe	C
Oseltamivir (*Tamiflu*)	Some minor skeletal abnormalities in animals	Caution*	C
Oxacillin	None known	Probably safe	B

3. Shown to be safe and effective for HIV-infected women at a single 200mg PO dose at start of labor.

Continued on next page.

Safety of Antimicrobial Drugs in Pregnancy

Drug	Toxicity in Pregnancy	Recommendation	FDA†
Oxytetracycline	Tooth discoloration and dysplasia, inhibition of bone growth in fetus; hepatic toxicity and azotemia with IV use in pregnant patients with decreased renal function or with overdosage	Contraindicated	D
Paromomycin (*Humatin*)	Poorly absorbed; toxicity in fetus unknown	Probably safe	C
Penicillin	None known	Probably safe	B
Pentamidine (*Pentam 300*, *NebuPent*)	Safety not established	Caution*	C
Permethrin (*Nix*, others)	Poorly absorbed; no known toxicity in fetus	Probably safe	B
Piperacillin (*Pipracil*)	None known	Probably safe	B
Piperacillin/ tazobactam (*Zosyn*)	None known	Probably safe	B
Posaconazole (*Noxafil*)	Teratogenic in animals	Caution*	C
Praziquantel (*Biltricide*)	Increased abortion rate in rats	Caution	B
Primaquine	Hemolysis in G-6-PD deficiency	Contraindicated	C
Pyrantel pamoate (*Antiminth*)	Absorbed in small amounts; no known toxicity in fetus	Probably safe	C
Pyrazinamide	Unknown	Caution*	C
Pyrethrins and piperonyl butoxide (*RID*, others)	Poorly absorbed; no known toxicity in fetus	Probably safe	C
Pyrimethamine (*Daraprim*)	Teratogenic in animals	Caution*; contraindicated during 1st trimester	C

* Use only for strong clinical indication in the absence of suitable alternative.
N/A = FDA pregnancy category not available

Continued on next page.

Safety of Antimicrobial Drugs in Pregnancy

Drug	Toxicity in Pregnancy	Recommendation	FDA†
Quinidine	Large doses can cause abortion	Probably safe	C
Quinine	Large doses can cause abortion; auditory nerve hypoplasia, deafness in fetus; visual changes, limb anomalies, visceral defects also reported	Caution*	C
Quinupristin/ dalfopristin (*Synercid*)	Unknown	Caution	B
Raltegravir (*Isentress*)	Fetal plasma concentrations are up to 2.5 times higher than maternal serum concentrations in animals	Caution*	C
Ribavirin (*Virazole, Rebetol*)	Mutagenic, teratogenic, embryocidal in nearly all species, and possibly carcinogenic in animals	Contraindicated	X
Rifabutin (*Mycobutin*)	Unknown	Caution	B
Rifampin (*Rifadin, Rimactane*)	Teratogenic in animals	Caution*	C
Rifapentine (*Priftin*)	Teratogenic in animals	Caution*	C
Rifaximin (*Xifaxan*)	Teratogenic in animals	Caution*	C
Rimantadine (*Flumadine*)	Embryotoxic in rats	Caution*	C
Ritonavir (*Norvir*)	Animal toxicity	Caution	B
Saquinavir (*Invirase*)	None known	Caution	B

Continued on next page.

Safety of Antimicrobial Drugs in Pregnancy

Drug	Toxicity in Pregnancy	Recommendation	FDA†
Sodium stibogluconate (*Pentostam*)	Not known	Caution*	N/A
Spectinomycin (*Trobicin*)	Unknown	Probably safe	B
Stavudine (d4T; *Zerit*)	Animal toxicity with high doses	Caution*	C
Streptomycin	Possible 8th-nerve toxicity in fetus; a few cases of ototoxicity reported	Contraindicated	D
Sulfonamides	Teratogenic in some animal studies; hemolysis in newborn with G-6-PD deficiency; increased risk of kernicterus in newborn	Caution*; contra-indicated at term	C
Suramin sodium (*Germanin*)	Teratogenic in mice	Caution*	N/A
Telbivudine (*Tyzeka*)	None known	Caution*	B
Telithromycin (*Ketek*)	None known	Caution*	C
Tenofovir (*Viread*)	None known	Caution	B
Tetracycline hydrochloride (*Sumycin*)	Tooth discoloration and dysplasia, inhibition of bone growth in fetus; hepatic toxicity and azotemia with IV use in pregnant patients with decreased renal function or with overdosage	Contraindicated	D
Thiabendazole (*Mintezol*)	None known	Caution*	C
Ticarcillin	None known	Probably safe	B
Ticarcillin/ clavulanic acid (*Timentin*)	None known	Probably safe	B

* Use only for strong clinical indication in the absence of suitable alternative.
N/A = FDA pregnancy category not available

Continued on next page.

Safety of Antimicrobial Drugs in Pregnancy

Drug	Toxicity in Pregnancy	Recommendation	FDA†
Tigecycline (*Tygacil*)	Decreased fetal weight and delays in bone ossification in animals	Caution*	D
Tinidazole (*Tindamax*)	Increased fetal mortality in rats	Caution*; contra-indicated during 1st trimester	C
Tobramycin	Possible 8th-nerve toxicity in fetus	Caution*	C
Trimethoprim (*Proloprim*)	Folate antagonism; teratogenic in rats	Caution*	C
Trimethoprim-sulfamethoxazole (*Bactrim*)	Same as sulfonamides and trimethoprim	Caution*; contra-indicated at term	C
Valacyclovir (*Valtrex*)	None known	Caution	B
Valganciclovir (*Valcyte*)	Teratogenic and embryo-toxic in animals	Caution*	C
Vancomycin (*Vancocin*)	Unknown – possible auditory and renal toxicity in fetus	Caution*	C
Voriconazole (*Vfend*)	Teratogenic and embryotoxic in animals	Contraindicated	D
Zalcitabine (ddC; *Hivid*)	Teratogenic and embryo-toxic in mice	Caution*	C
Zanamivir (*Relenza*)	None known	Caution*	C
Zidovudine (AZT; *Retrovir*)	Mutagenic *in vitro*	Caution*, [4]	C

4. Indicated to prevent HIV infection of fetus.

†FDA PREGNANCY CATEGORIES

Category	Interpretation
A	**Controlled studies show no risk** *Adequate, well-controlled studies in pregnant women have not shown an increased risk of fetal abnormalities*
B	**No evidence of risk in humans** *Animal studies have revealed no evidence of harm to the fetus. However, there are no adequate and well-controlled studies in pregnant women.* *or* *Animal studies have shown an adverse effect, but adequate and well-controlled studies in pregnant women have failed to demonstrate a risk to the fetus.*
C	**Risk cannot be ruled out** *Animal studies have shown an adverse effect and there are no adequate and well-controlled studies in pregnant women.* *or* *No animal studies have been conducted and there are no adequate and well-controlled studies in pregnant women.*
D	**Positive evidence of risk** *Studies, adequate well-controlled or observational, in pregnant women have demonstrated a risk to the fetus. However, the benefits of therapy may outweigh the potential risk.*
X	**Contraindicated in pregnancy** *Studies, adequate well-controlled or observational, in animals or pregnant women have demonstrated positive evidence of fetal abnormalities. The use of the product is contraindicated in women who are or may become pregnant.*

* Use only for strong clinical indication in the absence of suitable alternative.
N/A = FDA pregnancy category not available

A

abacavir – *Ziagen* (GlaxoSmithKline)
abacavir/lamivudine/zidovudine – *Trizivir* (GlaxoSmithKline)
Abelcet (Elan) – amphotericin B lipid complex
acyclovir – *Zovirax* (GlaxoSmithKline), others
adefovir – *Hepsera* (Gilead)
* *Aftate* (Schering) – tolnaftate
Agenerase (GlaxoSmithKline) – amprenavir
alatrofloxacin – *Trovan IV* (Pfizer)
albendazole – *Albenza* (GlaxoSmithKline)
Albenza (GlaxoSmithKline) – albendazole
Alferon N (Interferon Sciences) – interferon alfa-n3
Alinia (Romark) – nitazoxanide
amantadine – *Symmetrel* (Endo), others
AmBisome (Fujisawa) – amphotericin B liposomal
amikacin – *Amikin* (Bristol-Myers Squibb), others
* *Amikin* (Bristol-Myers Squibb) – amikacin
aminosalicylic acid – *Paser* (Jacobus)
amoxicillin – A*moxil* (GlaxoSmithKline), others
amoxicillin/clavulanic acid – *Augmentin* (GlaxoSmithKline), others
* *Amoxil* (GlaxoSmithKline) – amoxicillin
Amphotec (Sequus) – amphotericin B cholesteryl sulfate complex
amphotericin B – *Fungizone* (Bristol-Myers Squibb), others
amphotericin B cholesteryl sulfate complex – *Amphotec* (Sequus)
amphotericin B lipid complex – *Abelcet* (Elan)

---

* Also available generically.

§ Not commercially available. It may be obtained through compounding pharmacies. See footnote 4 on page 227.

† Available from the Centers for Disease Control and Prevention (CDC) Drug Service. See page 280.

• Not commercially available in the US.

‡ Available in the US only from the manufacturer.

Drug Trade Names

amphotericin B liposomal – *AmBisome* (Fujisawa)
ampicillin – *Principen* (Bristol-Myers Squibb), others
ampicillin/sulbactam – *Unasyn* (Pfizer), others
amprenavir – *Agenerase* (GlaxoSmithKline)
* *Ancef* (GlaxoSmithKline) – cefazolin
Ancobon (Roche) – flucytosine
anidulafungin – *Eraxis* (Pfizer)
† *Antiminth* (Pfizer) – pyrantel pamoate
Aptivus (Boehringer Ingelheim) – tipranavir
* *Aralen* (Sanofi) – chloroquine
§ *Arsobal* (Aventis, France) – melarsoprol
† artemether – *Artenam* (Arenco, Belgium)
atazanavir – *Reyataz* (Bristol-Myers Squibb)
atovaquone – *Mepron* (GlaxoSmithKline)
atovaquone/proguanil – *Malarone* (GlaxoSmithKline)
Atripla (Gilead/BMS) – efavirenz/emtricitabine/tenofovir
* *Augmentin* (GlaxoSmithKline) – amoxicillin/clavulanic acid
Avelox (Bayer) – moxifloxacin
Azactam (Bristol-Myers Squibb) – aztreonam
AZT – see zidovudine
azithromycin – *Zithromax* (Pfizer), *Zmax* (Pfizer), others
aztreonam – *Azactam* (Bristol-Myers Squibb)

B

* *Bactrim* (Roche) – trimethoprim/sulfamethoxazole

---

* Also available generically.
§ Not commercially available. It may be obtained through compounding pharmacies. See footnote 4 on page 227.
† Available from the Centers for Disease Control and Prevention (CDC) Drug Service. See page 280.
• Not commercially available in the US.
‡ Available in the US only from the manufacturer.

Baraclude (Bristol-Myers Squibb) – entecavir
Beepen-VK (GlaxoSmithKline) – penicillin V
§ benznidazole – *Rochagan* (Roche, Brazil)
* *Biaxin* (Abbott) – clarithromycin
Bicillin LA (King) – penicillin G benzathine
Biltricide (Bayer) – praziquantel
Bio-cef (Intl Ethic Lab) – cephalexin
† bithionol – *Bitin* (Tanabe, Japan)
† *Bitin* – bithionol (Tanabe, Japan)
Brodspec (Truxton) – tetracycline HCl
butoconazole – *Femstat* (Bayer), *Gynazole* (Ther-Rx)

C

Cancidas (Merck) – caspofungin
Capastat (Dura) – capreomycin
carbenicillin – *Geocillin* (Pfizer)
caspofungin – *Cancidas* (Merck)
Ceclor (Lilly) – cefaclor
cefaclor – *Ceclor* (Lilly)
Cedax (Biovail) – ceftibuten
cefadroxil – *Duricef* (Bristol-Myers Squibb), others
* *Cefadyl* (Bristol-Myers Squibb) – cephapirin
cefazolin – *Ancef* (GlaxoSmithKline), others
cefdinir – *Omnicef* (Abbott)
cefditoren – *Spectracef* (TAP)

---

* Also available generically.
§ Not commercially available. It may be obtained through compounding pharmacies. See footnote 4 on page 227.
† Available from the Centers for Disease Control and Prevention (CDC) Drug Service. See page 280.
• Not commercially available in the US.
‡ Available in the US only from the manufacturer.

Drug Trade Names

cefepime – *Maxipime* (Elan)
cefixime – *Suprax* (Lupin)
Cefizox (Fujisawa) – ceftizoxime
Cefobid (Pfizer) – cefoperazone
cefoperazone – *Cefobid* (Pfizer)
* *Cefotan* (AstraZeneca) – cefotetan
cefotaxime – *Claforan* (Aventis), others
cefotetan – *Cefotan* (AstraZeneca), others
cefoxitin – *Mefoxin* (Merck)
cefpodoxime – *Vantin* (Pharmacia), others
cefprozil – *Cefzil* (Bristol-Myers Squibb)
ceftazidime – *Fortaz, Tazicef* (GlaxoSmithKline), *Tazidime* (Lilly),
    others
ceftibuten – *Cedax* (Biovail)
* *Ceftin* (GlaxoSmithKline) – cefuroxime axetil
ceftizoxime – *Cefizox* (Fujisawa)
ceftriaxone – *Rocephin* (Roche), others
cefuroxime – *Zinacef* (GlaxoSmithKline), others
cefuroxime axetil – *Ceftin* (GlaxoSmithKline), others
Cefzil (Bristol-Myers Squibb) – cefprozil
cephalexin – *Keflex* (Middle Brook), others
cephapirin – *Cefadyl* (Bristol-Myers Squibb), others
cephradine – *Velosef* (Bristol-Myers Squibb), others
chloramphenicol – *Chloromycetin* (Pfizer), others
* *Chloromycetin* (Pfizer) – chloramphenicol
chloroquine – *Aralen* (Sanofi), others

---

* Also available generically.

§ Not commercially available. It may be obtained through compounding pharmacies. See footnote 4 on page 227.

† Available from the Centers for Disease Control and Prevention (CDC) Drug
Service. See page 280.

• Not commercially available in the US.

‡ Available in the US only from the manufacturer.

cidofovir – *Vistide* (Gilead)
* *Cipro* (Bayer) – ciprofloxacin
ciprofloxacin – *Cipro* (Bayer), others
* *Claforan* (Aventis) – cefotaxime
clarithromycin – *Biaxin* (Abbott), others
* *Cleocin* (Pfizer) – clindamycin
clindamycin – *Cleocin* (Pfizer), others
clofazimine – *Lamprene* (Novartis)
clotrimazole – *Mycelex* (Bayer), others
cloxacillin – generic
colistimethate – *Coly-Mycin* (Monarch)
Coly-Mycin (Monarch) – colistimethate
Combivir (GlaxoSmithKline) – lamivudine/zidovudine
* *Copegus* (Roche) – ribavirin
Cotrim (Teva) – trimethoprim/sulfamethoxazole
crotamiton – *Eurax* (Westwood-Squibb)
Crixivan (Merck) – indinavir
Cubicin (Cubist) – daptomycin
cycloserine – *Seromycin* (Lilly)
* *Cytovene* (Roche) – ganciclovir

D

ddC – see didanosine
ddI – see zalcitabine
dapsone – generic (Jacobus)

---

* Also available generically.
§ Not commercially available. It may be obtained through compounding pharmacies. See footnote 4 on page 227.
† Available from the Centers for Disease Control and Prevention (CDC) Drug Service. See page 280.
• Not commercially available in the US.
‡ Available in the US only from the manufacturer.

daptomycin – *Cubicin* (Cubist)
* *Daraprim* (GlaxoSmithKline) – pyrimethamine
darunavir – *Prezista* (Tibotec)
Declomycin (Lederle) – demeclocycline
delavirdine – *Rescriptor* (Pfizer)
demeclocycline – *Declomycin* (Lederle)
Denavir (Novartis) – penciclovir
dicloxacillin – *Dycill* (GlaxoSmithKline), others
didanosine – *Videx* (Bristol-Myers Squibb)
† diethylcarbamazine – *Hetrazan* (Lederle)
* *Diflucan* (Pfizer) – fluconazole
§ diloxanide furoate – *Furamide* (Boots, U.K.)
Doripenem – *Doribax* (Ortho McNeil)
Doribax (Ortho-McNeil) – doripenem
Doryx (Warner Chilcott) – doxycycline
doxycycline – *Vibramycin* (Pfizer), others
* *Duricef* (Bristol-Myers Squibb) – cefadroxil
* *Dycill* (GlaxoSmithKline) – dicloxacillin
Dynapen (Bristol-Myers Squibb) – dicloxacillin

E

E.E.S. (Abbott) – erythromycin
efavirenz – *Sustiva* (DuPont)
efavirenz/emtricitabine/tenofovir – *Atripla* (Gilead/BMS)
§ *Egaten* (Novartis) – triclabendazole

---

* Also available generically.
§ Not commercially available. It may be obtained through compounding pharmacies. See footnote 4 on page 227.
† Available from the Centers for Disease Control and Prevention (CDC) Drug Service. See page 280.
• Not commercially available in the US.
‡ Available in the US only from the manufacturer.

† eflornithine – *Ornidyl* (Aventis)
* *Elimite* (Allergan) – permethrin
emitricitabine – *Emtriva* (Gilead)
E-Mycin (Knoll) – erythromycin
enfuvirtide – *Fuzeon (*Trimeris-Roche)
entecavir – *Baraclude* (Bristol-Myers Squibb)
Epivir (GlaxoSmithKline) – lamivudine
Epzicom (GlaxoSmithKline) – abacavir/lamivudine
Eraxis (Pfizer) – anidulafungin
ertapenem – *Invanz* (Merck)
* *Ery-Tab* (Abbott) – erythromycin
* *ERYC* (Warner Chilcott) – erythromycin
* *Erythrocin* (Abbott) – erythromycin
erythromycin – *Erythrocin* (Abbott), others
erythromycin/sulfisoxazole – *Pediazole* (Ross/Abbott), others
Eryzole (Alra) – erythromycin/sulfisoxazole
ethambutol – *Myambutol* (Lederle), others
ethionamide – *Trecator-SC* (Wyeth)
Eurax (Westwood-Squibb) – crotamiton
Exelderm (Westwood-Squibb) – sulconazole

F

Factive (Oscient) – gemifloxacin
famciclovir – *Famvir* (GlaxoSmithKline)
Famvir (GlaxoSmithKline) – famciclovir

---

* Also available generically.
§ Not commercially available. It may be obtained through compounding pharmacies. See footnote 4 on page 227.
† Available from the Centers for Disease Control and Prevention (CDC) Drug Service. See page 280.
• Not commercially available in the US.
‡ Available in the US only from the manufacturer.

Fansidar (Roche) – pyrimethamine/sulfadoxine
Femstat (Bayer) – butoconazole
* *Flagyl* (Pfizer) – metronidazole
Floxin (Ortho-McNeil) – ofloxacin
fluconazole – *Diflucan* (Pfizer), others
flucytosine – *Ancobon* (Roche)
* *Flumadine* (Forest) – rimantadine
fomivirsen – *Vitravene* (Novartis)
* *Fortaz* (GlaxoSmithKline) – ceftazidime
fosamprenavir – *Lexiva* (GlaxoSmithKline)
foscarnet – *Foscavir* (AstraZeneca), others
* *Foscavir* (AstraZeneca) – foscarnet
fosfomycin – *Monurol* (Forest)
* *Fulvicin* (Schering) – griseofulvin
* *Fungizone* (Bristol-Myers Squibb) – amphotericin B
* *Furacin* (Roberts) – nitrofurazone
Furadantin (Dura) – nitrofurantoin
§ *Furamide* (Boots, U.K.) – diloxanide furoate
§ furazolidone – *Furoxone* (Roberts)
§ *Furoxone* (Roberts) – furazolidone

G

ganciclovir – *Cytovene* (Roche), others; *Vitrasert* (Bausch & Lomb)
* *Gantrisin* (Roche) – sulfisoxazole
* *Garamycin* (Schering) – gentamicin

---

* Also available generically.
§ Not commercially available. It may be obtained through compounding pharmacies. See footnote 4 on page 227.
† Available from the Centers for Disease Control and Prevention (CDC) Drug Service. See page 280.
• Not commercially available in the US.
‡ Available in the US only from the manufacturer.

gemifloxacin – *Factive* (Oscient)
gentamicin – *Garamycin* (Schering), others
Geocillin (Pfizer) – carbenicillin
§ *Glucantime* (Aventis, France) – meglumine antimoniate
* *Grifulvin V* (Ortho) – griseofulvin
griseofulvin – *Girifulvin V* (Ortho), others
* *Gris-PEG* (Allergan) – griseofulvin
Gynazole (Ther-Rx) – butoconazole

H

• *Halfan* (GlaxoSmithKline) – halofantrine
• halofantrine – *Halfan* (GlaxoSmithKline)
† *Hetrazan* (Lederle) – diethylcarbamazine
* *Hiprex* (Aventis) – methenamine hippurate
Hivid (Roche) – zalcitabine
Humatin (Monarch) – paromomycin
hydroxychloroquine – *Plaquenil* (Sanofi-Aventis)

I

imipenem/cilastatin – *Primaxin* (Merck)
imiquimod – *Aldara* (3M)
indinavir – *Crixivan* (Merck)
Infergen (Amgen) – interferon alfacon-1
Invanz (Merck) – ertapenem
interferon alfa-2a – *Roferon-A* (Roche)

---

* Also available generically.
§ Not commercially available. It may be obtained through compounding pharmacies. See footnote 4 on page 227.
† Available from the Centers for Disease Control and Prevention (CDC) Drug Service. See page 280.
• Not commercially available in the US.
‡ Available in the US only from the manufacturer.

interferon alfa-2a, pegylated – *Pegasys* (Roche)
interferon alfa-2b – *Intron A* (Schering)
interferon alfa-2b, pegylated – *PEG-Intron* (Schering)
interferon alfa-n3 – *Alferon N* (Interferon Sciences)
interferon alfacon-1 – *Infergen* (Amgen)
Intron A (Schering) – interferon alfa-2b
Invirase (Roche) – saquinavir
iodoquinol – *Yodoxin* (Glenwood), others
Isentress (Merck) – raltegravir
isoniazid – *Nydrazid* (Bristol-Myers Squibb), others
itraconazole – *Sporanox* (Janssen), others
ivermectin – *Stromectol* (Merck)

K

Kaletra (Abbott) – lopinavir/ritonavir
kanamycin – *Kantrex* (Bristol-Myers Squibb), others
* *Kantrex* (Bristol-Myers Squibb) – kanamycin
* *Keflex* (Dista) – cephalexin
Kefzol (Lilly) – cefazolin
Ketek (Aventis) – telithromycin
ketoconazole – *Nizoral* (Janssen), others

L

lamivudine – *Epivir*, *Epivir HBV* (GlaxoSmithKline)

---

* Also available generically.
§ Not commercially available. It may be obtained through compounding pharmacies. See footnote 4 on page 227.
† Available from the Centers for Disease Control and Prevention (CDC) Drug Service. See page 280.
• Not commercially available in the US.
‡ Available in the US only from the manufacturer.

lamivudine/zidovudine – *Combivir* (GlaxoSmithKline)
lamivudine/zidovudine/abacavir – *Trizivir* (GlaxoSmithKline)
† *Lampit* (Bayer, Germany) – nifurtimox
Lamprene (Novartis) – clofazimine
* *Lariam* (Roche) – mefloquine
levofloxacin – *Levaquin* (Ortho-McNeil)
Lincocin (Pfizer) – lincomycin
lincomycin – *Lincocin* (Pfizer), others
linezolid – *Zyvox* (Pfizer)
lopinavir/ritonavir – *Kaletra* (Abbott)
Lorabid (Lilly) – loracarbef
loracarbef – *Lorabid* (Lilly)

M

* *Macrobid* (Proctor & Gamble) – nitrofurantoin
* *Macrodantin* (Proctor & Gamble) – nitrofurantoin
Malarone (GlaxoSmithKline) – atovaquone/proguanil
malathion – *Ovide* (Taro)
* *Mandelamine* (Warner Chilcott) – methenamine mandelate
maraviroc – *Selzentry* (Pfizer)
Maxipime (Elan) – cefepime
mebendazole – *Vermox* (Janssen), others
mefloquine – *Lariam* (Roche), others
Mefoxin (Merck) – cefoxitin
§ meglumine antimoniate – *Glucantime* (Aventis, France)

---

* Also available generically.
§ Not commercially available. It may be obtained through compounding pharmacies. See footnote 4 on page 227.
† Available from the Centers for Disease Control and Prevention (CDC) Drug Service. See page 280.
• Not commercially available in the US.
‡ Available in the US only from the manufacturer.

† melarsoprol – *Arsobal* (Aventis, France)
Mepron (GlaxoSmithKline) – atovaquone
meropenem – *Merrem IV* (AstraZeneca)
Merrem IV (AstraZeneca) – meropenem
methenamine hippurate – *Hiprex* (Aventis), *Urex* (3M), others
methenamine mandelate – *Mandelamine* (Warner Chilcott), others
metronidazole – *Flagyl* (Searle), others
micafungin – *Mycamine* (Astellas)
miconazole – *Monistat* (Ortho-McNeil), others
§ miltefosine – *Impavido* (Zentaris, Geranay)
* *Minocin* (Wyeth) – minocycline
minocycline – *Minocin* (Wyeth), others
Mintezol (Merck) – thiabendazole
* *Monistat* (Ortho-McNeil) – miconazole
Monodox (Oclassen) – doxycycline
Monurol (Forest) – fosfomycin
moxifloxacin – *Avelox* (Bayer), *Vigamox* (Alcon)
Myambutol (X-Gen) – ethambutol
Mycamine (Astellas) – micafungin
* *Mycelex* (Bayer) – clotrimazole
Mycobutin (Pharmacia) – rifabutin
* *Mycostatin* (Bristol-Myers Squibb) – nystatin

N

nafcillin – *Nallpen* (Baxter)

---

* Also available generically.
§ Not commercially available. It may be obtained through compounding pharmacies. See footnote 4 on page 227.
† Available from the Centers for Disease Control and Prevention (CDC) Drug Service. See page 280.
• Not commercially available in the US.
‡ Available in the US only from the manufacturer.

nalidixic acid – *NegGram* (Sanofi), others
Nallpen (Baxter) – nafcillin
Natacyn (Alcon) – natamycin
natamycin – *Natacyn* (Alcon)
* *Nebcin* (Lilly) – tobramycin
* *NebuPent* (Fujisawa) – pentamidine
* *NegGram* (Sanofi) – nalidixic acid
nelfinavir – *Viracept* (Pfizer)
neomycin – generic
nevirapine – *Viramune* (Boehringer Ingelheim)
§ niclosamide – *Yomesan* (Bayer, Germany)
• nifurtimox – *Lampit* (Bayer, Germany)
nitazoxanide – *Alinia* (Romark)
nitrofurantoin – *Macrodantin* (Proctor & Gamble), others
nitrofurazone – *Furacin* (Roberts), others
* *Nix* (GlaxoSmithKline) – permethrin
* *Nizoral* (Janssen) – ketoconazole
norfloxacin – *Noroxin* (Merck)
Noroxin (Merck) – norfloxacin
Norvir (Abbott) – ritonavir
Noxafil (Schering-Plough) – posaconazole
* *Nydrazid* (Bristol-Myers Squibb) – isoniazid
nystatin – *Mycostatin* (Bristol-Myers Squibb), others
Nystex (Savage) – nystatin

---

* Also available generically.

§ Not commercially available. It may be obtained through compounding pharmacies. See footnote 4 on page 227.

† Available from the Centers for Disease Control and Prevention (CDC) Drug Service. See page 280.

• Not commercially available in the US.

‡ Available in the US only from the manufacturer.

O

ofloxacin – *Floxin* (Ortho-McNeil)
Omnicef (Abbott) – cefdinir
§ ornidazole – *Tiberal* (Hoffmann LaRoche, Switzerland)
† *Ornidyl* (Aventis) – eflornithine
oseltamivir – *Tamiflu* (Roche/Gilead)
Ovide (Medicis) – malathion
oxacillin – generic
§ oxamniquine – *Vansil* (Pfizer)
oxytetracycline – *Terramycin* (Pfizer)

P

§ *Paludrine* (Ayerst, Canada, ICI, U.K.) – proguanil
paromomycin – *Humatin* (Monarch)
Paser (Jacobus) – aminosalicylic acid
* *Pediazole* (Ross/Abbott) – erythromycin/sulfisoxazole
Pegasys (Roche) – pegylated interferon alfa 2a
PEG-Intron (Schering) – pegylated interferon alfa 2b
penciclovir – *Denavir* (Novartis)
penicillin G – generic, many manufacturers
penicillin G benzathine – *Bicillin LA* (King), *Permapen* (Pfizer)
penicillin G procaine – generic, many manufacturers
penicillin V – generic, many manufacturers
* *Pentam 300* (Fujisawa) – pentamidine

---

* Also available generically.
§ Not commercially available. It may be obtained through compounding pharmacies. See footnote 4 on page 227.
† Available from the Centers for Disease Control and Prevention (CDC) Drug Service. See page 280.
• Not commercially available in the US.
‡ Available in the US only from the manufacturer.

pentamidine isethionate – *Pentam 300* (Fujisawa), *NebuPent* (Fujisawa), others

† *Pentostam* (GlaxoSmithKline, U.K.) – sodium stibogluconate

Pen-V (Zenith Goldline) – penicillin V

Permapen (Pfizer) – penicillin G benzathine

permethrin – *Elimite* (Allergan), *Nix* (GlaxoSmithKline), others

piperacillin – *Pipracil* (Wyeth)

piperacillin/tazobactam – *Zosyn* (Wyeth)

Pipracil (Wyeth) – piperacillin

Plaquenil (Sanofi-Aventis) – hydroxychloroquine

polymyxin B – generic

posaconacole – *Noxafil* (Schering)

praziquantel – *Biltricide* (Bayer)

Priftin (Aventis) – rifapentine

primaquine phosphate (Sanofi) – generic

Primaxin (Merck) – imipenem/cilastatin sodium

* *Principen* (Bristol-Myers Squibb) – ampicillin

Prezista (Tibotec) – darunavir

§ proguanil – *Paludrine* (Ayerst, Canada; ICI, U.K.)

proguanil/atovaquone – *Malarone* (GlaxoSmithKline)

* *Proloprim* (GlaxoSmithKline) – trimethoprim

Pronto (Del) – pyrethrins with piperonyl butoxide

§ pyrantel pamoate – *Antiminth* (Pfizer), others

pyrazinamide – generic

pyrethrins with piperonyl butoxide – *RID* (Bayer), others

---

* Also available generically.

§ Not commercially available. It may be obtained through compounding pharmacies. See footnote 4 on page 227.

† Available from the Centers for Disease Control and Prevention (CDC) Drug Service. See page 280.

• Not commercially available in the US.

‡ Available in the US only from the manufacturer.

Drug Trade Names

pyrimethamine – *Daraprim* (GlaxoSmithKline)
pyrimethamine/sulfadoxine – *Fansidar* (Roche)

Q

Qualaquin (AR Scientific) – quinine sulfate
quinidine gluconate – generic
§ quinine dihydrochloride
quinine sulfate – *Qualaquin* (AR Scientific)
quinupristin/dalfopristin – *Synercid* (Aventis)

R

raltegravir – *Isentress* (Merck)
* *Rebetol* (Schering) – ribavirin
Rebetron (Schering) – ribavirin/interferon alfa-2b
Relenza (GlaxoSmithKline) – zanamivir
Rescriptor (Pfizer) – delavirdine
* *Retrovir* (GlaxoSmithKline) – zidovudine
ribavirin – *Virazole* (Valeant); *Rebetol* (Schering), *Copegus* (Roche),
    others
ribavirin/interferon alfa-2b – *Rebetron* (Schering)
* *RID* (Bayer) – pyrethrins with piperonyl butoxide
rifabutin – *Mycobutin* (Pfizer)
* *Rifadin* (Aventis) – rifampin
Rifamate (Aventis) – rifampin/isoniazid

---

* Also available generically.
§ Not commercially available. It may be obtained through compounding pharmacies. See footnote 4 on page 227.
† Available from the Centers for Disease Control and Prevention (CDC) Drug Service. See page 280.
• Not commercially available in the US.
‡ Available in the US only from the manufacturer.

rifampin – *Rimactane* (Novartis), *Rifadin* (Aventis), others
rifampin/isoniazid – *Rifamate* (Aventis)
rifapentine – *Priftin* (Aventis)
Rifater (Aventis) – rifampin/isoniazid/pyrazinamide
rifaximin – *Xifaxan* (Salix)
* *Rimactane* (Novartis) – rifampin
rimantadine – *Flumadine* (Forest), others
ritonavir – *Norvir* (Abbott)
ritonavir/lopinavir – *Kaletra* (Abbott)
* *Rocephin* (Roche) – ceftriaxone
§ *Rochagan* (Roche, Brazil) – benznidazole
Roferon-A (Roche) – interferon alfa-2a
‡ *Rovamycine* (Aventis) – spiramycin

S

saquinavir – *Invirase* (Roche)
Selzentry (Pfizer) – maraviroc
* *Septra* (GlaxoSmithKline) – trimethoprim/sulfamethoxazole
Seromycin (Lilly) – cycloserine
Sertaconazole – *Ertaczo* (Ortho Neutrogena)
† sodium stibogluconate – *Pentostam* (GlaxoSmithKline, U.K.)
spectinomycin – *Trobicin* (Pfizer)
Spectracef (Cornerstone) – cefditoren
‡ spiramycin – *Rovamycine* (Aventis)
* *Sporanox* (Janssen) – itraconazole

---

* Also available generically.

§ Not commercially available. It may be obtained through compounding pharmacies. See footnote 4 on page 227.

† Available from the Centers for Disease Control and Prevention (CDC) Drug Service. See page 280.

• Not commercially available in the US.

‡ Available in the US only from the manufacturer.

stavudine – *Zerit* (Bristol-Myers Squibb)
streptomycin – generic
Stromectol (Merck) – ivermectin
sulconazole – *Exelderm* (Westwood-Squibb)
Sulfatrim (Actavis Mid Atlantic) – trimethoprim/sulfamethoxazole
sulfisoxazole – *Gantrisin* (Roche), others
* *Sumycin* (Bristol-Myers Squibb) – tetracycline HCl
Suprax (Lupin) – cefixime
† suramin – (Bayer, Germany)
Sustiva (Bristol-Myers Squibb) – efavirenz
* *Symmetrel* (Endo) – amantadine
Synercid (Aventis) – quinupristin/dalfopristin

T

Tamiflu (Roche/Gilead) – oseltamivir
* *Tazicef* (GlaxoSmithKline) – ceftazidime
**Tazidime* (Lilly) – ceftazidime
telbivudine – *Tyzeka* (Novartis/Idenix)
telithromycin – *Ketek* (Aventis)
tenofovir – *Viread* (Gilead)
Terramycin (Pfizer) – oxytetracycline
Tetracon (Consolidated Midland) – tetracycline HCl
tetracycline HCl – *Sumycin* (Bristol-Myers Squibb), others
thiabendazole – *Mintezol* (Merck)
§ *Tiberal* (Hoffmann LaRoche, Switzerland) – ornidazole

---

* Also available generically.
§ Not commercially available. It may be obtained through compounding pharmacies. See footnote 4 on page 227.
† Available from the Centers for Disease Control and Prevention (CDC) Drug Service. See page 280.
• Not commercially available in the US.
‡ Available in the US only from the manufacturer.

Ticar (GlaxoSmithKline) – ticarcillin

ticarcillin – *Ticar* (GlaxoSmithKline)

ticarcillin/clavulanic acid – *Timentin* (GlaxoSmithKline)

tigecycline – *Tygacil* (Wyeth)

Timentin (GlaxoSmithKline) – ticarcillin/clavulanic acid

Tindamax (Presutti) – tinidazole

tinidazole – *Tindamax* (Presutti)

tioconazole – *Vagistat* (Bristol-Myers Squibb)

tipranavir – *Aptivus* (Boehringer Ingelheim)

tobramycin – *Nebcin* (Lilly), others

tolnaftate – *Aftate* (Schering), others

Trecator-SC (Wyeth) – ethionamide

§ triclabendazole – *Egaten* (Novartis)

trifluridine – *Viroptic* (GlaxoSmithKline), and others

trimethoprim – *Proloprim* (GlaxoSmithKline), others

trimethoprim-sulfamethoxazole – *Bactrim* (Roche), *Septra* (GlaxoSmithKline), others

Trimox (Bristol-Myers Squibb) – amoxicillin

Trimpex (Roche) – trimethoprim

* *Triple Sulfa* (Allscripts) – trisulfapyrimidines

trisulfapyrimidines – *Triple Sulfa* (Allscripts), others

Trizivir (GlaxoSmithKline) – abacavir/lamivudine/zidovudine

Trobicin (Pfizer) – spectinomycin

Trovan (Pfizer) – trovafloxacin

Truvada (Gilead) – emitricitabine/tenofovir

Truxazole (Truxton) – sulfisoxazole

---

* Also available generically.

§ Not commercially available. It may be obtained through compounding pharmacies. See footnote 4 on page 227.

† Available from the Centers for Disease Control and Prevention (CDC) Drug Service. See page 280.

• Not commercially available in the US.

‡ Available in the US only from the manufacturer.

Drug Trade Names

Truxcillin VK (Truxton) – penicillin V
Tygacil (Wyeth) – tigecycline
Tyzeka (Novartis/Idenix) – telbivudine

U

* *Unasyn* (Pfizer) – ampicillin/sulbactam
* *Urex* (Virco) – methenamine hippurate

V

Vagistat (Bristol-Myers Squibb) – tioconazole
valacyclovir – *Valtrex* (GlaxoSmithKline)
Valcyte (Roche) – valganciclovir
valganciclovir – *Valcyte* (Roche)
Valtrex (GlaxoSmithKline) – valacyclovir
* *Vancocin* (Lilly) – vancomycin
vancomycin – *Vancocin* (Lilly), others
§ *Vansil* (Pfizer) – oxamniquine
* *Vantin* (Pfizer) – cefpodoxime
Veetids (Bristol-Myers Squibb) – penicillin V
* *Velosef* (Bristol-Myers Squibb) – cephradine
* *Vermox* (Janssen) – mebendazole
Vfend (Pfizer) – voriconazole
* *Vibramycin* (Pfizer) – doxycycline
* *Vibra-Tabs* (Pfizer) – doxycycline

---

* Also available generically.
§ Not commercially available. It may be obtained through compounding pharmacies. See footnote 4 on page 227.
† Available from the Centers for Disease Control and Prevention (CDC) Drug Service. See page 280.
• Not commercially available in the US.
‡ Available in the US only from the manufacturer.

vidarabine – generic
Videx (Bristol-Myers Squibb) – didanosine
Vigamox (Alcon) – moxifloxacin
Viracept (Pfizer) – nelfinavir
Viramune (Boehringer Ingelheim) – nevirapine
Virazole (Valeant) – ribavirin
Viread (Gilead) – tenofovir
Viroptic (GlaxoSmithKline) – trifluridine
Vistide (Gilead) – cidofovir
Vitrasert (Bausch & Lomb) – ganciclovir
Vitravene (Novartis) – fomivirsen
voriconazole – *Vfend* (Pfizer)

W

* *Wesmycin* (Wesley) – tetracycline HCl

X

Xifaxan (Salix) – Rifamaxin

Y

* *Yodoxin* (Glenwood) – iodoquinol
§ *Yomesan* (Bayer, Germany) – niclosamide

---

* Also available generically.
§ Not commercially available. It may be obtained through compounding pharmacies. See footnote 4 on page 227.
† Available from the Centers for Disease Control and Prevention (CDC) Drug Service. See page 280.
• Not commercially available in the US.
‡ Available in the US only from the manufacturer.

Z

zalcitabine – *Hivid* (Roche)
zanamivir – *Relenza* (GlaxoSmithKline)
Zerit (Bristol-Myers Squibb) – stavudine
Ziagen (GlaxoSmithKline) – abacavir
zidovudine – *Retrovir* (GlaxoSmithKline)
zidovudine/lamivudine – *Combivir* (GlaxoSmithKline)
zidovudine/lamivudine/abacavir – *Trizivir* (GlaxoSmithKline)
* *Zinacef* (GlaxoSmithKline) – cefuroxime
* *Zithromax* (Pfizer) – azithromycin
* *Zmax* (Pfizer) – azithromycin
Zosyn (Wyeth) – piperacillin/tazobactam
* *Zovirax* (GlaxoSmithKline) – acyclovir
Zyvox (Pfizer) – linezolid

---

* Also available generically.
§ Not commercially available. It may be obtained through compounding pharmacies. See footnote 4 on page 227.
† Available from the Centers for Disease Control and Prevention (CDC) Drug Service. See page 280.
• Not commercially available in the US.
‡ Available in the US only from the manufacturer.

DOSAGE OF ANTIMICROBIAL AGENTS

In choosing the dosage of an antimicrobial drug, the physician must consider the site of infection, the identity and antimicrobial susceptibility of the infecting organism, the possible toxicity of the drug of choice, and the condition of the patient, with special attention to renal function. This article and the table that follows on page 420 offer some guidelines for determining antimicrobial dosage, but dosage recommendations taken out of context of the clinical situation may be misleading.

RENAL INSUFFICIENCY — Antimicrobial drugs excreted through the urinary tract may be toxic for patients with renal insufficiency if they are given in usual therapeutic doses, because serum concentrations in these patients may become dangerously high. Nephrotoxic and ototoxic drugs such as gentamicin or other aminoglycosides may damage the kidney, further decreasing the excretion of these drugs, leading to higher serum concentrations that may be ototoxic and may cause additional renal damage. In patients with renal insufficiency, therefore, an antimicrobial drug with minimal nephrotoxicity, such as a beta-lactam, is preferred. When nephrotoxic drugs must be used, renal function should be monitored. Measurements of serum creatinine or blood urea nitrogen (BUN) concentrations are useful as indices of renal function, but are not as accurate as measurements of creatinine clearance; serum creatinine and BUN concentrations may be normal even with significant loss of renal function.

In renal insufficiency, control of serum concentrations of potentially toxic drugs can be achieved either by varying the dose or by varying the interval between doses. Serum antimicrobial concentrations should be measured whenever possible; rigid adherence to any dosage regimen can result in either inadequate or toxic serum concentrations in patients with renal insufficiency, particularly when renal function is changing rapidly.

Continuous renal replacement therapies (CRRTs) are increasingly being used to treat critically ill patients with acute or chronic renal failure.

Dosage of Antimicrobial Agents

There are several methods, including continuous arteriovenous hemofiltration (CAVH), continuous venovenous hemofiltration (CVVH), continuous venovenous hemodialysis (CVVHD), and continuous venovenous hemodialfiltration (CVVHDF). Dosing for CRRT depends on the method of renal replacement therapy used, flow rate and filter type.

CHILDREN'S DOSAGE — Many antimicrobial drugs have such a broad therapeutic index that it makes no difference in practice if children's dosage is based on weight or on surface area. Where dosage considerations are important in preventing severe toxic effects, as with the aminoglycosides, recommendations for safe usage are derived primarily from experience with dosage based on weight.

ONCE-DAILY AMINOGLYCOSIDES — In certain categories of patients once-daily doses of gentamicin, tobramycin and amikacin are as effective for many indications as multiple daily doses and are equally or less nephrotoxic. Monitoring 24-hour trough drug levels is recommended to minimize the risk of toxicity. Once-daily doses of aminoglycosides are not recommended for treatment of endocarditis and should be used cautiously in the elderly, immunocompromised patients and those with renal insufficiency.

THE TABLE — **Dosage** – The recommendations in the table that follows are based on the judgment of Medical Letter consultants. In some cases they differ from the manufacturer's recommendations, partly because clinical experience reported after the labeling is approved is not always reflected by an appropriate change in the manufacturer's recommendations. The range of dosage specified for some drugs may not include relatively rare indications. In general, lower doses are sufficient for treatment of urinary tract infection, and higher doses are recommended for such severe infections as meningitis, endocarditis and the sepsis syndrome. Doses for CRRTs represent the full range recommended for various types of CRRT, and are based on dialysate flow/ultrafiltration rates of ≥ 1L/hr.

Interval – More than one interval between doses is recommended for some drugs. In general, the longer intervals should be used for infections of the urinary tract and for intramuscular administration. Recommendations are made in hours, but many oral drugs can be given three or four times during the daytime for convenience. For maximum absorption, which is often not necessary, most oral antibiotics should be given at least 30 minutes before or two hours after a meal.

ANTIMICROBIAL DRUG DOSAGE†

| | Adults | | Children | |
	Oral	Parenteral	Oral	Parenteral
Abacavir	300 mg q12h or 600 mg q24h		8 mg/kg q12h	
Abacavir/ lamivudine	600 mg/300 mg q24h			
Acyclovir	200 mg 5x/d or 400 mg q8h[1]	5-15 mg/kg q8h	20 mg/kg q6h	5-20 mg/kg q8h
Adefovir	10 mg q24h			
Albendazole	400 mg q12-24h		10-15 mg/kg q24h	
Amantadine	100 mg q12-24h		4.4 mg/kg q12-24h	
Amikacin		5 mg/kg q8h, 7.5 mg/kg q12h or 15-20 mg/kg q24h[3]		5 mg/kg q8h or 7.5 mg/kg q12h[3]
Aminosalicylic acid	8-12 g div q12-8h		200-300 mg/kg div q12-6h	
Amoxicillin	250-500 mg q8h or 500-875 mg q12h[4]		6.6-13.3 mg/kg q8h or 15 mg/kg q12h[4]	
Amoxicillin/ clavulanic acid	250-500 mg[5] q8h or 500-875 mg[5] q12h or 2000 mg[5] q12h		6.6-13.3 mg/kg[5] q8h or 12.5-45 mg/kg[5] q12h	
Amphotericin B		0.3-1.0 mg/kg[6] q24h		0.3-1.0 mg/kg[6] q24h
Ampho B cholesteryl sulfate complex (Amphotec)		3-4 mg/kg q24h		3-4 mg/kg q24h
Ampho B lipid complex (Abelcet)		5 mg/kg q24h		5 mg/kg q24h

† Dosage recommendations are also included in some articles within this handbook. Certain factors, such as site of infection, susceptibility of infecting organism and concomitant use of interacting drugs, need to be considered when dosing antimicrobial drugs.
1. For treatment of initial genital herpes. For suppression of genital herpes, 400 mg q12h is used. For treatment of varicella, 800 mg q6h and for zoster, 800 mg 5 times daily every 4 hours are recommended.
2. For patients on hemodialysis, dose is 10 mg q7 days, given after hemodialysis.
3. For information on once-daily dosing, see page 418. For renal failure give full dose once, then monitor levels.

Usual Maximum Dose/Day	Adult Dosage in Renal Failure For Creatinine Clearance (mL/min)			Dose for CRRTs	Extra Dose After Hemodialysis
	80-50	50-10	<10		
600 mg	Change not required				no
600 mg/ 300 mg	No change	Not recommended			
4 g oral 60 mg/kg IV	No change	IV: q12-24h	PO: 200 mg q12h IV:50% of dose		yes
10 mg	10 mg q24h	10 mg q48-72h	Unknown		yes[2]
800 mg	Change not required				no
200 mg	100 mg q12-24h	100-200 mg q24-48h	200 mg q7d		no
1.5 g	5-7.5 mg/kg q12h	5-7.5 mg/kg q24-36h	see foot-note 3	q24h, monitor levels	yes
12 g	Unknown	Unknown	Not recom-mended		yes (50% of dose)
3 g[4]	250-500 mg q8h	250-500 mg q12h	250-500 mg q24h	250-500 mg q24h	yes
4 g	No change	250-500 mg[5] q12h	250-500 mg[5] q24h	250-500 mg[5] q24h	yes
1 mg/kg[6]	Change not required[7]				no
7.5mg/kg	Unknown				
5 mg/kg	Unknown				no

CRRTs: Continuous renal replacement therapies. See also pages 417–418.
4. Doses up to 4 g/d (80-90 mg/kg/d, divided q12h in children) are sometimes used for infections with intermediately-resistant pneumococcus. An extended-release formulation *(Moxatag* 775 mg q24h) is approved for treatment of pharyngitis or tonsilllitis caused by *Streptococcus pyogenes.*
5. Dosage based on amoxicillin content. In order to ensure the proper amount of clavulanic acid, the use of half or multiple tablets is not recommended (unless using *Augmentin XR*).
6. Or up to 1.5 mg/kg given every other day. Given IV, over a period of two to four hours.
7. A pre- and post-dose IV bolus of 500 mL normal saline may decrease renal toxicity.

Continued on next page.

ANTIMICROBIAL DRUG DOSAGE† (continued)

| | Adults | | Children | |
	Oral	Parenteral	Oral	Parenteral
Ampho B liposomal (AmBisome)		3-5 mg/kg q24h		3-5 mg/kg q24h
Ampicillin	250-500 mg q6h	1-2 g q4-6h	12.5-25 mg/kg q6h	25-50 mg/kg q6h[8]
Ampicillin/ sulbactam		1.5-3 g[9] q6h		50-100 mg/kg[9] q6h
Amprenavir[10]	1200 mg q12h		20 mg/kg q12h[11] or 15 mg/kg q8h[11]	
Anidulafungin		100-200mg day 1, then 50-100 mg q24h		0.75-1.5[12] mg/kg q24h
Atazanavir	400 mg q24h[13]			
Atovaquone	750 mg q12h[14]		30 mg/kg q24h[15]	
Atovaquone/ proguanil	1000 mg/400 mg q24h[16]		See foot- note 17	
Azithromycin	250-1000 mg[18] q24h or 2 g once[18]	500 mg q24h	5-12 mg/kg[18] q24h	
Aztreonam[10]		1-2 g q6-8h		30-120 mg/kg q6-8h
Capreomycin		15 mg/kg q24h		15-30 mg/kg q24h
Carbenicillin indanyl sodium	1-2 tabs[19] q6h		7.5-12.5 mg/kg q12h	

8. For meningitis in children caused by ampicillin-sensitive *H. influenzae* type b, Medical Letter consultants recommend up to 400 mg/kg/d. Meningitis should be treated q4h.
9. Combination formulation: 1.5-g vial contains 1 g ampicillin/500 mg sulbactam; 3-g vial contains 2 g ampicillin/1 g sulbactam.
10. Dosage adjustment may be necessary in patients with hepatic dysfunction.
11. Using capsules. Also available in solution: 22.5 mg/kg q12h or 17 mg/kg q8h (max. 2800 mg/d).
12. Safety and effectiveness not established in children. Concentrations and exposures following adminis- tration of these maintenance doses in children 2-17 yrs old were similar to those observed in adults receiving maintenance doses of 50 and 100 mg/d.
13. For treatment-experienced patients or those taking efavirenz or tenofovir, the recommended dose is 300 mg taken once daily with 100 mg of ritonavir.
14. For treatment of *Pneumocystis jiroveci* pneumonia (PCP). The dose for prevention of PCP is 1500 mg once daily.

Usual Maximum Dose/Day	Adult Dosage in Renal Failure For Creatinine Clearance (mL/min)			Dose for CRRTs	Extra Dose After Hemodialysis
	80-50	50-10	<10		
6 mg/kg	Unknown				no
12 g	0.5-2 g q6h	0.5-2 g q8h	0.5-2 g q12h	0.5-2g q8h	yes
12 g	No change	1.5-3g q8-12h	1.5-3g q24h	3gIV q8-12h	yes
2400 mg	Change not required				
100 mg	Change not required				no
400 mg	Change not required				
1500 mg	Change not required				
1000 mg/ 400 mg	No change	CrCl <30mL/min not recommended			no
500 mg	Change not required				
8 g	No change	500-1000 mg q8h	250-500 mg q8h	1-2g IV q12h	yes
1 g	No change	7.5 mg/kg q24-48h	7.5 mg/kg q72h		
3 g	See package insert				

CRRTs: Continuous renal replacement therapies. See also pages 417–418.
15. For infants 1-3 months and children older than 24 months of age.The recommended dose for children 4-24 months of age is up to 45 mg/kg once daily.
16. Dosage for treatment of malaria. For prevention of malaria, dose is 250 mg/100 mg once daily. Each adult tablet contains 250 mg atovaquone/100 mg proguanil.
17. For pediatric dosing, see Drugs for Parasitic Infections (Malaria) page 246.
18. For adults: 500 mg on day 1 and 250 mg/d on days 2-5; urethritis and cervicitis: 1 g once for *C. trachomatis,* 2 g once for *N. gonorrhoeae;* MAC prophylaxis: 1200 mg once/week; MAC treatment: 600 mg once daily (with ethambutol). For children: pharyngitis/tonsillitis: 12 mg/kg once a day for 5 days; acute otitis media: 10 mg/kg on day 1 and 5 mg/kg on days 2 to 5 or single-dose 30 mg/kg or 10 mg/kg once daily for 3 days (max = 1500mg). Extended-release oral suspension *(Zmax)* is given as 2 g once for treatment of adults with acute bacterial sinusitis or mild-moderate CAP.
19. Tablets contain 382 mg of carbenicillin.

Continued on next page.

ANTIMICROBIAL DRUG DOSAGE† (continued)

| | Adults | | Children | |
	Oral	Parenteral	Oral	Parenteral
Caspofungin[10]		70 mg day 1, then 50 mg q24h[20,21]		See foot-note 22
Cefaclor	250-500 mg q8h or 375-500 mg ER q12h		6.6-13.3 mg/kg q8h	
Cefadroxil	0.5-1 g q12-24h		15 mg/kg q12h	
Cefazolin		500 mg-2 g q6-8h		25-100 mg/kg/d, div q6-8h
Cefdinir	300 mg q12h or 600 mg q24h		7 mg/kg q12h or 14 mg/kg q24h	
Cefditoren	200-400 mg q12h		See foot-note 23	
Cefepime		1-2 g q8-12h		50 mg/kg q8-12h
Cefixime	200 mg q12h or 400 mg q24h		4 mg/kg q12h or 8 mg/kg q24h	
Cefoperazone[10]		500 mg-4 g q6-12h		25-100 mg/kg q12h
Cefotaxime		1-2 g q4-12h		50-200 mg/kg/d, div q4-6h
Cefotetan		500 mg-3 g q12h		20-40 mg/kg q12h[24]
Cefoxitin		1-3 g q4-6h		80-160 mg/kg/d, div q4-6h
Cefpodoxime	100-400 mg q12h		10 mg/kg q24h or 5 mg/kg q12h	

20. Loading dose not needed for treatment of esophageal candidiasis.
21. For patients with moderate hepatic insufficiency (Child-Pugh score 7-9) the daily dose should be reduced to 35 mg following the standard 70 mg loading dose on day 1.
22. Not approved for use in children. Limited experience in clinical trials with children 2-11 yrs: 70 mg/m² on day 1 (max 70 mg), then 50 mg/m²/day (max 50 mg).

Usual Maximum Dose/Day	Adult Dosage in Renal Failure For Creatinine Clearance (mL/min)			Dose for CRRTs	Extra Dose After Hemodialysis
	80-50	50-10	<10		
50 mg	Change not required				no
2 g	No change	No change	50% of dose		yes
2 g	500 mg q12-24h	500 mg q12-24h	500 mg q36h		yes
6 g	1 g q8h	1 g q8-12h	1 g q24h	1-2g IV q12h	yes
600 mg	No change	CrCl <30mL/min 300 mg q24h			yes
800 mg	No change	200 mg q12-24h	Unknown		
6 g	2 g q8-12h	1-2 g q12-24h	500 mg-1 g q24h	1-2g IV q12h	yes
400 mg	200-400 mg q24h	200-400 mg q24h	200 mg q24h		no
12 g	Change not required				no*
12 g	No change	1-2 g q6-12h	1-2 g q12-24h	1-2 g IV q8-12h	yes
6 g	0.5-3g q12h	0.5-3g q12-24h	0.5-3g q48h	750 mg IV q12h	yes
12 g	1-2 g q8h	1-2 g q8-12h	0.5-1 g q12-24h	1-2g q8-12h	yes
800 mg	200-400 mg q12h	CrCl <30 mL/min 200-400 mg q24h			yes

CRRTs: Continuous renal replacement therapies. See also pages 417–418.
* But give usual dose after dialysis.
23. Has not been studied in children. Use adult dosage in adolescents ≥12 years of age.
24. Not approved for use in children. Dosage recommended by the Committee on Infectious Diseases of the American Academy of Pediatrics.

Continued on next page.

ANTIMICROBIAL DRUG DOSAGE† (continued)

| | Adults | | Children | |
	Oral	Parenteral	Oral	Parenteral
Cefprozil	250-500 mg q12h		15 mg/kg q12h	
Ceftazidime		250 mg-2 g q8-12h		30-50 mg/kg q8h
Ceftibuten	400 mg q24h		9 mg/kg q24h	
Ceftizoxime		500 mg-4 g q8-12h		50 mg/kg q6-8h
Ceftriaxone		1-2 g q12-24h		50-100 mg/kg/d, div q12-24h
Cefuroxime		750 mg-1.5 g q6-8h		50-150 mg/kg/d, div q6-8h
Cefuroxime axetil	125-500 mg q12h		10-15 mg/kg q12h	
Cephalexin	250 mg-1 g q6h		6.25-25 mg/kg q6h	
Cephradine	250-500 mg q6-12h		6.25-25 mg/kg q6h or 12.5-50 mg/kg q12h	
Chloram-phenicol[10]		12.5-25 mg/kg[25] q6h		12.5-25 mg/kg[25] q6h
Chloroquine	See foot-note 26		See foot-note 26	
Cidofovir		5 mg/kg once/wk x2, then 5 mg/kg every other wk[27]		
Ciprofloxacin	250-750 mg q12h or 1000 mg q24h[28]	200-400 mg q8-12h	10-20 mg/kg[29] q12h	6-10 mg/kg[29] q8-12h

25. IV administration; dosage should be adjusted according to serum concentration.
26. For specific dosing information, see Drugs for Parasitic Infections (Malaria), page 246.
27. For CMV. Initiation of therapy contraindicated in patients with serum creatinine >1.5 mg/dL, creatinine clearance ≤55 mL/min or urine protein ≥100 mg/dL. If serum creatinine increases by 0.3-0.4 mg/dL above baseline, decrease dose to 3 mg/kg. Discontinue for increases ≥0.5 mg/dL. Administer with probenecid and hydration before and after infusion.

Usual Maximum Dose/Day	Adult Dosage in Renal Failure For Creatinine Clearance (mL/min)			Dose for CRRTs	Extra Dose After Hemodialysis
	80-50	50-10	<10		
1000 mg	No change	CrCl <30 mL/min 250-500 mg q24h			yes
6 g	0.5-2 g q8-12h	q12-24h	q24-48h	1-2g IV q12h	yes
400 mg	No change	100-200 mg q24h	100 mg q24h		no*
12 g	0.5-1.5 g q8h	0.25-1 g q12h	0.25-1 g q24-48h	0.25-1g q12h	yes
4 g	Change not required				no
9 g	0.75-1.5g q8h	0.75-1.5g q8-12h	0.75-1.5g q24h	0.75-1.5g IV q12h	yes
1 g	Change not required		250 mg q24h		yes
4 g	No change	0.25-1 g q8-12h	0.25-1 g q12-24h		yes
4 g	No change	50% of dose	25% of dose		yes
4 g	Change not required				no*
	No change	No change	50% of usual dose		no
	See footnote 27				
1.5 g	No change	CrCl <30 mL/min 200-400 mg IV or 250-500 mg PO q18-24h		200-400mg IV q12h	no*

CRRTs: Continuous renal replacement therapies. See also pages 417–418.
* But give usual dose after dialysis.
28. Extended-release formulation for treatment of UTI.
29. For PEP of inhalation anthrax oral dose is 15 mg/kg (max 500 mg) and IV dose is 10 mg/kg (max 400 mg).

Continued on next page.

ANTIMICROBIAL DRUG DOSAGE† (continued)

| | **Adults** | | **Children** | |
	Oral	Parenteral	Oral	Parenteral
Clarithromycin	250-500 mg q12h or 1000 mg q24h[30]		7.5 mg/kg q12h	
Clindamycin[10]	150-450 mg q6h-8h	300-900 mg q6h-8h	2-8 mg/kg q6h-8h	2.5-10 mg/kg q6h
Colistin (colistimethate sodium)		2.5-5 mg/kg/d, div in 2-4 doses		2.5-5 mg/kg/d, div in 2-4 doses
Cycloserine[32]	250-500 mg q12h		5-10 mg/kg q12h	
Dapsone[33]	100 mg q24h		2 mg/kg q24h	
Daptomycin		4-6 mg/kg q24h		
Darunavir/ ritonavir	600 mg/100 mg q12h			
Delavirdine	400 mg tid			
Dicloxacillin	125-1000 mg q6h		3.125-6.25 mg/kg q6h	
Didanosine	>60 kg: 400 mg q24h[34] <60 kg: 250 mg q24h[34]		≤8 mos: 100 mg/m^2 >8 mos: 120 mg/m^2 q12h[34]	
Doripenem		500 mg q8h		

30. Extended-release formulation, approved for sinusitis, acute exacerbation of chronic bronchitis, and community-acquired pneumonia.
31. Based on serum creatinine: 1.3-1.5 mg/dL, dose 2.5-3.8 mg/kg/d divided q12h; 1.6-2.5 mg/dL, dose 2.5 mg/kg/d q24h; 2.6-4 mg/dL, dose 1.5 mg/kg q36h.
32. Monitor concentrations, toxicity increases markedly above 30 mcg/mL. ATS/CDC/IDSA recommend not using in patients with CrCl <50 mL/min unless on HD.
33. Dosage for prophylaxis of *Pneumocystis jiroveci* pneumonia (PCP). Adult dosage can be changed to 50 mg daily or 200 mg weekly if given with weekly pyrimethamine and leucovorin.

Usual Maximum Dose/Day	Adult Dosage in Renal Failure For Creatinine Clearance (mL/min)			Dose for CRRTs	Extra Dose After Hemodialysis
	80-50	50-10	<10		
1 g	No change	q24h	Unknown		
4.8 g	Change not required				no
5 mg/kg	See footnote 31				
1 g	No change	q12-24h[32]	q24h[32]		
100 mg	No change	No change	Unknown		
	No change	CrCl<30 mL/min 4-6 mg/kg q48h		4-6 mg/kg q24-48h	no*
1200 mg	Change not required				
1.2 g	Change not required				no
4 g	Change not required				no
400 mg	No change	≥60kg: 125-200 mg q24h[35] <60kg: 125 mg q24h[35]	125 mg q24h[35] Not recc.	75-100 mg q24h[35]	yes
1.5 g	No change	250 mg q8-12h	Unknown		

CRRTs: Continuous renal replacement therapies. See also pages 417–418.
* But give usual dose after dialysis.
34. Refers to delayed-release capsules for adults and pediatric powder for oral solution for childern.
35. Dosage in renal failure refers to delayed-release capsules. Dose for CRRTs refers to pediatric powder for oral solution.

Continued on next page.

ANTIMICROBIAL DRUG DOSAGE† (continued)

| | Adults | | Children | |
	Oral	Parenteral	Oral	Parenteral
Doxycycline	100 mg q12-24h	100 mg q12-24h	2.2 mg/kg[36] q12-24h	2.2 mg/kg[36] q12-24h
Efavirenz	600 mg q24h		200-400 mg q24h	
Efavirenz/ emtricitabine/ tenofovir	600 mg/200 mg/ 300 mg q24h			
Emtricitabine	200 mg q24h[37]		3-6mg/kg (solution) q24h	
Emtricitabine/ tenofovir	200 mg/300 mg q24h			
Enfuvirtide		90 mg SC q12h		≥6 yrs: 2 mg/kg SC q12h
Entecavir	0.5 mg q24h[38]			
Ertapenem		1 g q24h		15 mg/kg q12h[24]
Erythromycin	250-500 mg q6h	250 mg-1 g IV[40] q6h	7.5-12.5 mg/kg q6h	3.75-12.5 mg/kg IV[40] q6h
Ethambutol	15-25 mg/kg q24h or 50 mg/kg 2-3x/wk		15-25 mg/kg q24h[41] or 50 mg/kg 2x/wk	
Ethionamide	250-500 mg q12h		7.5-10 mg/kg q12h	
Famciclovir	500 mg q8h[42]			
Fluconazole	50-800 mg q24h	100-800 mg q24h	3-12 mg/kg q24h	3-12 mg/kg q24h

36. Not recommended for children less than eight years old.
37. Dosage for capsules. For solution dosage is: 240 mg q24h; for CrCl 50-10 mL/min 80-120 mg q24h; for CrCl <10mL/min 60 mg q24h.
38. Dose for nucleoside-naive patients ≥16 years old. For patients refractory to lamivudine, regular dosage is 1 mg once daily and dosage in renal failure is CrCl 50-10: 0.3-0.5 mg q24h; CrCl <10: 0.1 mg q24h.
39. If the 500-mg dose is given within 6 hours prior to HD, a supplemental dose of 150 mg is recommended after HD. If the 500-mg dose is given >6 hours before HD, no supplemental dose is needed.

Usual Maximum Dose/Day	Adult Dosage in Renal Failure For Creatinine Clearance (mL/min)			Dose for CRRTs	Extra Dose After Hemodialysis
	80-50	50-10	<10		
200 mg	Change not required				no
600 mg	Change not required				
600 mg/ 200 mg/ 300 mg	No change	Not recommended			
200 mg	No change	200 mg q48-72h[37]	200 mg q96h[37]	200 mg q48-72h	no*
200 mg/ 300 mg	No change	CrCl 30-49 mL/min: q48h CrCl <30 mL/min: not recommended			
180 mg	No change	CrCl ≥35 mL/min: No change CrCl <35 mL/min: Unknown			
1 mg	No change	0.15-0.25 mg[38] q24h	0.05 mg[38] q24h		no*
1 g	No change	CrCl <30 mL/ min: 500 mg q24h	500 mg q24h		yes[39]
4 g	Change not required				no
2.5 g	No change	20 mg/kg q24-36h	20 mg/kg q48h		no*
1 g	No change	No change	250-500 mg q24h		no
1.5 g	500 mg q12h	500 mg q24h	Not recommended		yes
800 mg	No change	100-800 mg q48h	100-800 mg q72h	400-800 mg q24h	yes

CRRTs: Continuous renal replacement therapies. See also pages 417–418.
* But give usual dose after dialysis.
40. By slow infusion to minimize thrombophlebitis.
41. Not recommended in children whose visual acuity cannot be monitored (<6 years old).
42. For herpes zoster. For first episode genital herpes, the dosage is 250 mg q8h. For genital herpes recurrence, it is 125 mg q12h. For suppression of genital herpes, it is 250 mg q12h.

Continued on next page.

ANTIMICROBIAL DRUG DOSAGE† (continued)

| | Adults | | Children | |
	Oral	Parenteral	Oral	Parenteral
Flucytosine	12.5-37.5 mg/kg q6h		12.5-37.5 mg/kg q6h	
Fosampren-avir[10]	1400 mg q12h[43]		30mg/kg[44] q12h	
Foscarnet		60 mg/kg q8h or 90 mg/kg q12h[45]		
Fosfomycin	3 g once			
Furazolidone	100 mg q6h		5-8 mg/kg/d div q6h	
Ganciclovir	1 g q8h	5 mg/kg[46] q12h		5 mg/kg[46] q12h
Gemifloxacin	320 mg q24h		See foot-note 47	
Gentamicin		1-2.5 mg/kg q8h or 5-7 mg/kg q24h[3]		1-2.5 mg/kg q8h[3]
Griseofulvin microsize ultra-microsize	500-1000 mg q24h 330-750 mg q24h		10-20 mg/kg/d div q12-24h 5-15 mg/kg/d div q12-24h	
Imipenem/cilastin		250 mg-1 g q6-8h		15-25 mg/kg q6h
Indinavir	800 mg q8h[48]		500 mg/m² q8h	

43. For therapy-naive patients. May also be given as 1,400 mg once daily with ritonavir 200 mg once daily or 700 mg twice daily with ritonavir 100 mg twice daily. The dose for protease inhibitor-experienced patients is 700 mg bid with ritonavir 100 mg bid.
44. For therapy-naive patients ≥ 2 years old. A dose of 18 mg/kg q 12h with ritonavir 3 mg/kg q12h is recommended for therapy-experienced patients ≥ 6 years old and is an alternative for therapy-naive patients > 6 years old.
45. For induction therapy of CMV, given over at least one hour; for maintenance, 90-120 mg/kg daily over two hours. For HSV or VZV, 40 mg/kg q8h.
46. Dosage for CMV induction (give IV at constant rate over one hour); for IV maintenance without renal failure: 5 mg/kg once daily 7 days/week or 6 mg/kg once daily 5 days/week; for IV maintenance with renal failure: induction dose is reduced by half.

Usual Maximum Dose/Day	Adult Dosage in Renal Failure For Creatinine Clearance (mL/min)			Dose for CRRTs	Extra Dose After Hemodialysis
	80-50	50-10	<10		
150 mg/kg	No change	12.5-37.5 mg/kg q12-24h	12.5-37.5 mg/kg q24-48h	12.5-37.5 mg/kg q12-24h	yes
2.8 g	Change not required				
	See package insert				
3 g	Change not required				yes
400 mg	Unknown				
10 mg/kg IV	2.5 mg/kg[46] IV q12h	1.25-2.5 IV mg/kg[46] q24h	1.25 mg/kg[46] IV 3x/wk	1.25-5 mg/kg IV q24h	no*
3 g PO	0.5-1 g PO tid	0.5-1 g PO q24h	500 mg PO 3x/wk		no*
320 mg	No change	160 mg q24h	160 mg q24h		no*
	1.5 mg/kg q8-12h	1.5 mg/kg q12-24h	See foot-note 3		yes
1 g	Change not required				
750 mg	Change not required				
4 g	250-500 mg q6-8h	250-500 mg q8-12h	250-500 mg q12h	500 mg IV q8-12h	yes
	Change not required				

CRRTs: Continuous renal replacement therapies. See also pages 417–418.
* But give usual dose after dialysis.
47. According to The American Academy of Pediatrics, although fluoroquinolones are generally contra-indicated in children <18 years old, their use may be justified in special circumstances, such as when no other oral agent is available.
48. Dose adjustment is necessary when administered with other drugs including delavirdine, efavirenz, lopinavir/ritonavir and ritonavir.

Continued on next page.

ANTIMICROBIAL DRUG DOSAGE† (continued)

| | Adults | | Children | |
	Oral	Parenteral	Oral	Parenteral
Interferon alfa-2a, 2b pegylated, alfa-2b pegylated, alfa-2a		3 MIU 3x/wk SC or IM[49] 1 mcg/kg SC q wk 180 mcg SC q wk		See foot-note 49
Isoniazid[10]	300 mg q24h		10-20 mg/kg q24h	
Itraconazole	100-200 mg q12-24h	200 mg q12h x 4 then 200 mg q24h	5 mg/kg q24h	
Ivermectin	200 mcg/kg q24h		200 mcg/kg q24h	
Kanamycin		5 mg/kg q8h or 7.5 mg/kg q12h		5 mg/kg q8h or 7.5 mg/kg q12h
Ketoconazole	200-400 mg q12-24h		3.3-6.6 mg/kg q24h	
Lamivudine[50]	150 mg q12h or 300 mg q24h		4 mg/kg q12h	
Levofloxacin	250-750 mg q24h	250-750 mg q24h	See foot-note 47	
Lincomycin	500 mg q6-8h	600 mg-1g[52] q8-12h	30-60 mg/kg/d, div q6-8h	10-20 mg/kg/d, div q8-12h
Linezolid	400-600 mg q12h	600 mg q12h	10 mg/kg[53] q8h	10 mg/kg[53] q8h

49. For chronic hepatitis C in adults. For acute hepatitis C in adults the dosage is 5 MIU 24h x 3 weeks, then TIW. For chronic hepatitis B the dosage of interferon alfa-2b is 5 MIU 24h or 10 MIU TIW for adults and for children it is 3-6 MIU/m² TIW.
50. For treatment of HIV. For treatment of hepatitis B, the dose of lamivudine is 100 mg/d in patients with Normal renal function and dosage in renal failure is CrCl 50-15: 100 mg x 1, then 25-50 mg/d; CrCl <15: 35 mg x 1, then 10-15 mg/d.

| Usual Maximum Dose/Day | Adult Dosage in Renal Failure For Creatinine Clearance (mL/min) | | | Dose for CRRTs | Extra Dose After Hemodialysis |
	80-50	50-10	<10		
3 MIU	Change not required				
	No change	Use caution			
	No change	Use caution			
300 mg	Change not required				no*
400 mg	Change not required; but IV not recommended for CrCl <30 mL/min				
	Unknown				
1.5 g	5-7.5 mg/kg q24h	5-7.5 mg/kg q24-72h	See foot-note 3		yes
400 mg	Change not required				
300 mg	No change	150 mg q24h or 150 mg once, then 100 mg q24h	50-150 mg once, then 25-50 mg q24h	100-150 mg q24h	no
750 mg	No change	see foot-note 51	Unknown	250-500 mg q24h	no
8 g	No change	Severe renal impairment: 25%-30% usual dose			
1200 mg	Change not required				no*

CRRTs: Continuous renal replacement therapies. See also pages 417–418.
* But give usual dose after dialysis.
51. CrCl 20-49 mL/min: 250 mg q24h or 500 mg once, then 250 mg q24h or 750 mg q48h. CrCl 10-19 mL/min: 250 mg q48h or 500 mg once, then 250 mg q48h or 750 mg once, then 500 mg q48h.
52. For life-threatening infections, dosage may be increased to a maximum of 8 g/d.
53. For children up to 11 years of age. Pediatric patients ≥12 years should receive 600 mg q12h.

Continued on next page.

ANTIMICROBIAL DRUG DOSAGE† (continued)

| | Adults | | Children | |
	Oral	Parenteral	Oral	Parenteral
Lopinavir/ ritonavir	400 mg/ 100 mg q12h[54] or 800 mg/ 200 mg q24h[55]		7-15 kg: 12/3 mg/kg q12h[54] 15-40 kg: 10/2.5 mg/kg q12h[54]	
Loracarbef	200-400 mg q12-24h		7.5-15 mg/kg q12h	
Maraviroc	300 mg q12h			
Mebendazole	100-200 mg q12h		100-200 mg q12h	
Mefloquine	1250 mg once[56]		15 mg/kg once[56]	
Meropenem		1-2 g q8h		20-40 mg/kg q8h
Methenamine hippurate	1 g q12h		12.5-25 mg/kg q12h	
Methenamine mandelate	1 g q6h		12.5-18.75 mg/kg q6h	
Metroni- dazole[10]	500 mg q6-8h[57]	500 mg q6-8h[57]	7.5 mg/kg q6-8h[57]	7.5 mg/kg q6-8h[57]
Micafungin		150 mg q24h[58]		
Minocycline	200 mg x1, then 100 mg q12h		4 mg/kg x1, 2 mg/kg q12h[36]	
Moxifloxacin[10]	400 mg q24h	400 mg q24h	See foot- note 47	
Nafcillin		500 mg-2 g q4-6h		25-50 mg/kg q6h
Nalidixic acid	1 g q6h		≥ 3 mos: 55 mg/kg/d div q6h	

54. A dose increase is necessary if coadministered with nevirapine or efavirenz in treatment-experienced patients when reduced susceptibility to lopinavir is suspected.
55. For treatment-naive patients. Should not be administered as once/d regimen in combination with efavirenz, nevirapine, amprenavir or nelfinavir.
56. Dosage for treatment of malaria; given as 750 mg followed 12 hrs later by 500 mg for adults and 15 mg/kg followed 12 hrs later by 10 mg/kg for children. Dosage for once/wk prophylaxis of malaria; adults, 250 mg; children , 5 mg/kg (<5 kg), 1/8 tab (5-10 kg), 1/4 tab (11-20 kg), 1/2 tab (21-30 kg), 3/4 tab (31-45 kg), 1 tab (>45 kg).

Usual Maximum Dose/Day	Adult Dosage in Renal Failure For Creatinine Clearance (mL/min)			Dose for CRRTs	Extra Dose After Hemodialysis
	80-50	50-10	<10		
800 mg/ 200 mg	Change not required				
800 mg	No change	200-400 mg q24h	200-400 mg q3-5 days		yes
600 mg	No change	See footnote 89			
400 mg	Unknown				
1250 mg	Unknown				
6 g	No change	0.5-1 g q12h	0.5 g q24h	1 g IV q12h	no*
4 g	No change	Not recommended			
4 g	No change	Not recommended			
4 g	No change	No change	500 mg q12h		no*
	Change not required				
400 mg	Change not required				
400 mg	Change not required				
12 g	Change not required				no
4 g	No change	No change	Not recommended		

CRRTs: Continuous renal replacement therapies. See also pages 417–418.
* But give usual dose after dialysis.
57. Dosage for anaerobic bacterial infections. For antiparasitic dosages, see Drugs for Parasitic Infections, page 225.
58. For treatment of esophageal candidiasis. The dose for prophylaxis of *Candida* infections in HSCT is 50 mg/d.

Continued on next page.

ANTIMICROBIAL DRUG DOSAGE† (continued)

| | Adults | | Children | |
	Oral	Parenteral	Oral	Parenteral
Nelfinavir[10]	750 mg q8h or 1250 mg q12h		25-30 mg/kg q8h	
Nevirapine	200 mg/d x14, followed by 200 mg bid		<8 yrs: 4 mg/kd/d x14, followed by 7 mg/kg bid ≥8 yrs: 4 mg/kd/d x14, followed by 4 mg/kg bid	
Nitazoxanide	500 mg q12h		1-3 yrs: 100 mg q12h 4-11 yrs: 200 mg q12h	
Nitrofurantoin	50-100 mg q6h		1.25-1.75 mg/kg q6h	
Norfloxacin	400 mg q12h		See foot- note 47	
Ofloxacin	200-400 mg q12h	200-400 mg q12h	See foot- note 47	
Oseltamivir	75 mg q12h[59]		≤15 kg: 30 mg q12h 16-23 kg: 45 mg q12h 24-40 kg: 60 mg q12h >40 kg: 75 mg q12h	
Oxacillin	500 mg-1 g q6h	500 mg-2 g q4-6h	12.5-25 mg/kg q6h	25-50 mg/kg q6h
Paromomycin	25-35 mg/kg/d div q8h		25-35 mg/kg/d div q8h	
Penicillin G		1.2-30 million U/d, div q2-12h[60]		100,000- 250,000 U/d, div q2-12h[60]
Penicillin V	250-500 mg q6-8h		6.25-12.5 mg/kg q6h	
Pentamidine		4 mg/kg[62] q24h		4 mg/kg[62] q24h
Piperacillin		2-4 g q4-6h		200-300 mg/kg/d, div q4-6h

59. For treatment of influenza. For influenza prophylaxis dosage is 75 mg q24h for patients with normal renal function and 75 mg q48h or 30 mg q24h for patients with CrCl 10-30 mL/min.
60. The interval between parenteral doses can be as short as 2 hours for initial intravenous treatment of meningococcemia, or as long as 12 hours between intramuscular doses of penicillin G procaine.
61. Patients with severe renal insufficiency should be given no more than one third to one half the maximum daily dosage, i.e., instead of giving 30 million units per day, 10-15 million units could be given. Patients on lower doses usually tolerate full dosage even with severe renal insufficiency.

Usual Maximum Dose/Day	Adult Dosage in Renal Failure For Creatinine Clearance (mL/min)			Dose for CRRTs	Extra Dose After Hemodialysis
	80-50	50-10	<10		
2.5 g	Change not required				
400 mg	Change not required				yes
1 g	Use with caution				
400 mg	No change	Not recommended			
800 mg	No change	CrCl <30 mL/min 400 mg q24h			no
800 mg	No change	200-400 mg q24h	100-200 mg q24h		no
150 mg	No change	CrCl 10-30 mL/min q24h[59]	Unknown		
12 g	Change not required				no
	Unknown				
30 million U	Change not required		See foot-note 61	1-2 million U q4h	yes
3 g	Change not required				
	4 mg/kg q24h	4 mg/kg q24-36h	4 mg/kg q48h		no
24 g	No change	3-4 g q6-8h	3-4 g q12h		yes

CRRTs: Continuous renal replacement therapies. See also pages 417–418.
* But give usual dose after dialysis.
62. For treatment of PCP. For prophylaxis of PCP, the dosage for adults and children ≥5 years is 300 mg inhaled monthly via nebulizer.

Continued on next page.

ANTIMICROBIAL DRUG DOSAGE† (continued)

| | **Adults** | | **Children** | |
	Oral	Parenteral	Oral	Parenteral
Piperacillin/ tazobactam[63]		3.375 g q6h or 4.5 g q6-8h		240 mg/kg/d piperacillin div q8h
Polymyxin B		2.5-3mg/kg/d q24h or div q12h[64]		≥ 2 yrs: 2.5-3mg/kg/d < 2 yrs: 2.5-4 mg/kg/d q24h or div q12h[64]
Posaconazole	200 mg q8h or 400 mg q12h		≥13 yrs: 200 mg q8h or 400 mg q12h	
Praziquantel	20-25 mg/kg q8-12h		20-25 mg/kg q8-12h	
Primaquine	30 mg base q24h		0.6 mg base/kg q24h	
Pyrantel pamoate	11 mg/kg		11 mg/kg	
Pyrazinamide	15-30 mg/kg q24h		15-30 mg/kg q24h	
Pyrimethamine	25-100 mg[65] q24h		0.5-1 mg/kg[65] q12h	
Pyrimethamine/ sulfadoxine	75/1500 mg once		See footnote 66	
Quinidine gluconate		10 mg/kg then[67] 0.02 mg/kg/min		10 mg/kg then[67] 0.02 mg/kg/min
Quinine sulfate	650 mg q8h		10 mg/kg q8h	
Quinupristin/ dalfopristin		7.5 mg/kg q8-12h		7.5 mg/kg q8-12h
Raltegravir	400 mg q12h			

63. Combination formulation: A 2.25-g vial contains 2 g piperacillin/250 mg tazobactam; a 3.375-g vial contains 3 g piperacillin/375 mg tazobactam; a 4.5-g vial contains 4 g piperacillin/500 mg tazobactam.
64. Should be given as single dose q24h unless unable to tolerate fluid load; then can divide q12h (1 mg = 10,000 U).
65. For treatment of toxoplasmosis. Leucovorin should be administered with pyrimethamine.
66. Each tablet contains 25 mg pyrimethamine/500 mg sulfadoxine. Pediatric dose: <1 yr: 1/4 tab; 1-3 yrs: 1/2 tab; 4-8 yrs: 1 tab; 9-14 yrs: 2 tabs.

| Usual Maximum Dose/Day | Adult Dosage in Renal Failure For Creatinine Clearance (mL/min) | | | Dose for CRRTs | Extra Dose After Hemodialysis |
	80-50	50-10	<10		
18 g	No change	2.25-3.375 g q6h	2.25 g q6-8h	4.5 g IV q8-12h	yes
3 mg/kg	No change	2.5-3 mg/kg once, then 1-1.5 mg/kg q24h (CrCl 30-50 mL/min) or q48h-72 (CrCl <30 mL/min)	anuric patients 1 mg/kg q5 days		
800 mg	Change not required				
	Change not required				
30 mg base	Change not required				
1 g	Unknown				
2 g	Change not required				
100 mg	Change not required				no
75/1500 mg	Use with caution				
600 mg	No change	No change	75% of usual dose		yes
	No change	650 mg q8-12h	650 mg q24h		no*
Unknown	Change not required				
800 mg	Change not required				

CRRTs: Continuous renal replacement therapies. See also pages 417–418.
* But give usual dose after dialysis.
67. Loading dose should be decreased or omitted in patients who have received quinine or mefloquine. If >48 hours IV treatment required, dose should be reduced by 30-50%.

Continued on next page.

ANTIMICROBIAL DRUG DOSAGE† (continued)

| | Adults | | Children | |
	Oral	Parenteral	Oral	Parenteral
Ribavirin	75 kg: 400 mg q AM and 600 mg q PM >75 kg: 600 mg bid			
Rifabutin	150 mg q12h or 300 mg q24h		5-20 mg/kg/d	
Rifampin[10]	600 mg q24h[68]	600 mg q24h	10-20 mg/kg q24h[68]	10-20 mg/kg q24h
Rifampin/ isoniazid[69]	600/300 mg[69] q24h			
Rifampin/ isoniazid/pyra- zinamide[69]	≤44 kg: 4 tabs[70] 45-54 kg: 5 tabs 55-90 kg: 6 tabs			
Rifapentine	600 mg once wkly			
Rifaximin	200 mg q8h		≥12 yrs: 200 mg q8h	
Rimantadine[10]	100 mg q12h		5 mg/kg once	
Ritonavir[10]	600 mg q12h[71]		400 mg/m^2 q12h	
Saquinavir/ ritonavir	1000 mg/100 mg q12h			
Spectinomycin		2-4 g once		< 45 kg: 40 mg/kg once
Stavudine[10]	≥60 kg: 40 mg q12h or 100 mg q24h[72] <60 kg: 30 mg q12h or 75 mg q24h[72]		≥30 kg: 30 mg q12h <30 kg: 1 mg/kg q12h	
Streptomycin		15-30 mg/kg q24h[73] or 25-30 mg/kg 2-3x/wk		20-40 mg/kg q24h[73]

68. For meningococcal carriers, dosage is 600 mg bid x 2 days for adults, 10 mg/kg q12h x 2 days for children more than one month old, and 5 mg/kg q12h x 2 days for infants less than one month old.
69. Pyridoxine 10-25 mg should be added to prevent neuropathy in malnourished or pregnant patients and those with HIV infection, alcoholism or diabetes.
70. Each tablet contains rifampin 120 mg, isoniazid 50 mg, and pyrazinamide 300 mg. For patients >90 kg - 6 tabs plus additional pyrazinamide to achieve total of 20-25 mg/kg/d.
71. When used in combination with other protease inhibitors the ritonavir dose is 100-400 mg PO b.i.d.

Usual Maximum Dose/Day	Adult Dosage in Renal Failure For Creatinine Clearance (mL/min)			Dose for CRRTs	Extra Dose After Hemodialysis
	80-50	50-10	<10		
1200 mg	No change	Not recommended			
300 mg	Change not required				no
600 mg	Change not required				
600/300 mg	Change not required				
	Change not required				
600 mg	Change not required				
600 mg	Change not required				
200 mg	No change	No change	100 mg q24h		no
1200 mg	No change	No change	100 mg q24h		no
2000 mg/ 200 mg	Change not required				
	No change	Not recommended			
80 mg	No change	20 mg q12-24h or 50 mg q24-48h[72] 15 mg q12-24h or 37.5 mg q24-48h[72]	Not recc. if not on HD		See foot-note 72
1-2 g	q24h	q24-72h	q72-96h		yes

CRRTs: Continuous renal replacement therapies. See also pages 417–418.
*But give usual dose after dialysis.
72. Dose for extended-release capsules *(Zerit XR)*. Hemodialysis patients: ≥60 kg, 20 mg q24h or 50 mg q48h *(Zerit XR)*; <60 kg, 15 mg q24h or 37.5 mg q48h *(Zerit XR)* administered after hemodialysis and at the same time of day on non-dialysis days.
73. Given IM for tuberculosis. Dose for endocarditis: 500 mg-1 g q12h.

Continued on next page.

ANTIMICROBIAL DRUG DOSAGE† (continued)

	Adults		Children	
	Oral	Parenteral	Oral	Parenteral
Sulfadiazine[74]	1-1.5 g q6h		25-50 mg/kg q6h	
Sulfisoxazole	500 mg-1 g q6h	25 mg/kg q6h	150 mg/kg/d div q4-6h	100 mg/kg/d div q6-8h
Telbivudine	600 mg q24h			
Telithromycin	800 mg q24h			
Tenofovir	300 mg q24h		2-8 yrs: 8 mg/kg q 24h > 8 yrs: 210 mg/m^2 q 24h	
Terbinafine	250 mg q24h			
Tetracy-cline[76]	250-500 mg q6h		6.25-12.5 mg/kg q6h[36]	
Thiabendazole	50 mg/kg/d div q12h		50 mg/kg/d div q12h	
Ticarcillin		200-300 mg/kg/d div q4-6h		200-300 mg/kg/d div q4-6h
Ticarcillin/ clavulanic acid[77]		3.1 g q4-6h		200-300 mg/kg/d div q4-6h
Tigecycline[10]		100 mg x1, then 50 mg q12h		See foot-note 36
Tinidazole	2 g q24h[78]		50 mg/kg q24h[78]	
Tipranavir/ ritonavir	500/200 mg q12h			
Tobramycin		1-2.5 mg/kg q8h or 5-7 mg/kg q24h[3]		1-2.5 mg/kg q8h[3]

74. Given in conjunction with pyrimethamine for toxoplasmosis.
75. For patients with CrCl <30 mL/min and coexisting hepatic impairment the dose should be 400 mg once daily. Patients on hemodialysis: 600 mg should be given after dialysis on dialysis days.
76. Tetracycline or oxytetracycline. The oral dose of demeclocycline for adults is 600 mg daily in two to four divided doses.

Usual Maximum Dose/Day	Adult Dosage in Renal Failure For Creatinine Clearance (mL/min)			Dose for CRRTs	Extra Dose After Hemodialysis
	80-50	50-10	<10		
8 g	Unknown				
8 g	0.5-1 g q6-8h	0.5-1 g q8-12h	0.5-1 g q12-24h		yes
600 mg	No change	600 mg q48-72h	600 mg q96h		no*
800 mg	No change	CrCl < 30 mL/min 600 mg q24h[75]			no[75]
300 mg	No change	CrCl 30-49 mL/min 300 mg q48h CrCl 10-29 mL/min 300 mg 2x/wk	300 mg q7days		
250 mg	No change	Not recommended			
2 g	No change	250-500 mg q12-24h	250-500 mg q24h		no
3 g	Unknown; use with caution				
24 g	2-3 g q4-6h	2-3 g q6-8h	2 g q12h		yes
24 g	No change	2 g q4-8h	2 g q12h		yes
	Change not required				
2 g	Change not required				yes
1 g/400 mg	Change not required				
	1.5 mg/kg q8-12h	1.5 mg/kg q12-24h	See foot-note 3		yes

CRRTs: Continuous renal replacement therapies. See also pages 417–418.
*But give usual dose after dialysis.
77. Combination formulation: a 3.1-g vial contains 3 g ticarcillin/100 mg clavulanic acid.
78. For 3-5 days for amebiasis. For treatment of giardiasis and trichomoniasis, the dose is 2 g once.

Continued on next page.

ANTIMICROBIAL DRUG DOSAGE† (continued)

	Adults		Children	
	Oral	Parenteral	Oral	Parenteral
Trimethoprim	100 mg q12h or 200 mg q24h		2 mg/kg q12h	
Trimethoprim-sulfamethox-azole (TMP-SMX)	1 SS tab[79] q6h or 2 SS tabs q12h[79]	4-5 mg/kg (TMP) q6-12h	4-5 mg/kg (TMP) q6h	4-5 mg/kg (TMP) q6-12h
Valacyclovir	1 g q8h[81]			
Valganciclovir	Induction: 900 mg q12h Maintenance: 900 mg q24h		See foot-note 23	
Vancomycin	125-500 mg q6h[83]	15 mg/kg IV q12h[82]	12.5 mg/kg q6h[83]	10-15 mg/kg IV q6h[82,84]
Voriconazole	≥40 kg: 200 mg bid[85] <40 kg: 100 mg bid[85]	Loading: 6 mg/kg q12h x2 Maintenance: 4 mg/kg q12h[86]	See foot-note 87	
Zalcitabine (ddC)	0.75 mg q8h		0.005 to 0.01 mg/kg q8h	
Zanamivir	10 mg q12h by inhalation		>7 yrs: 10 mg q12h by inhalation	
Zidovudine[10] (AZT)	200 mg q8h or 300 mg q12h		160 mg/m² q8h or 180-240 mg/m² q12h	
Zidovudine/lamivudine	300/150 mg q12h		>12 yrs: 300/150 mg q12h	
Zidovudine/lamivudine/abacavir	300/150/300 mg q12h			

79. Each SS tablet contains 80 mg trimethoprim and 400 mg sulfamethoxazole. Double-strength tablets are also available; the usual dosage of these is 1 tablet q12h. Suspension contains 40 mg trimethoprim and 200 mg sulfamethoxazole per 5 mL.
80. The usual maximum daily dose is 4 tablets orally or 1200 mg trimethoprim with 6000 mg sulfamethoxazole IV.
81. For herpes zoster. For a first episode of genital herpes, the dosage is 1 g q12h. For recurrence of genital herpes, it is 500 mg q12h. For suppression of genital herpes, it is 1 g q24h.
82. Vancomycin should be infused over a period of at least 60 minutes.
83. Only for treatment of pseudomembranous colitis.
84. Sixty mg/kg/d may be needed for staphylococcal central-nervous-system infections.
85. IV loading dose of 6 mg/kg q12h x 2 doses is recommended prior to oral maintenance. Dose may be increased to 300 mg q12h (if ≥40 kg) and 150 mg q12h (if <40 kg).

Usual Maximum Dose/Day	Adult Dosage in Renal Failure For Creatinine Clearance (mL/min)			Dose for CRRTs	Extra Dose After Hemodialysis
	80-50	50-10	<10		
200 mg	No change	q18h	q24h		yes
See footnote 80	4-5 mg/kg (TMP) q6-12h	50% of dose	Not recommended		yes
3 g	1 g q8h	1 g q12-24h	500 mg q24h	500 mg q24h	
1800 mg	Induction: No change Maintenance: No change	450 mg q12-48h 450 mg q24h-2 wks	Not recommended Not recommended		
	1 g q12-24h	1 g q24h	Full dose x1, then per levels		yes
	Change not required	Change not required for oral voriconazole[88]			
2.25 mg	No change	0.75 mg q12h	0.75 mg q24h		
20 mg		Change not required			
600 mg	No change	No change	100 mg q6-8h	100 mg q8h	no*
600/ 300 mg	No change	Not recommended			
600/300/ 600 mg	No change	Not recommended			

CRRTs: Continuous renal replacement therapies. See also pages 417–418.

* But give usual dose after dialysis.

86. In patients also taking phenytoin, maintenance dose should be increased to 5 mg/kg/q12h IV or 400 mg q12h PO.

87. Not approved for use in children <12 yrs. Adult dosage has been effective in children (TJ Walsh et al, Pediatr Infect Dis J 2002; 21:240).

88. Cyclodextrin (IV vehicle) accumulates in patients with CrCl <50 mL/min. Oral voriconazole is recommended in these patients.

89. Dosage with strong CYP3A inhibitors is 150 mg q12h, and with CYP3A inducers is 600 mg q12h. Patients with CrCl <50 mL/min who receive maraviroc with a CYP3A inhibitor may have an increased risk of adverse effects.

INDEX

Note: Page numbers in bold type indicate major references

Index

Index

Index

Index

Index

Index

Index

Index

Index

Index

Index

Index

Index

Index

TABLE INDEX

Table Index